Prosodic Features and Prosodic Structu

Prosodic Features and Prosodic Structure

The Phonology of Suprasegmentals

ANTHONY FOX

OXFORD

UNIVERSITY PRESS

*This book has been printed digitally and produced in a standard specification
in order to ensure its continuing availability*

OXFORD
UNIVERSITY PRESS

Great Clarendon Street, Oxford OX2 6DP

Oxford University Press is a department of the University of Oxford.
It furthers the University's objective of excellence in research, scholarship,
and education by publishing worldwide in

Oxford New York

Auckland Cape Town Dar es Salaam Hong Kong Karachi
Kuala Lumpur Madrid Melbourne Mexico City Nairobi
New Delhi Shanghai Taipei Toronto
With offices in
Argentina Austria Brazil Chile Czech Republic France Greece
Guatemala Hungary Italy Japan South Korea Poland Portugal
Singapore Switzerland Thailand Turkey Ukraine Vietnam

Oxford is a registered trade mark of Oxford University Press
in the UK and in certain other countries

Published in the United States
by Oxford University Press Inc., New York

© Anthony Fox 2000

The moral rights of the author have been asserted

Database right Oxford University Press (maker)

Reprinted 2007

ISBN 978-0-19-925396-8

Preface

This book has a number of aims. At one level, it can be seen as a survey of different approaches to the phonological description of the prosodic features of speech, which it is hoped will prove useful to readers seeking a detailed account of theory in this area. In this capacity, of course, it cannot be exhaustive; the literature on these features is vast and beyond the scope of any one book to encompass. Inevitably, therefore, I have been forced to be selective, pursuing only those lines of enquiry which seem to me to offer a significant contribution to our understanding of these features, and especially those which are compatible with the overall conception that informs the book as a whole. If readers find that their favourite model is given short shrift—a number of prominent theories, for example Lexical Phonology, have been virtually ignored—this is not because the theory is necessarily dismissed as invalid, but merely because its contribution may not be specific to the major theme of the book. One currently important and increasingly popular framework—Optimality Theory—has similarly not been pursued in detail, since, whatever its claims, its value for the understanding of the phenomena discussed here is as yet uncertain.

On the other hand, the reader will find that the chronological net is cast fairly wide. I have attempted not only to describe currently accepted or popular models, but to lay the foundations for this description by examining their antecedents, the earlier concepts and frameworks which may now be considered superseded, or even quaint. These are included not merely as an historical exercise, but rather to demonstrate that the issues currently under discussion are not the creation of current linguists but are intrinsic to the phenomena themselves, and indeed that the insights offered in earlier frameworks may have something to offer modern linguists. Much as we would like to think otherwise, research in our field is not a simple linear progression towards an ever greater understanding of linguistic phenomena and increasingly adequate models. More than once we find that earlier insights are lost when the overall models in which they are expressed are rejected, only to be reinvented later and proclaimed as new discoveries. It is in part to highlight this phenomenon and to instil a due sense of humility in current practitioners that such a broad chronological brush has been employed.

But the book aims to do more than provide a survey. It attempts to draw together various strands from the research into these phenomena and to weave them into a more coherent fabric, which is presented in the final chapter but adumbrated at many earlier points. I do not presume to present a fully articulated theory, still less a formal model, but rather a general view of prosodic organization which reflects the conviction that this organization is not the mere co-occurrence and co-incidence of independent features, but rather constitutes an integrated whole: a *structure*. It is only in terms of this structure that the individual features can be interpreted.

I am happy to acknowledge my gratitude to a number of people. Frances Morphy and John Davey of Oxford University Press for their encouragement; anonymous readers for initial remarks on the proposal; and Alan Cruttenden for more detailed and helpful comments on the text. However, none of these can be blamed for the weaknesses and errors that doubtless remain. Finally, I should like to thank my colleagues in the Department of Linguistics and Phonetics at the University of Leeds for making it possible for me to be relieved of teaching and administrative chores for a semester, and John Macklin, Cowdray Professor of Spanish at Leeds, for using his good offices to obtain funding for teaching replacement.

Leeds, June 1999   A.F.

Contents

1

Introduction

1.1 The Nature of Prosodic Features

This book is concerned with the linguistic description of the so-called 'prosodic' features of speech, which are generally taken to include length, accent and stress, tone, intonation, and potentially a few others. The description and the definition of these features have always been something of a problem for linguists; for many years, and especially in the formative period of modern linguistic theory in the second quarter of the twentieth century, the study of these features suffered from relative neglect. With some exceptions, phonological descriptions were based primarily on 'segments'—vowels and consonants—and prosodic features were either ignored or forced into an inappropriate segmental mould. In recent years this imbalance has been redressed, and several phonological theories are now available which are not merely more sympathetic to prosodic features but are even largely based upon them. However, it remains the case that there is no universal consensus among phonologists about either the nature of prosodic features themselves or the general framework for their description, and it is difficult to obtain a clear picture of the field as a whole. The purpose of this book is to examine the nature of these features, and to consider some of the principles on which such a framework can be based.

It is necessary to clarify at the outset a number of the basic assumptions on which this enterprise rests, and to explain some terminological usages which might otherwise give rise to misunderstandings. We may begin with the term 'prosodic' itself. The reference and scope of this term is a theoretical question, and not one which can be dealt with summarily. The Greek προσῳδία (*prosodía*), from which it is derived, is a musical term which appears to signify something like 'song sung to music' or 'sung accompaniment', implying that prosody is the musical accompaniment to the words themselves.[1] In more recent usage the term has come to refer to the principles of versification, covering such things as rhythmical patterns, rhyming schemes and verse structure, but in linguistic contexts it is more frequently encountered with a different, if related, meaning, referring, as mentioned above, to such characteristics of utterances as stress and intonation, and, moreover, in prose rather than in verse. A precise

---

[1] However, the term was not restricted to features of pitch; it also included the 'breathings' of classical Greek, graphic marks which indicate the presence or absence of the glottal fricative or aspiration.

characterization of the scope and current linguistic meaning of 'prosody', and its delimitation from other related terms, is, however, difficult to achieve.

It is perhaps understandable that the description of speech has traditionally been largely in terms of segmental features, that is, the vowels and consonants or their attributes; it is these, after all, that are represented in spelling and that are responsible for distinguishing words from one another. Prosodic features, at once more elusive and apparently less significant, are easily ignored, and their contribution underestimated. The classical structuralist schools of phonology based their theories primarily on the *phoneme* as the basic distinctive segmental unit. In so far as features such as stress and intonation were considered at all, it was largely in terms of a phoneme-based, and therefore segmental, phonology. In American structuralist phonology, these features were seen as rather special kinds of phonemes: *suprasegmental phonemes*, which were considered to be located 'on top of' segmental phonemes. Prague School phonologists were characteristically less rigorous, and they had a rather more flexible conception of the structure of speech which allowed them to treat prosodic features separately from segments, but they offered no coherent framework for the description of such features. Classical Generative Phonology adopted uncritically the Bloomfieldian conception of suprasegmental features as attributes of segmental units, and although this model devoted considerable attention to the formalization of the processes of stress assignment, it failed to advance our understanding of the nature or real role of prosodic features. More has been achieved by recent models, collectively termed 'non-linear', since they have explicitly adopted more complex, multi-dimensional frameworks which do more justice to prosodies. We are now in a better position, therefore, to evaluate the nature and role of these features.

Although the terms 'suprasegmental' and 'prosodic' to a large extent coincide in their scope and reference, it is nevertheless sometimes useful, and desirable, to distinguish them. To begin with, a simple dichotomy 'segmental' vs. 'suprasegmental' does not do justice to the richness of phonological structure 'above' the segment; as we shall see, this structure is complex, involving a variety of different dimensions, and prosodic features cannot simply be seen as features which are superimposed on segments. More importantly, a distinction can be made between 'suprasegmental' as a mode of description on the one hand and 'prosodic' as a kind of feature on the other. In other words, we may use the term 'suprasegmental' to refer to a particular formalization in which a phonological feature or process is conceived of in non-segmental terms; in theory any phonological feature can be analysed in this way, whether it is prosodic or not. The term 'prosodic', on the other hand, can be applied to certain features of utterances regardless of how they are formalized; prosodic features can, in principle, be analysed segmentally as well as suprasegmentally. To give a more concrete example, in some theoretical frameworks features such as nasality or voice may be treated suprasegmentally, as having extent beyond the limits of a single segment.[2] In the usage adopted here, however, such features are not prosodic, even though they may be amenable to suprasegmental analysis.

1.2 The Phonetic Basis

We still need to clarify the nature of prosodic features themselves, and in particular to establish what they have in common and in what ways they differ, collectively, from other features of speech. One approach here is to seek to identify prosodic features *phonetically*, by establishing phonetic criteria for grouping together such features as length, accent, intonation, and tone—to mention just the main categories of prosodic features that will be discussed in this book— and distinguishing them from segments or segmental features such as place and manner of articulation.

In terms of their physiological or acoustic attributes, these features appear to form a very disparate group. Though tone and intonation clearly have considerable phonetic affinity, since they exploit the same phonetic parameter of pitch, the mechanisms involved here are quite different from those of accent or stress, while it is very difficult to provide a consistent phonetic characterization of length at all (see 2.1, below). Moreover, from a phonetic point of view such features do not appear to be very different from so-called segmental features, such as voice. We are also not able to isolate prosodic features in terms of the speech chain (Denes and Pinson, 1993), that is, the different phases of the speech process—articulation, sound, perception—since both prosodic and non-prosodic features are involved at every stage.

It is nevertheless possible to separate prosodic and non-prosodic features from one another in terms of other phonetic criteria. It is convenient to distinguish three components of the physiology of speaking: the *subglottal* component, the *larynx*, and the *supralaryngeal* component (Abercrombie, 1967: 21–2; Lieberman and Blumstein, 1988). The first of these, consisting of the lungs, trachea, and associated muscles, produces and regulates the pulmonic air-stream which is utilized for normal speech; the second provides voice and other laryngeal features of speech, and also regulates the pitch; the third, consisting of the various airways and cavities of the pharynx, mouth, and nose, and the associated muscles, especially those of the tongue, acts as a kind of variable filter, modifying the air-stream so as to produce the wide range of sounds required for speech.

Most of the segmental features of speech are produced by the supralaryngeal component. Place and manner of articulation depend on the postures and movements of the tongue, velum, jaw, and so on. The one exception to this

---

[2] This applies especially to two theoretical frameworks: Firthian Prosodic Analysis and Autosegmental Phonology. The former uses the term 'prosody' to refer to *any* feature that is treated non-segmentally (see 1.3, below).

generalization is voice, which, as we have noted, is generated in the larynx, along with other laryngeal features such as aspiration and glottalization.[3] By contrast, prosodic features can be seen *primarily* as the result of laryngeal or subglottal activity. Tone and intonation are based on pitch, which is controlled by the laryngeal muscles, while accentual features are often attributed to the activity of the respiratory muscles.[4]

We thus have a phonetic basis for distinguishing prosodic from non-prosodic features of speech in the component of the speech process where the features can be localized. The one exception is the larynx, which appears to have both a segmental and a prosodic role. On the one hand the larynx is responsible for the production of voice, aspiration, and glottalization, which are considered to be properties of segments; on the other hand it is responsible for the control of voice pitch, which is considered to be a prosodic feature. Thus, although we can provide a phonetic definition of prosodic features as those features which are not localized in the supralaryngeal component, it is not quite adequate, since it does not distinguish between prosodic and non-prosodic laryngeal features. We therefore need to invoke further criteria in order to define these features satisfactorily.

It will be noted, however, that despite the inadequacy of this phonetic definition, it does provide some insights into the nature of prosodic features. From a phonetic point of view, speech sounds can be regarded as modifications of an air-stream, the latter being, in the majority of cases, pulmonic, i.e. produced by the lungs. This air-stream is first modified by the larynx, which selectively converts the aperiodic air-flow into a periodic one, giving voiceless and voiced sounds, and these are further modified by the various supralaryngeal parts of the vocal tract. There is a sense, therefore, in which the laryngeal and subglottal components are more basic than the supralaryngeal, and the subglottal component is more basic than the laryngeal. Since the prosodic features are associated with the latter two, and segmental features primarily with the supralaryngeal component, we could consider prosodic features to be similarly more fundamental, in the sense that segmental features involve the modification of an air-stream which is already specified for prosodic features.

1.3 The Phonological Basis

We have seen that in principle prosodic features have different phonetic characteristics from segmental features, but they cannot be defined solely in phonetic

---

[3] For the purposes of phonetic classification, the glottis is conventionally treated as a place of articulation comparable to those of the supralaryngeal component, so that [h] and [ʔ] are merely a glottal fricative and glottal plosive, respectively. Their status is actually slightly different from other sounds, however, as they can be seen as properties of the *source* rather than of the supralaryngeal filter.

[4] As we shall see in Ch. 3, the phonetic basis of accent is in reality rather more complex than this, though this does not affect the basic point being made here.

terms. In their treatment of these features, phoneticians themselves acknowledge this, and generally have recourse to phonological principles. For Fry (1968), prosodic features can only be identified according to their linguistic role; thus, 'only those distinctions which have linguistic relevance are classed as prosodic features in a particular language'.[5] Crystal (1969: 5) claims that 'we may define prosodic systems as sets of mutually defining *phonological* features which have an essentially variable relationship to the words selected, as opposed to those features . . . which have a direct and identifying relationship to such words' (emphasis added).[6]

The main distinguishing characteristic of prosodic, as opposed to segmental, features is that they apply to larger domains than the individual segment. Lehiste (1970: 1) describes them as 'features whose domain extends over more than one segment' and (1970: 2–3) 'features whose arrangement in contrastive patterns in the time dimension is not restricted to single segments defined by their phonetic quality'. Laver (1994: 152) similarly characterizes them as 'all factors which can potentially be prolonged beyond the domain of the segment'. Together with this—though whether as a consequence of the larger domain or a cause of it is unclear—goes the fact that the linguistic distinctions involved here are of a different kind from those of segments: they are not only *paradigmatic* but also *syntagmatic*.[7] As Lehiste notes (1970: 2), these features 'are established by a comparison of items in sequence (i.e. syntagmatic comparison), whereas segmental features can be defined without reference to the sequence of segments in which the segment appears, and their presence can be established either by inspection or paradigmatic comparison'. Ladefoged (1975: 14) likewise remarks that 'all the suprasegmental features are characterized by the fact that they must be described in relation to other items in the same utterance'.

The relationship between segmental and prosodic features may also be viewed somewhat differently from a phonological perspective. We have already concluded that, phonetically speaking, prosodic features are more basic than supralaryngeal features, since they are part of the process of speech production—the 'source' rather than the 'filter'. From a phonological point of view, however, the reverse may be the case; prosodic features are often seen as modifications of segments. This view reflects the assumed greater contribution of segmental features to distinguishing meaning, and hence their greater phono-

---

[5] Curiously, Fry opposes 'prosodic' to 'phonological', the latter term apparently referring only to segmental phonemes. However, 'linguistic relevance' is evidently broader, and it is possible—in Fry's terms—for features to be linguistically relevant without being phonological.

[6] Crystal's definition is unsatisfactory, as it implies that prosodic features are not inherent in the words of a language. This may be true of intonation, but certainly not of accentual or tonal features. It is true that such features are frequently modified in connected speech, but then so are non-prosodic properties such as voicing and supralaryngeal features.

[7] For the source of this distinction see Saussure, 1967 [1916]: 170–5, though his term is 'associative' rather than 'paradigmatic'.

logical significance; from this perspective, prosodic features are merely secondary modifications.

In general, it is this latter view of prosodic features—as secondary modifications of segmental features—that is found in the discussions of the major phonological schools. Indeed, Bloomfield (1935: 109) explicitly describes prosodic features as *modifications* of the 'typical actions of the vocal organs'; he includes here length, loudness and pitch. These features are also described as *secondary phonemes*, the defining characteristic of which being that they 'are not part of any simple meaningful speech-form taken by itself, but appear only when two or more are combined into a larger form, or else when speech-forms are used in certain ways—especially as sentences' (p. 90). However, though prosodic features are usually secondary, this is not always the case; Bloomfield remarks (p. 109) that although pitch is secondary in English it is used as a primary phoneme in Chinese; duration is similarly a primary phoneme in German. Hence, it would appear that prosodic features are primary if they have a word-distinguishing function.[8]

Prague School linguists make no attempt to apply the same categories to prosodic and segmental features, as their functions are different. Trubetzkoy (1935: 24) gives a clear definition: 'by *prosodic features* are meant those properties of syllables by means of which they are marked as parts of rhythmic–melodic units. Here belong length, intensity, pitch, melody, etc. For phonology these properties can naturally only be taken into account if they are "phonologically relevant", i.e. if they form "phonological oppositions".'[9] As the vehicle for prosodic features Trubetzkoy recognizes the 'Silbenträger' (syllable-bearer), which is usually the vowel, but in later work (Trubetzkoy, 1939: 166) he emphasizes that 'the prosodic features belong not to the vowels as such but to the syllables'. In some cases, it is not the syllable that bears the prosodic features but only part of it: the mora.[10] In any case, prosodic features are clearly distinguished from phonemes.

A somewhat different approach is found in the works of American phonemicists. Though referring to prosodic features as 'modifications of the segmental sounds', Bloch and Trager (1942: 41) apply the same analytical procedures to these features as to segmental phonemes—establishment of contrasts, classing similar features together where they are in complementary distribution—and designate the resulting entities *prosodic* or *suprasegmental phonemes*. Though recognizing that such features as intonation have larger scope than the segment,

---

[8] We cannot really speak of a *phonological* function here, since this would imply that only word-distinguishing features are phonologically relevant. This is, indeed, Bloomfield's view; he regards English intonational differences as 'non-distinctive but socially effective'; they 'border most closely on genuine linguistic distinctions' (1935: 114). What counts as phonological is more broadly defined in the present book; at least some intonational distinctions may be considered phonological (see Ch. 5).

[9] Here and passim translations by AF.

[10] For further discussion of the mora see 2.5.4 and 2.8.3.

'they are analyzed and classified like other features of pronunciation, except that in arranging and comparing forms we must use whole sentences in place of isolated words' (p. 42). The reduction of prosodic features to the same status as segmental features is taken still further in works such as Trager and Smith (1951), where the relationships between the different kinds of phonemes are summarized thus (p. 52): 'vowel, consonant, and stress phonemes have allophones statable in terms of position in the sequence; plus juncture and pitch phonemes have allophones statable in terms of stress sequences; terminal junctures have allophones statable in terms of the pitch preceding them'. The different kinds of phonemes are thus differentiated primarily in terms of their distribution.

Jakobson's theory of distinctive features builds on the Prague tradition rather than the American view, so that prosodic features are regarded as a separate category, though co-occurring with segmental features. A distinction is made between 'inherent' and 'prosodic' features, where 'the latter are superposed upon the former and are lumped together with them into phonemes' (Jakobson, Fant, Halle, 1951: 13). The basis of the distinction is variously characterized; inherent features are said to be 'definable without any reference to the sequence' while prosodic features 'can be defined only with reference to the time series'. Alternatively, it is claimed that 'a prosodic feature is displayed only by those phonemes which form the crest of a syllable and it may be defined only with reference to the relief of the syllable or of the syllable chain, whereas the inherent feature is displayed by phonemes irrespective of their role in the relief of the syllable, and the definition of such a feature does not refer to the relief of the syllable or of the syllable chain' (Jakobson and Halle, 1956: 22). A distinction is also made between *intersyllabic* and *intrasyllabic* prosodic features, according to the 'frame of reference' of the feature. In the former case, 'the crest of one syllable is compared with the crests of other syllables within the same sequence', while in the latter 'an instant pertaining to the crest may be compared with other instants of the same crest or with the subsequent slope' (ibid.).[11] Though there are some differences of emphasis in these different definitions and categories, there is no contradiction; prosodic features characterize a larger entity than the segmental phoneme—either a syllable or part of a syllable—and their identification also requires a stretch of speech longer than an individual phoneme, since the phonological contrasts involved are syntagmatic (*in praesentia*—between one part of the utterance and another), rather than paradigmatic (*in absentia*—between an occurring item and a non-occurring item).

There is thus a difference of opinion, among scholars in the structuralist paradigm, as to whether prosodic features should be accorded a different status from segmental phonemes or features. The majority of scholars outside the American

---

[11] This somewhat impenetrable formulation is introduced to deal with cases where one part of a syllable is prosodically different from another, as with a falling or rising tone or with cases where either the first or the second mora of a syllable can be accented (see 2.5.2).

structuralist tradition assign these features to a separate category, but the distinction is minimized by American scholars, who attempt to reduce all contrasting features to the same phonemic status. On the other hand, for those scholars who identify a separate category, there is something of a consensus as to the basis of the distinction: prosodic features extend over more than one phoneme and, phonologically, they involve syntagmatic as well as paradigmatic contrasts.

One structuralist school which adopts a different approach to this question is that of Firthian Prosodic Analysis. Firth (1948) rejects the phoneme as excessively paradigmatic, and refers much of the phonetic content of utterances to the syntagmatic dimension, as 'properties of the sentence or word'. He thus distinguishes *prosodies* from *phonematic units*, but these two categories are not to be identified with prosodic features and phonemes in the sense discussed by other scholars. According to Robins (1957), both of these are abstractions from the phonic data, but of different kinds. Phonematic units are 'those features or aspects of the phonic material which are best regarded as referable to minimal segments, having serial order in relation to each other in structures'; prosodies, on the other hand, 'are, by definition, of more than one segment in scope or domain of relevance, and may in fact belong to structures of any length'. Though these categories may appear to be parallel to 'phonemes' and 'prosodic features', they are in fact quite different, since Firth's prosodies may not only include much of the phonic material which would by other scholars be regarded as segmental, but they are also potentially highly abstract, including, in Firth's original proposal at least, patterns of syllable structure such as CV. The phonematic units cannot, therefore, be identified with phonemes, partly because they are, in effect, merely what is left in particular segmental positions when the prosodies have been extracted, and partly because the basis on which they are established is quite different from that of phonemes; they do not depend on principles such as complementary distribution and contrast.

Although Firth includes such features as stress, tone, and intonation among his prosodies—inevitably, since, as other scholars have concluded, they are 'of more than one segment in scope or domain of relevance'—it is clear that his approach cannot be applied in the present context, since he does not distinguish such features from laryngeal features such as voice and aspiration, and supralaryngeal features such as palatalization, velarization, retroflexion, etc.; all of these may be—and regularly are—treated as prosodies. In terms of the terminological framework presented above, a Firthian description would be characterized as suprasegmental rather than prosodic. Nevertheless, something of the spirit of Firth's approach, and in particular his emphasis on the syntagmatic dimension, will be found to underlie the present book, as will be evident from the discussion in the following chapters.

Some of the characteristics of Firthian Prosodic Analysis are also found in more recent theories, especially Autosegmental Phonology. As in Firth's approach, there is a recognition that an utterance does not need to be treated as the concatenation of segmental units, but can be analysed in terms of a number of quasi-independent simultaneous parameters. Although originally devised to accommodate tone (see 4.4, below), autosegmental representations have been extended to cover traditionally segmental features, including such phenomena as vowel harmony. Again, in the present terminology such treatment of features is considered to be suprasegmental rather than prosodic, and this approach is therefore not the subject of the present discussion, but some of the non-linear assumptions of autosegmental phonology are adopted in this book.

As we have noted, it is possible to define prosodic features in part phonetically and in part in terms of their phonological characteristics, in particular with reference to their non-segmental domain and their syntagmatic basis. But this conclusion has wider repercussions, since it obliges us to consider the nature and organization of the phonological structure of which such features can be said to be a part. It implies that, far from being merely a string of segmental phonemes, utterances are phonologically complex, with a variety of simultaneous dimensions. As we shall see in detail in later chapters, the prosodic structure of utterances is here assumed to be best represented on several 'levels', which are, however, not merely independent 'tiers', synchronized in some way with one another, but are more closely interdependent, together forming an integrated hierarchical structure. This structure in turn forms the framework, the basic organizing principle, for the segmental features of utterances. The best way of characterizing prosodic features—at least initially—is to regard them as those features which constitute or are part of this structural framework. This characterization is, of course, both incomplete and ambiguous, and we shall need both to clarify and to develop it as we proceed.

1.4 The Scope of Prosodic Features

Although we have so far attempted to characterize the prosodic features in general terms, and the major features involved—length and rhythm, accent and stress, tone and intonation—have been enumerated, no definitive list has been given. This is deliberate, since it is, in fact, difficult to produce such a list; even if we are able to define these features adequately, it is not necessarily possible to circumscribe them neatly, for a number of reasons.

In the first place, few, if any, features are simple and one-dimensional. Features such as tone and intonation may be said to involve only a single parameter—here the pitch of the voice—while others, such as rhythm, are not definable in such terms. Rhythm is a complex feature involving accent, length, and tempo, while accent is itself not definable in terms of a single parameter (see Chapter 3, below). In fact, even apparently simple features such as tone and intonation involve more than one dimension; neither is necessarily neatly separable from features of accent and voice quality. As a result, it is not possible to determine how many individual prosodic features should be recognized. Though the prosodic features of speech may ultimately be specified in terms of a small number of acoustic parameters, such as length, pitch and intensity, these are, of course, *phonetic* parameters, and the matter is different with the *phonological* features with which we are here concerned.

A further difficulty is that prosodic features have a clear affinity with *paralinguistic* features, and it is difficult to establish the boundary between them. Paralinguistic features have been defined as 'all those non-linguistic, non-verbal features (both vocal and non-vocal) which participants manipulate in conversation', while 'vocal paralinguistic features would include all activities which are usually loosely referred to as contributing to "tone of voice"' (Laver and Hutcheson, 1972: 13). But there is really no clear dividing line between paralinguistic features, so defined, on the one hand and prosodic features on the other; 'tone of voice' is expressed as much by prosodic features such as intonation as by paralinguistic features such as voice-quality, and indeed both pitch and voice-quality may have both linguistic and non-linguistic functions.

This lack of discreteness is recognized by Crystal and Quirk (1964: 12), who acknowledge that they 'are using the expressions "prosodic" and "paralinguistic" to denote a scale which has at its "most prosodic" end systems of features (for example, intonation contours) which can fairly easily be integrated with other aspects of linguistic structure, while at the "most paralinguistic" end there are features most obviously remote from the possibility of integration with the linguistic structure proper (tremulous voice or clicks of annoyance, for example).' They therefore concede that 'there is no question of a sharp division between the two'.

For these reasons, a definitive list of prosodic features is hardly possible. Nevertheless, Crystal and Quirk (1964) give a composite list including both prosodic and paralinguistic features, which comprises (from the most prosodic to the most paralinguistic) tone, tempo, prominence, pitch range, rhythmicality, tension, quality, qualification, pause, and vocalization. Crystal (1969) gives a slightly different list for English, and is prepared to separate prosodic and paralinguistic features. Under the former heading come (again in the direction from 'most linguistic' to 'least linguistic') pitch direction, pitch range, pause, loudness, tempo, and rhythmicality, while 'tension' is considered to fall in both the prosodic and paralinguistic categories.

It would hardly be possible, within the confines of this book, to deal in detail with such a wide range of potential features, especially since the linguistic role of a number of them is difficult to establish. We are able, however, to identify a much smaller set of 'core' prosodic features, whose linguistic role is more clearly demonstrable. Sweet (1906) recognizes primarily length, stress and pitch, with voice-quality as a secondary feature; Lehiste (1970) similarly has three chapters, devoted to 'Quantity', 'Tonal Features', and 'Stress'. In the present book, prosodic features are discussed under four main headings: 'Length', 'Accent', 'Tone', and 'Intonation', but this does not imply that these are the only features to be recognized, and other features are considered where appropriate (rhythm, for example, is discussed under length, while voice-quality is dealt with under tone). These features are identified here not only because they are the most 'linguistic' of the prosodic features but also because they are the major components of prosodic structure.

2

Length

2.1 Introduction: The Nature and Status of Length

Of all the prosodic features, length appears—at first sight at least—to be conceptually the simplest and least controversial. Speaking is a time-dependent activity;
utterances take place in real time, and although articulatory events are not necessarily discrete—articulations overlap and some events are simultaneous rather
than successive—there is nevertheless a temporal order to both the production
and the perception of the speech signal. Thus, any part of this signal will occupy
a finite portion of time, which can be measured, and the length of any such part
is simply the time taken to utter it.

As soon as we attempt to make any kind of generalizations about length,
however, and especially when we take account of its functional role, many complexities and difficulties arise. In the first place, the length of speech sounds is
highly variable; not only do different sounds differ in their length, but even what
we take to be the 'same' sound may occupy very different amounts of time under different circumstances and in different contexts. The factors at work here
are many and various: the nature of the sound itself, the number and character
of the surrounding sounds, the position of the sound in the word or syllable in
which it occurs, the speed and style of utterance, and so on.[1]

For example, different sound types characteristically have different *intrinsic*
lengths, which are typical values for the sound type in question, though in all
cases such differences are relative rather than absolute. Labial consonants, for
example, are usually longer than alveolars or velars, and voiceless stops are longer than voiceless fricatives (Laver, 1994: 434–5); open vowels tend to be longer
than close ones (Lehiste, 1970: 18–27). Overlaid on these universal tenden-
cies—and in practice often difficult to separate from them—are the different
length characteristics of sounds in different languages; 'long' vowels in German,
for example, tend to be relatively longer than their English counterparts
(Delattre, 1965: 63).

To these intrinsic properties of length we must add the *extrinsic* or contextu-
ally determined ones, which again are subject to language-specific variations.

---

[1] For detailed reviews of the role of such factors, see especially Lehiste (1970: ch. 2) and Laver
(1994: ch. 14).

Some of these properties depend on surrounding sound types (it is well known, for example, that English vowels are shorter before voiceless consonants than before voiced ones), others merely on the position in the sequence or syllable (intervocalic consonants are usually shorter than initial or final ones). Other prosodic features also play a part: the length of a sound may be different according to whether the syllable in which it occurs is stressed or not, or, in tone-languages, on the particular tone with which the syllable is uttered. In Mandarin Chinese, for example, the vowel of a syllable uttered with the third (low) tone is longer than that of a syllable with the fourth (falling) tone. Other, more obvious, factors which influence length are the number of sounds in the syllable or word (the more sounds there are, the shorter they become), the speed of utterance (the faster the speed, the shorter the sounds), and so on. The majority of these factors are mechanical and of no phonological significance, though deciding which of them have a phonological role may often be difficult.

There are also a number of more basic general problems of a theoretical and practical nature which impinge on the study of length. First, length differs significantly from many other sound attributes; it is not a qualitative feature of the production or perception of sounds comparable to, for example, tongue height or nasality. The latter are articulatory or acoustic properties, which are detectable throughout the sounds concerned, unlike length, which cannot be identified by sampling the sound at any point, and can only be established for the sound as a whole, and in relation to other sounds. Moreover, the actual phonetic 'content' of length is not a single definable phonetic attribute but is dependent on the other attributes of the sound. For example, a long [a:] and a long [i:] do not share any phonetic property as such; the [:] of the transcription is not a consistent, phonetically definable property (which would be the case with, say, nasalization or lip rounding), but has to be interpreted differently in each case. Phonetically, its properties are those of the sound—here [a] or [i]—which it accompanies. It is therefore a *diacritic* feature, in the sense that it is only interpretable with reference to the sound with which it occurs.[2] On a more practical level, a further problem relates to the *measurement* of length. Speech is not as readily segmentable as our phonetic transcriptions imply, and the boundaries between sounds are seldom clearcut. Exactly what we measure and where we measure from and to are by no means trivial matters. Hence Fry (1968: 386) can write that 'the measurement of length in itself presents no difficulty . . . . The problem in duration is only in knowing what to measure.'

From a phonological perspective, too, a major problem is again the fact that

---

[2] The meaning of the term 'diacritic' here is not to be confused with its use in referring to additional marks added to symbols in a transcription; in the usage intended here it refers to a property of the *sound itself*, though again one which is only interpretable in terms of another property of which it is a modification (cf. Trask, 1996: 110, where the present usage is described as 'rare').

length is not simply an attribute of phonological units on a par with features of vowel quality, such as height, backness, and lip-rounding. These features provide phonological distinctions such as 'high' vs. 'low', 'back' vs. 'front', 'rounded' vs. 'unrounded', and so on, which serve to oppose one phonological entity to another. While length distinctions may be interpreted in a similar way, giving oppositions between 'long' and 'short' vowels and consonants (see 2.4.3, below), there is a complication here, inasmuch as such differences of length can only be realized in terms of differences in the time dimension, and hence have potential implications for the phonological *structure* of the words in which these sounds occur. Putting this more technically, we can say that length is ambivalent with regard to its role in *paradigmatic* and *syntagmatic* relations,[3] i.e. it may function both in an opposition such as 'long' vs. 'short' and *simultaneously* in a contrast between, for example, 'one unit' and 'two units'. This ambivalence allows for radically different theoretical interpretations of length by different scholars, as we shall see below.

In the context of the theme of the present book, one final question must also be asked: to what extent is it legitimate to regard length as a *prosodic* feature in the sense in which this term has been defined in Chapter 1? The question is pertinent, since length is often considered solely in relation to individual phonological *segments*, such as vowels (and, less often, consonants), and segmental features are in principle not prosodic. Apart from the fact that length is traditionally grouped together with 'pitch' and 'stress' as a suprasegmental feature,[4] there are more important reasons for regarding it as legitimately prosodic. First, length has, as we have observed, implications for *temporal structure*, and is therefore involved in the phonological organization of the utterance as a whole; second, length is by no means restricted to segments, but may apply to other, larger, units of the utterance, such as the syllable, as we shall see later in this chapter; third, length has, as we have noted, close relations with other features, such as accent, whose prosodic credentials are not in doubt. In spite of the predominant attribution of length to segments, therefore, we are justified in concluding that it, too, has prosodic status.

Our task in the present chapter is twofold. First, we must attempt to identify and clarify the nature and phonological role of length in the light of the various considerations presented above. Second, we must consider some of the characteristics of a model of prosodic features and prosodic structure which is able to accommodate length in a satisfactory way.

---

[3] Saussure, 1967 [1916]: 170–5.

[4] See, for example, Sweet (1906), who groups together quantity and stress, as well as other features, as aspects of speech 'synthesis', and Lehiste (1970), who has three central chapters, devoted to 'Quantity', 'Tonal Features' and 'Stress'.

2.2 Background to the Study of Length

2.2.1 THE CLASSICAL TRADITION

Current conceptions of language did not arise in a vacuum; they must be seen against the background of traditional views, most of which come from the study of the classical languages, Greek and Latin. The grammarians of the ancient world already appreciated that there were length distinctions in their languages[5] and that these distinctions were of linguistic importance, and the tradition that followed them has maintained and extended this knowledge. The orthographies of Greek and Latin represent length only unsystematically, if at all; in Classical Greek, separate letters are provided—though only from the end of the fifth century BC—for long vowels in the case of ω (*o-mega* = 'big o') and η (*eta*), which are distinct from the short vowels o (*o-micron* = 'little o') and ε (*e-psilon* = 'plain e'), but long and short α, ι and υ ('a', 'i' and 'u') are not distinguished; in Latin, differences of vowel length are not normally indicated in the standard orthography at all, though occasionally long vowels are written double or with a diacritic (Gildersleve and Lodge, 1895: 7). Nevertheless, such differences can be of lexical and grammatical significance: Latin *lĕgō* ('I gather') is distinct from *lēgō* ('I bequeath') and *Rōmă* ('Rome') is distinct from *Rōmā* ('from Rome')— long and short vowels are here indicated by ‾ and ˘ respectively.

Length is also one of the determining factors in the placement of the Latin word-accent: in polysyllabic words the accent falls on the penultimate syllable if it is 'long', but on the antepenultimate syllable if the penultimate syllable is 'short'. A 'long' syllable is defined as one containing a long vowel, or a short vowel followed by more than one consonant, and a 'short' syllable as one containing a short vowel followed by not more than one consonant.[6] Thus, the first syllable is accented in *'dŏmĭnŭs* ('lord') or *'īnsŭlă* ('island'), and the second in *nā'tūră* ('nature') or *mă'gĭstĕr* ('master'). In addition, length is of particular importance for verse structure, which is based on quantitative relations rather than, as in English, on accentual patterns.[7] The Latin hexameter, for example, contains six rhythmical 'feet', in which a foot containing one long and two short syllables (‾ ˘ ˘, a 'dactyl') is equivalent to, and may be replaced by, a foot with two long syllables (‾ ‾, a 'spondee') in most positions in the line.

All these matters have long been familiar to classical scholars, and are part of the European linguistic tradition. This tradition has also engendered a misconception, however. As noted above, the 'long' syllable, in both the rules for locating the accent and in the metrical patterns, does not need to contain a 'long' vowel; a 'short' vowel followed by more than one consonant will do just as well

---

[5] On vowel length in Greek and Latin see Allen (1965, ch. 3; 1968, ch. 3; 1973).
[6] For further discussion of Latin syllable length using the concept of the *mora* see 2.5.4, below.
[7] It is likely that quantitative verse nevertheless had an accentual ictus. On quantitative verse see Allen (1964).

(see 2.5.3, below). Thus, *mă'gĭstĕr* ('master') contains only short vowels, but the accent is on the penultimate syllable because this syllable is 'long' (the vowel is followed by two consonants); similarly the first syllable of *căstră* ('camp') counts as 'long' for metrical purposes, even though its vowel is short. In both cases the length of the syllable derives from the presence of a consonant cluster following the vowel rather than from the length of the vowel itself. Syllables containing a long vowel are said to be long 'by nature'; those containing a short vowel followed by more than one consonant are said to be long 'by convention' or 'by position'.[8] In the latter case, of course, the *vowel* still remains short, though the *syllable* counts as long for metrical purposes and for determining the position of the accent. In the course of the transmission of the grammatical tradition, however, the idea that the syllable is long 'by position' has been reinterpreted to mean that the short vowel is actually *lengthened* in this position, which is, of course, not the case. This misunderstanding was widespread among mediaeval grammarians, and some present-day writers on the classical languages have continued to perpetuate it.[9]

Though in some ways merely a naive lapse, resulting from the uncritical transmission of a tradition, this misconception is of some interest as a revealing symptom of the complexities and ambiguities of the phenomenon of length itself. We have already noted some of these complexities, in particular the fact that length has implications for syllable structure, and that it can apply to both segments and syllables. These are precisely the sorts of difficulties that are involved in the misunderstandings of classical grammarians, who failed to distinguish vowel length from syllable length, and to disentangle the length of a vowel from the structural complexity of the syllable of which it is a part. Since much of the subsequent theoretical discussion surrounding length is concerned with precisely these matters, these confusions offer, in retrospect, an important pointer to some of the major issues involved here.

2.2.2 EARLY PHONETICIANS

Practical phoneticians at the end of the nineteenth century drew attention to the inadequacies of the traditional approach to length. Most influential here was the work of Sweet, whose *Handbook of Phonetics* (1877) contains for the first time remarks on length which are based on observation rather than inherited wisdom and go beyond the traditional distinction between 'long' and 'short' vowels. Sweet stands in the tradition of the 'English School' of phonetics, but his prede-

---

[8] The Greek terms (used, for example, by Dionysius Thrax) are φύσει ('by nature') and θέσει, which translates as either 'by convention' or 'by position'. Latin grammarians used the terms *natura* and *positu* or *positione* (cf. Allen, 1973).

[9] For example, we read in Raven's *Greek Metre* (1962: 23), that 'any vowel which is short by nature *becomes long* by position when immediately followed by a double consonant (ζ, ξ, ψ), or by two or more consonants together' (emphasis added).

cessors in this tradition, such as Ellis (1848), still discuss length in traditional terms. Sweet's originality was acknowledged by his successors; Meyer (1903: 1) notes that 'Sweet is the first of the modern phoneticians to give information on the length of sounds which more or less does justice to the real facts'.[10]

Sweet despised the mere 'paper phonetics' of the philologists, and he provides a notation system which is able to distinguish five degrees of length (though he does concede that for practical purposes three degrees, or even two, are usually sufficient). He also presents an original description of length in English which takes into account the influence of the following consonant on the length of the vowel. He recognizes three degrees for both vowels and consonants: 'long', 'half-long' and 'short'. His 'long' vowels correspond to the traditional long vowels when in final position or when followed by a voiced consonant, for example in such words as *sir* or *hard*;[11] 'half-long' vowels correspond to traditional long vowels when followed by a voiceless consonant (*heart*), or to traditional short vowels before a voiced consonant (*bud*); his 'short' vowels correspond to traditional short vowels before voiceless consonants (*hit*). Similarly, consonants are 'long' when they are voiceless after a short vowel (*hit*), 'half-long' when they are voiced after a half-long vowel (*bud*), and 'short' when they are voiced after a long vowel (*hard*) or voiceless after a half-long vowel (*heart*). Sweet also notes differences of consonant length in clusters, e.g. the *l* of *build* versus that of *built*, or the *n* of *pens* versus that of *pence* (cf. Jespersen, 1913: 180).

Sweet's categories, however pertinent they may be from a phonetic point of view, clearly cut across not only the traditional distinctions but also what would later be recognized as the phonologically relevant categories of length in English. His influence was considerable, and is noticeable in the work of subsequent writers on phonetics, such as Sievers (1893) and Jespersen (1913). The former observes, for example, the different lengths of [aː] in German words such as *Zahl*, *zahle*, and *zahlende*; the latter adopts Sweet's five degrees of length, and his analysis of English vowel and consonant length, and notes the different lengths of [uː] in English *gloom, gloomy, gloomily*, or of [iː] in *feel, feeling, feelingly* (Jespersen, 1913: 180). Of significance, too, is Jespersen's distinction between 'external' and 'internal' determination of length, which amounts to a recognition of the distinction between phonologically relevant and irrelevant length distinctions.[12]

---

[10] Translation by AF.

[11] Sweet is, of course, describing an r-less pronunciation in which words like 'hard' and 'heart' have a long vowel and no r-sound.

[12] For Jespersen, the former is 'dependent on purely external phonetic conditions . . . for which rules can be established (stress, position in the syllable, context)' whereas the latter depends 'on internal circumstances, so that the quantity is an equally important component of the words and can be used to distinguish meaning just as well as the sound components themselves' (1913: 182)—translation by AF.

2.2.3 EARLY EXPERIMENTAL PHONETICS

Several experimental studies of the length of speech sounds had been carried out in the latter half of the nineteenth century, for example by the Austrian physiologist Brücke, author of a standard work on phonetics (Brücke, 1856), but such work was greatly enhanced in the last decade of the century by the rise of Experimental Phonetics, which applied newly invented instruments to the study of spoken language. Although these instruments were primitive by modern standards, one feature of speech that was relatively easy to record by these means was the length of the sounds. For the most part, such studies, for example by phoneticians such as Viëtor (1894), are concerned with measuring the exact quantitative relationships between the traditional 'long' and 'short' vowels. This is usually done by means of a 'graphic method' which involves producing a visual rather than an acoustic recording of the pronunciation of individual words, measuring the length of the visual traces of vowels, and averaging several such measurements. Most impressive among these experimental studies are those of Meyer (1903), who undertook a detailed investigation of the length of various English sounds. Meyer's work entailed very considerable labour, with 4,800 measurements of individual sounds in a variety of contexts, in 393 one-syllable and 141 two-syllable words. Since Meyer's work was so thorough and reliable (and also perhaps because it would have been excessively time-consuming to replicate it), he was still being cited as the definitive source of data on length 30 years later.

The results of these experimental investigations were very revealing, if unsurprising. They were able to demonstrate the inadequacy of the traditional distinction between 'short' and 'long' vowels, since many more distinctions were found to occur. Indeed, even the five degrees recognized by Sweet were found to be quite insufficient to cover the wide divergence of length found in different contexts. Thus, if Sweet despised 'paper phonetics' and trusted his ears, experimental phoneticians in their turn despised the 'ear phonetics' of Sweet, and preferred the more 'objective' evidence of machines.

2.2.4 THE PHONETICS AND PHONOLOGY OF LENGTH

It will be clear from the foregoing discussion that some considerable progress had been made by phoneticians at the end of the nineteenth century and the beginning of the twentieth in overcoming the limitations of the classical tradition. It was widely recognized that the length of sounds was a rather more complex matter than merely a distinction between 'long' and 'short' vowels, and that many more—indeed, indefinitely many—degrees of length could be recognized, especially with the use of experimental methods.

From our present perspective, however, an important element appears to be missing from these early treatments of the topic: the phonological dimension.

There was at this time no explicit recognition of phonological concepts; though such ideas had already been foreshadowed, explicit phonological theories had to await the development of structuralist approaches in the coming decades of the twentieth century. Thus, in spite of the detailed observations made by both practical and experimental phoneticians, without phonological concepts it is impossible to order and interpret the observations in what we would now consider to be a linguistically significant way. We may certainly detect in Sweet's statement that it is usually necessary to recognize only two or three degrees an embryonic, and intuitive, phonology, but his analysis of length in English shows that his approach is really phonetic rather than phonological. Jespersen's recognition of 'external' and 'internal' length is likewise indicative of an understanding of the difference between phonetic and phonological aspects of the phenomenon, but these ideas were not immediately taken up.

Explicit phonological concepts were introduced into the discussion from the late 1920s, initially in the work of the Prague School and subsequently by scholars in other theoretical frameworks, and these will be examined in detail in this chapter. Such phonological considerations do not, of course, render phonetic description such as that discussed above either irrelevant or useless. Rather they provide a framework for the interpretation of phonetic observations in terms of their linguistic relevance and role. Thus, both practical and experimental investigations of length have continued with increasing sophistication, usually with an awareness—not always manifested in the early work outlined above—of the linguistic significance of the phenomena under investigation.

Although our main focus in this chapter is on the phonology of length, we must therefore not lose sight of the fact that such phonetic investigation has continued, and that account must be taken of its findings at appropriate points in the discussion.

2.3 Preliminaries to the Phonology of Length

2.3.1 PHONOLOGICAL PERSPECTIVES ON LENGTH

The introduction of a phonological perspective into the consideration of length is not without its difficulties, not least because the different schools and traditions of phonological theory give rather divergent, and often incompatible, interpretations of the phenomenon. But the linguistic role of length itself also provides sufficient ambiguity and uncertainty to ensure that there is no single and simple solution to the problems posed. We have already noted (2.1, above) that length has an ambivalent phonological status: on the one hand it can be regarded as participating in paradigmatic contrasts such as 'short' vs. 'long', but such contrasts are inevitably manifested along the time dimension, and are thus susceptible to a syntagmatic interpretation in terms of different numbers or arrangements of units. We may thus initially identify two different perspectives to the study of length: a *paradigmatic* and a *syntagmatic* interpretation.

However, both of these, and the latter in particular, comprise a variety of theoretical positions; a syntagmatic view may be confined to seeing long sounds as sequences of short ones, or it may take rather more account of the context in which the sounds occur. We shall see, therefore, that there is a range of theoretical interpretations of length which embraces narrower or wider aspects of the context, seeing length in progressively less segmental and more prosodic terms; indeed we may see a *prosodic* interpretation as effectively a third general orientation.

It must be stressed, however, that these different approaches to length are not necessarily mutually exclusive, and that they can be seen as representing not theories of length as such but rather dimensions along which length can be interpreted. As a result, these categories may cut across the different 'schools'; a number of theoretical frameworks allow different aspects of the phenomenon to be dealt with in different ways. Nor is the progression from 'paradigmatic' through 'syntagmatic' to 'prosodic' necessarily a chronological one: several different perspectives are represented in current theories. Our aim in this discussion is thus to consider the nature of the phenomenon of length itself rather than merely the specific approaches of the different 'schools'.

2.3.2 THE PHONOLOGICAL ROLE OF LENGTH

Although the theoretical interpretations of length may differ, the starting point for most discussions is generally the same: the lexically or grammatically significant distinction found in many languages between 'long' and 'short' sounds, especially vowels. In Japanese, for example, we encounter pairs such as /isso/ ('rather') vs. /isso:/ ('more'), or /soko/ ('bottom') vs. /soko:/ ('conduct'), while in Finnish we find sets such as /tule/ ('come') vs. /tule:/ ('comes') vs. /tu:le:/ ('it blows').[13] Similar distinctions are reported for consonants, though they are evidently somewhat less common. In Hungarian, for example, there are distinctions such as those given in Fig. 2.1.

Fig. 2.1 hal   *hal* ('fish')   vs. hal: *hall* ('hears')
         lap   *lap* ('sheet of paper')   vs. lap: *lapp* ('Laplander')
         fø:t *föt* ('chief thing', acc.)   vs. fø:t: *fött* ('cooked')

In some languages, such as Mixe (Hoogshagen, 1959) and Estonian, more than two degrees of length are noted. The examples of Fig. 2.2 are from Estonian, which distinguishes three degrees in both vowels and consonants (Ariste, 1939).

Fig. 2.2 sada   *sada*   ('100')   kapi   *kabi*   ('hoof')
         sa:da   *saada* ('send')   kap:i   *kapi*   ('wardrobe')
         sa::da *saada* ('to get')   kap::i *kappi* ('wardrobe', partitive singular)

---

[13] Data from Jones (1967: 120–1).

Although these cases provide straightforward evidence for the phonological relevance of length, this does not determine the actual theoretical interpretation, and, as we shall see in the course of this chapter, the same phenomenon may be susceptible to several different analyses. There are also many cases where the interpretation is complicated by other factors or problems. We may find, for example, that although there are length distinctions, they are relatively marginal, and do not characterize the system as a whole. This is the case with French, where length plays a part in the vowel system, but only in a few cases such as [ɛ] vs. [ɛ:] in *mettre* vs. *maître*. In other languages there may be length distinctions, but it is difficult to localize them; in Icelandic, Swedish, and other Scandinavian languages, for example, there is a reciprocal relationship between the vowel and consonant length within the syllable, such that a long vowel is followed by a short consonant, and vice versa. It is a moot point in such cases whether it is the length of the vowel or that of the consonant that is phonologically significant, and different views are held.[14]

A different complication is provided by languages such as English or German, where there are length differences in the vowels, but they are generally accompanied by other differences; the 'short' vowels are considerably more 'lax' and centralised than the 'long' ones, and it is therefore unclear whether it is length or some other phonetic feature such as 'tension' that should be regarded as the primary distinctive feature in these contrasts.[15]

In yet another group of languages, there are relationships between length, accentuation and pitch, for example in the 'tonal accents' or 'intonations' of Lithuanian and Serbo–Croat. Here there are pitch differences traditionally ascribed to different kinds of accents, which in turn depend on the lengths of the syllables. In such cases, it is difficult to separate the phonological role of length from that of these other features.[16]

A different kind of issue is raised by the relationship between length and syllable structure, as in the Latin examples given in 2.2.1, above. We noted that Latin syllables are considered 'long' not merely when they contain a long vowel but also when they contain a short vowel followed by more than one consonant, and this situation is found in many other languages, too. In these cases there is therefore some sort of equivalence between vowel length and certain syllable structures, but the nature of this equivalence, and of the categories required to account for it, is again the subject of different interpretations.

Finally, we may recall that it is not merely segments but also syllables and other 'higher' units that may differ in length. As we noted in 2.2.2, early writers on the subject, such as Sievers and Jespersen, drew attention to the different lengths of syllables in such words as *gloom*, *gloomy*, and *gloomily*. More striking is the example given by Scott (1940) of the distinction between the two utter-

---

[14] For discussion of this case see 2.6.3.2, below.
[15] See 2.4.3/2.4.4, below, for further discussion.   [16] See 4.7.3, below.

ances *Take Grey to London* and *Take Greater London*, which are identical in their segmental structure but nevertheless different in the patterning of length in the syllables they contain. Such examples are indicative of wider questions relating to the timing of syllables, and the rhythm of utterances as a whole, which a comprehensive theory of the phonology of length must attempt to address.

2.3.3 A NOTE ON TERMINOLOGY

Ideally, our terminological framework should reflect the conceptual framework, but this is not always so in the case of 'length', a term which is often applied indiscriminately in a phonetic and phonological sense, and also in relation to different kinds of units. Some consensus has been achieved with the designation of 'phonetic' length, i.e. the absolute physical length of a sound or syllable, for which we may use the term *duration*. The duration of a sound is measured in absolute terms, viz. in milliseconds or centiseconds, with no phonological implications. This would in principle leave the term *length* free for phonological use. However, a further term is also available here: *quantity*, which has traditionally been used in relation to metrical values in classical verse, but has also been widely applied more generally. One proposal here is that of Allen (1973), who suggests restricting 'length' to segmental phonology and using 'quantity' for syllabic length, but this terminological scheme, though laudable, is seldom observed. The term *weight* is also in use in relation to syllable length, as discussed in 2.6.2, below. On a purely terminological level, some difficulty is created by the absence of suitable adjectives; 'length' provides us with the terms *long* and *short*, and 'weight' gives us *heavy* and *light*, but there are no corresponding terms for 'duration' or 'quantity', so that we must again have recourse to 'long' and 'short', perhaps with qualifications such as 'phonologically long', 'phonetically short', and so on. When we add to this the different usage in different theoretical and descriptive traditions, the interpretation of the terminology used is clearly a highly context-sensitive matter.

2.4 The Paradigmatic Interpretation of Length

2.4.1 INTRODUCTION

From a phonological perspective, significant length differences, such as those cited in 2.3.2, can be resolved into a distinction between 'long' and 'short' sounds (and possibly, as in the case of languages such as Estonian, more than two such degrees). This is perhaps the most obvious and natural analysis, but there are others, and we must here consider whether this approach is able to accommodate phonologically significant length phenomena in a satisfactory way.

A major contribution here, all the more significant for being the first explicitly articulated phonological theory of length, was made from the early 1930s onwards by linguists of the Prague School, especially its principal members, Roman Jakobson and Nikolai Trubetzkoy.[17] Initially, this did not result in a simplification of the field, but rather the reverse: their discussions can be said to have identified—one might perhaps say created—what was to become known as the 'quantity problem' (cf. Trubetzkoy, 1938; Fischer-Jørgensen, 1940–1). The radical stance adopted by these scholars, following the theoretical precepts of the Prague position through to their logical conclusions, established a framework which was to dominate, albeit briefly, the immediate post-war discussion of these matters on the continent of Europe. The approach of these scholars can be called 'paradigmatic', inasmuch as the main focus of their work is the exploration of the nature and role of distinctive phonological *oppositions*.[18]

The nature of the paradigmatic distinctions involving length is also explored further in Jakobson's extension and development of the Prague School theory of oppositions into Distinctive Feature theory, which underlies much current phonology, especially in a generative framework.

2.4.2 LENGTH AND PHONOLOGICAL OPPOSITIONS

2.4.2.1 Phonological Relevance

From the point of view of a functional theory of phonological oppositions, an initial question to be addressed relates to the phonological *relevance* of a feature, that is, whether it has a distinctive phonological function at all. In the case of length, Trubetzkoy (1938) observes that all phonemes of a language must occupy time if they are to exist at all, hence the possession of a basic unit of length by a phoneme cannot in itself be phonologically relevant. From this it follows that an apparent opposition of length between two phonemes, one of which merely possesses this basic amount of length, cannot in fact be interpreted as such, since we cannot have an opposition involving a phonologically irrelevant feature, and the opposition must be reanalysed in some other terms. The difficulties that this conclusion creates for the phonological description of length are the essential ingredients of the 'quantity problem'.

There are different ways in which such apparent length contrasts may be analysed, depending on the language in question. One possibility is to treat 'long' vowels as having a bipartite structure, with two phonemes (a 'polyphon-

---

[17] The major works relevant for this discussion are Jakobson, 1931 and 1937; Trubetzkoy, 1935, 1936, 1938, and 1939. It is not always easy to separate out the individual contributions of each of these scholars, as there was considerable mutual influence.

[18] Prague School terminology distinguishes 'opposition' from 'contrast', the former being paradigmatic, the latter syntagmatic. Thus, English *bit* and *pit* give an *opposition* between /b/ and /p/, while 'import (noun) and im'port (verb), which differ in the location of the accent, constitute a *contrast*. No such distinction is made elsewhere, for example in American structuralist theory, the term *contrast* being used for the Prague 'opposition'.

ematic' interpretation). According to Trubetzkoy, this 'analytic' approach to length is justifiable under certain conditions which will be considered below (2.5.2). In these cases the syllable, or rather the 'Silbenträger' (the syllable 'bearer' or nucleus) is divided into two parts or *moras*. Languages where this is possible are *mora languages*, as it is the mora, rather than the syllable, which carries the prosodic features of the language. Since this approach is essentially syntagmatic, discussion of its implications will be postponed until later.

In languages where this analytic approach is not available it is the *syllable*, rather than the mora, that is of prosodic significance; such languages are therefore termed *syllable languages*. Since length itself cannot be the relevant feature in an opposition, in these languages it must be interpreted in some other way. Two possible analyses are proposed, according to whether we take the 'long' or the 'short' length to be basic, and this is determined by an appeal to *markedness*. In any opposition one value, or *term*, is considered to be 'marked', the other 'unmarked'. The precise interpretation of the concept of markedness is rather variable, but the implication is that the 'marked' term possesses some specific phonetic feature that the 'unmarked' term lacks, and that it is in some sense less expected or usual, and therefore all the more significant and meaningful. However, for Trubetzkoy the test of which term is unmarked or marked is the appearance of the term in question in a position where the opposition is inoperative, or *neutralized*; in this position it is the unmarked term which is assumed to occur.

In the matter of length, Trubetzkoy identifies two different cases, according to whether it is the 'short' or the 'long' vowel—it is usually a vowel that we are concerned with here—that is unmarked, and these two cases demand a different interpretation of the apparent opposition between 'short' and 'long'.

2.4.2.2 'Extendibility'

The first case is that in which it is the 'short' vowel that is unmarked. According to Trubetzkoy (1939: 175), this is true of colloquial Czech, which has no length opposition in initial vowels; the opposition is neutralized in this position, and the vowel that appears here is the *short* one. Since the unmarked value of length (here 'short') is not phonologically relevant, the 'long' vowel cannot be regarded as phonologically long in opposition to it. How, then, can the opposition be characterized?

The solution here is to replace length by *extendibility* as the phonologically relevant feature. This is clarified and justified by Trubetzkoy (1938) using a geometrical analogy. He argues that the 'short' vs. 'long' distinction here is equivalent *not* to the geometrical distinction between two *lines* of different length (since the 'short' vowel has no length, phonologically speaking), but to the distinction between a *point* and a *line*, since a geometrical point, like an unmarked 'short' vowel, has no length; it merely has location. A line is distinguished from a point not by its greater length (a point cannot be regarded as 'shorter' than a line, since length is not a property of a point at all) but by the fact that it *has extent* as a property, and is therefore *extendible*.[19] The opposition is therefore not one of length but of extendibility.

The terminological shift from 'long' to 'extendible' may seem to be slight and over-subtle. Nevertheless, it has some significant consequences, notably that length *as such* is excluded from phonological relevance. From this, Trubetzkoy is able to draw an important general conclusion, as we shall see shortly.

2.4.2.3 'Contact'

There is another case, however: a language where the unmarked value of the opposition is the 'long' term. An example of such a language is English, where short vowels (other than [ə]) do not occur in final open syllables; vowels in this position are always long (e.g. in *buffalo, andante*, etc.). Again, therefore, the opposition is neutralized, but here it is in favour of the 'long' vowel. As before, the length of the vowel cannot be phonologically relevant, and the apparent opposition with the 'short' vowels must be interpreted differently. Here, Trubetzkoy's solution is to regard the 'short' vowels (which only occur before a consonant) as being *cut off* by the following consonant, while the 'long' vowels continue unchecked. The opposition is therefore one of *contact* between the vowel and the consonant: between 'close' and 'loose' contact. The implication is that the vowel is or is not cut off at the moment of its maximum intensity.[20]

2.4.2.4 Length, Stress, and 'Intensity'

One of the implications of the functional basis of Prague School phonology is that the phonetic content of oppositions is less significant than the oppositions themselves. This means that the phonetic features which exercise a given function may vary from case to case, and may therefore be complementary in their use. Consequently, length may be seen merely as one of several features which fulfil a given function.

We have already identified different roles for length in the realization of oppositions in different languages. In the case of Czech, as we have seen, it is claimed that length may be involved in realizing the opposition between 'extendible' and 'non-extendible' (though 'length' as such is not the phonologically relevant feature). Trubetzkoy claims further that this opposition can be generalized with such features as stress ('Druckstärke') as the realization of an opposition of *intensity*, i.e. that 'extendible' and 'stressed' are alternative ways of indicating intensity. Hence, according to Trubetzkoy, in languages where length

---

[19] The German term is *dehnungsfähig*.

[20] The German term for this opposition is *Silbenschnittkorrelation* ('syllable cut correlation'). This distinction did not originate with Trubetzkoy; it appears to go back to Sievers (5th edn., 1901: 222), who speaks of 'strong' and 'weak cut-off' (*stark geschnittener Akzent, schwach geschnittener Akzent*) in relation to accentuation. Trubetzkoy's terms may have been adopted from Jespersen (e.g. *Elementarbuch*, 1912: 153), who uses the terms *fester Anschluß* and *loser Anschluß*.

functions as a marker of intensity, no other phonologically relevant intensity factor, such as stress, can co-occur with it. In some cases, such as Tamale, stress is simply absent; in others (such as Czech, Icelandic, or Hungarian), stress features may be present, but the position of the stressed syllable is fixed and hence it cannot be distinctive; in still others (such as Latin), stress is not fixed, but its position is predictable from other features (cf. the accentuation rules given in 2.2.1), and hence again it does not fulfil a distinctive function.

Length may also be subordinate to stress in the sense that length distinctions are only found in stressed syllables, but not unstressed ones. Jakobson (1937) suggests that it is in these cases that the 'contact' opposition operates, with 'long' as the unmarked term (the 'extendibility' opposition, with 'short' as the unmarked term, will then apply in cases where length is *not* subordinate to stress).

2.4.2.5 Paradigmatic Functions of Length

Thus, in Prague School terms, the phonetic property of length can be interpreted paradigmatically in two ways, according to the different functions that it fulfils. (This is in addition to the 'analytic' approach to length, which will be considered below.) A 'long' vowel can be:

(i) the realization of 'extendibility', i.e. it is opposed to a non-extendible basic length; this in turn is a manifestation of 'intensity'

(ii) as 'loose contact', the normal expression of an unobstructed vowel, i.e. it is opposed to a vowel that is cut off by the following consonant.

It will be noted that in neither case does Trubetzkoy consider length *itself* to be distinctive or phonologically relevant. Measurable differences in the length of sounds are regarded as the reflection of some other property: 'the opposition between short and long sounds in languages with internally determined quantity is always merely the phonetic expression of some deeper phonological opposition'.[21] This effectively excludes length from any phonological relevance in language, and allows Trubetzkoy to draw the ultimate conclusion that *the linguistic system has in principle no temporal dimension*, 'for *langue* is in itself timeless'.[22]

This conclusion is, in fact, entirely in keeping with the Saussurean roots of Prague theory. Saussure's conception of 'language' is as an inventory of items shared by the speech community rather than as a set of structural principles. Hence even the sentence is not part of 'langue' but of 'parole', the actual language use of the individual speaker. Trubetzkoy's conclusion that there is no temporal element to the linguistic system reflects this view, as, indeed, does the paradigmatic focus of Prague School theory as a whole.

---

[21] *Der Gegensatz zwischen kurzen und langen Lauten in Sprachen mit innerlich bestimmter Quantität* [*ist*] *immer nur der phonetische Ausdruck irgendeines tiefer liegenden phonologischen Gegensatzes.* Note that the distinction between 'internally' and 'externally' determined length is from Jespersen.

[22] *Denn das Sprachgebilde ("la langue") ist an und für sich zeitlos.*

2.4.2.6 Criticism and Evaluation

The stature and influence of Jakobson and Trubetzkoy were doubtless among the factors that helped to ensure that the views put forward by these scholars were taken seriously by other European linguists, particularly those who were sympathetic to the Prague orientation. We thus find interpretations of the role of length in a number of languages which seek to apply these principles. Richter (1938), for example, investigates length in Italian, in pairs such as *matto* ('mad') vs. *amato* ('loved'), and comes to the conclusion that the distinction is not one of length as such, which is found to be unreliable here, but rather of *extendibility*, as prescribed by Trubetzkoy. In an investigation of length in Icelandic, Bergsveinsson (1941) similarly concludes that the difference between 'long' and 'short' vowels lies in the nature of the *contact* with the following consonant— again entirely in accord with Trubetzkoy's precepts.

These confirmations of the Prague School position are more than outweighed by negative responses, however. With regard to 'extendibility', it is pointed out by Forchhammer (1939) that this cannot be a phonologically relevant feature because it is unusable by the hearer: one cannot tell whether a sound is 'extendible' by listening to it, since extendibility is a potential, not an actual, property. As far as the feature of 'contact' is concerned, the arguments are more empirically testable, and a number of investigators have attempted to determine its phonetic correlates. The majority of those who have examined the issue (e.g. van Wijk, 1940; Fischer-Jørgensen, 1940–1) have found little or no evidence for any phonetic feature of 'Silbenschnitt', and have remained sceptical. Von Essen (1962) claims to have found a phonetic difference here, though not quite of the kind predicted by Trubetzkoy, since the cut-off in both 'short' and 'long' cases is found to be *after* the maximum of the vowel. On the other hand, Lehiste (1970) reports that experimentally cutting off the *beginning* of a 'long' vowel leads to the perception of the 'short' one, demonstrating that the kind of 'contact' with the *following* consonant cannot be responsible for the difference. The phonetic case for Trubetzkoy's interpretation is therefore clearly not a strong one.

In the wake of Trubetzkoy's claims, a number of other phoneticians explored the phonetic correlates of length in some detail,[23] and their studies show an awareness of the need to relate quantitative measurements to qualitative linguistic categories, but there is little phonetic evidence to support the categories themselves. A number of phoneticians and linguists (e.g. Linke, 1939; Laziczius, 1939) feel obliged to deplore Trubetzkoy's apparent indifference to the phonetic basis of the categories he postulates.[24]

One attempt to reconcile the phonetic and phonological aspects of length which deserves a mention here, if only because it enjoyed some support at the

[23] In addition to those just mentioned, we may note the contributions of Ariste (1939), Durand (1939, 1946), and Linke (1939), among others.

[24] Trubetzkoy was notoriously hostile to phonetic criteria in phonology, though his attitude was by no means typical of Prague School linguists.

time from several of the phoneticians and linguists discussed here, is that of Zwirner's 'phonometry' (1932, 1939). Zwirner's method is to measure the phonetic realizations of specific phonological categories (in this case the lengths of 'short' and 'long' phonemes) and to derive a statistical norm for each. Though there are found to be overlaps between the 'scatters' of values for each phoneme, the norms themselves are clearly distinct. Trubetzkoy himself (1939: 10–12) rejects such a procedure, as it replaces linguistically significant categories by purely statistical ones, but a number of linguists of the day saw this as a means of reconciling the phonological and phonetic perspectives on length.

As for Trubetzkoy's general conclusion that the linguistic system has no temporal dimension, this has, understandably, not generally been accepted by linguists. As the Hungarian linguist Gyula Laziczius remarks (1939), 'length cannot be excluded from the quantity question'.[25] On the other hand, if we follow Trubetzkoy in taking the non-temporal nature of *langue* as axiomatic we could, with Naert (1943), interpret length as a *quality* rather than as *quantity*, and therefore consider it to have no temporal implications, though what is gained by this terminological sleight of hand is difficult to assess. There would appear to be no legitimate reason to follow either Saussure or Trubetzkoy in this approach.[26]

2.4.3   THE DISTINCTIVE FEATURES OF LENGTH

2.4.3.1   Introduction

Given a paradigmatic interpretation of length, there are different ways of characterizing the distinction phonetically. The traditional view has, of course, been that there are 'long' and 'short' sounds, but alternative interpretations are possible here, especially in those cases where distinctions of length are not the only differences between the sounds. Even in the nineteenth century, alternative dimensions along which vowel sounds may differ were discussed, apart from the usual ones involving tongue position. One possible parameter here is the *shape* of the tongue; Bell (1867) describes this in terms of the categories 'primary' and 'wide' and, following him, Sweet (1877) uses the terms 'narrow' and 'wide'. Sweet (1906: 19–20) describes the distinction as follows: 'in forming narrow vowels there is a feeling of tenseness in that part of the tongue where the vowel is formed, the surface of the tongue being made more convex than in its natural "wide" shape, in which it is relaxed and flattened. This convexity of the tongue naturally narrows the passage—whence the name'. The exact interpretation of this is not completely clear, but among the 'wide' vowels given by Sweet are the English vowels of *bit, men, man, put,* and *not*; among the 'narrow' vowels are

---

[25] *Das Quantum [ist] nicht aus der Lautquantitätsfrage zu entfernen.*
[26] Anderson (1984) has attempted to revive several of Trubetzkoy's notions on length, reinterpreting them within a very different theoretical framework.

those of *sir, air, law*. The distinction has therefore usually been taken to refer to pairs of vowels such as those of English *bid* vs. *bead, cam* vs. *calm, pull* vs. *pool* and so on, which have traditionally been regarded as differing in length. Because of the difficulties involved in defining and identifying this distinction, it was abandoned in the British phonetic tradition (see Catford, 1977: 204). Jones (1956: 39–40) rejects it, and describes vowels in terms of tongue position, lip position, and length. Others, however, have maintained the distinction, under different terminological guises.

Prague School theory is concerned to identify the features of phonemes which serve to differentiate them, but, in its classical form, it does not regard these features as phonological units as such, and their phonetic nature is in any case subordinated to the phonological oppositions. However, Jakobson's later work extends and develops some of the Prague principles in a number of radical ways; in his theory of distinctive features, phonemes are seen merely as 'bundles' of concurrent features (cf. Jakobson, Fant, and Halle, 1952; Jakobson and Halle, 1956). The phonetic definition of the features therefore becomes of paramount importance, and a more explicit characterization is required.

The status of 'length' in distinctive feature theory is, however, somewhat ambivalent. Early statements of the theory (e.g. Jakobson, Fant, and Halle, 1952) do not include 'length' as a feature. However, later publications (e.g. Jakobson and Halle, 1956) do recognize 'quantity' as a 'prosodic feature' alongside 'tone' and 'force', and accord it some status, either as the *length* feature (corresponding to Trubetzkoy's 'extendibility') or as the *contact* feature (Trubetzkoy's 'Silben-schnitt'). As in the original Prague theory, length is seen as having a close relationship to intensity, so that it becomes redundant in cases where stress is distinctive. Certainly, their relationship 'seems to indicate that the prosodic distinctive features utilizing intensity and those utilizing time tend to merge' (Jakobson and Halle, 1956: 25). However, for the most part, it is not 'length' as such that is regarded as phonologically distinctive, but other features.

2.4.3.2 'Tense' vs. 'Lax'

The most widely accepted feature to cover length distinctions, especially in English, is 'tension', with a distinctive feature [±tense]. 'Tense' implies 'long', since 'the heightened subglottal air pressure in the production of tense vowels is indissolubly paired with a longer duration. As has been repeatedly stated by different observers, the tense vowels are necessarily lengthened in comparison with the corresponding lax phonemes' (Jakobson, Fant, and Halle, 1952: 58). This feature is explicitly linked to Bell's and Sweet's distinction between 'primary'/ 'narrow' and 'wide' (Jakobson and Halle, 1964: 96).

The feature [±tense] is also adopted by Chomsky and Halle (1968), and they use it to characterize the distinction between the traditional 'long' and 'short' vowels of English or German, e.g. *ihre* vs. *irre, Huhne* vs. *Hunne*, etc. They group the 'tense'/'lax' distinction under 'manner of articulation features', and have a separate feature of 'length' under the heading 'prosodic features', but the latter category, along with other prosodic features, is simply ignored. In keeping with the original Prague view that the unmarked term for English vowels is long, Chomsky and Halle's marking conventions also assume that [+tense] is the un-marked value for this feature,[27] though the conventions are intended to be uni-versal, and not restricted to English. As far as the phonetic definition of 'tension' is concerned, Chomsky and Halle (p. 324) consider that [+tense] segments 'are executed with a greater deviation from the neutral or rest position of the vocal tract' than [–tense] ones.

Some aspects of this use of [±tense] may, however, be questioned. In the first place, the phonetic definition is not very satisfactory, since the 'neutral or rest position' is not always the same for different languages;[28] second, 'tension' is inadequate as a distinctive feature, since its identification by listeners is unreli-able; third, even if we accept this feature for English, in which 'long' and 'short' vowels are qualitatively different, it will not do for languages where this is not so. As Lass (1984: 92) concludes, 'as far as I can tell, there are no qualities attrib-utable to [+tense] that can't be reduced to the traditional dimensions of height, backness and duration. The feature [±tense] can probably be discarded'.

2.4.3.3 'Advanced Tongue Root'

Another feature that has been used to characterize differences of a similar sort to those we have been considering so far is *Advanced Tongue Root* (ATR) (Halle and Stevens, 1969). This, too, has been invoked in cases such as the English vowel pairs in *bead* and *bed*, etc. A phonetic description of ATR is given by Laver (1994: 141–2): 'this has the effect of enlarging the middle and lower phar-ynx, and gives the longitudinal profile of the root of the tongue a tighter curve than it has in its neutral configuration'. The significance of this is that in a number of languages, especially in West Africa, there are sets of vowels differing in this feature which take part in vowel harmony processes. In one dialect of Akan, for example, there are the sets of Fig. 2.3 (Durand, 1990: 46).

Fig. 2.3   [+ATR]   [−ATR]

i	u	ɪ	ʊ
e	o	ɛ	ɔ
ɜ		a	

These pairings look remarkably like those of, say, English or German, but Ladefoged and Maddieson (1996: 302–6) demonstrate convincingly that, although this feature seems justified for the languages in question, where the distinction

---

[27] This is prescribed by the rule [*u* tense] → [+tense].

[28] A useful test here is the 'hesitation vowel' used by speakers, and this is different even for speak-ers of different varieties of English. While speakers from England generally use a central [ə]-like vowel (usually written 'er'), many Scots use a front [e]-like vowel.

appears to be an autonomous one, the apparently similar phenomenon of English is merely the concomitant of other distinctions.

2.4.3.4 'Long' vs. 'Short'

In spite of the conclusions reached by Trubetzkoy and other Prague linguists that length has no real phonological status and is therefore not a feature of 'langue', and also despite the use of [±tense] to cover a number of phenomena associated with length, there is apparently still much to be said for the recognition of *length itself* as the relevant feature in a paradigmatic treatment of these oppositions, and in fact this feature has continued to be used; many descriptions of languages where length appears to have some phonological role are content to make an explicit distinction between 'short' and 'long' in the vowel system. This may be done informally, by simply recognizing a category of long vowels and providing a suitable notation, or formally, by using the feature [±long]. It should also be noted that the status of both [±tense] and [±long] has continued to be unclear, even in Generative Phonology. Though, as we have seen, the former is used to the exclusion of the latter by Chomsky and Halle (1968), Halle (1977) reintroduces [±long] alongside [±tense] to account for the stressing of syllables which do not contain an underlying 'tense' vowel (revealed by the lack of diphthongization), as in *Alabama*, or *soprano*. In their revision of Chomsky and Halle's description of English phonology, Halle and Mohanan (1985) go further, and eliminate [±tense] altogether from underlying representations of vowels, so that 'tension' becomes a predictable, and superficial, consequence of underlying length, rather than the other way round.[29]

2.4.4 QUALITY VS. QUANTITY

The foregoing discussion of the distinctive features of length raises more general questions about the phonetic nature of the paradigmatic distinction between 'long' and 'short' which are not confined to this particular theoretical framework. Regardless of how we interpret this distinction phonologically, whether in terms of 'tension', 'length', or some other feature, there is clear evidence that, in a language such as English, the difference between 'long' and 'short' vowels is not exclusively one of *quantity*, but also involves *quality*; in articulatory terms the 'short' vowels generally have a more centralized articulation.

This fact has a number of implications, even for purely descriptive and pedagogical work, since it is reflected in practical matters such as transcription systems. In the case of English, the question raised is whether the 'short' and 'long' vowels are best represented by distinct symbols, reflecting their different qualities, or by the same symbols with a differentiating length mark (:), reflecting the

---

[29] Halle and Mohanan do not use the feature [±long], however, since they adopt the autosegmental notation for length, which associates a 'short' segment to a single 'skeleton slot' and a 'long' segment to two such slots (see 2.7, below).

different quantities. The former style of transcription can be called 'qualitative', the latter 'quantitative' (Abercrombie, 1964: 26). In works on British English, a 'qualitative' transcription has been used by, for example, Ward (1939), while Jones (1956, and elsewhere) generally uses a 'quantitative' transcription in his publications. There is also a third possibility, which represents *both* quantity *and* quality, and, though this could be seen as phonologically redundant, it has become effectively standard for British English following its use by Gimson (1980). Examples of these different approaches are given in Fig. 2.4 (note that the precise symbol shapes are subject to some variation, e.g. [æ] vs. [a], [ɑ] vs. [ʊ], or [ɪ] vs. [ı], but this does not affect the principle at issue here).

Fig. 2.4	'Qualitative'	'Quantitative'	Both
'ship'	ı	i	ı
'sheep'	i	iː	iː
'look'	ʊ	u	ʊ
'Luke'	u	uː	uː
'cot'	ɒ	ɔ	ɒ
'caught'	ɔ	ɔː	ɔː
'at'	a	a	a
'art'	ɑ	aː	ɑː

The choice among these different systems is not determined by 'accuracy' or 'truth', of course, nor does it really reflect a different phonological analysis, since the symbols are representations of the same set of phonemes. Nevertheless, the different systems do appear to reflect different assumptions as to what is significant in the distinctions, and the issue therefore raises broader questions. Though the phonological issues in the quality/quantity debate may be unresolvable, Gimson (1945–9) reports on experiments which demonstrate the higher priority given to quality in the perception of these contrasts by listeners, and this may therefore be taken as providing support for the 'qualitative' approach.[30]

The choice of symbols may also be influenced by the nature of the system as a whole. The vowel system of a major variety of Standard German resembles that of English in having comparable pairs differing in both quality and quantity, as illustrated in Fig. 2.5.

Fig. 2.5	bieten	('to offer')	vs.	bitten	('to ask')	/iː /	vs.	/ı/
	beten	('to pray')	vs.	Betten	('beds')	/eː /	vs.	/ɛ/
	hüten	('to look after')	vs.	Hütten	('huts')	/yː /	vs.	/ʏ/
	Höhle	('cave')	vs.	Hölle	('hell')	/øː /	vs.	/œ/
	spuken	('to haunt')	vs.	spucken	('to spit')	/uː /	vs.	/ʊ/
	Ofen	('stove')	vs.	offen	('open')	/oː /	vs.	/ɔ/
	lahm	('lame')	vs.	Lamm	('lamb')	/aː /	vs.	/a/

---

[30] For a useful discussion of the issues here see Abercrombie (1964: 24–31).

As in English, either a quantitative or a qualitative transcription can be employed here. However, the quantitative pairing of vowels pervades the whole German system, embracing virtually all of the vowels, as indicated in Fig. 2.6.[31] A purely qualitative transcription (i.e. one omitting all of the length marks in Fig. 2.5), while not precluding such an arrangement, would fail to bring out the significance of the quantitative pairings for the system as a whole.[32]

Fig. 2.6

	Front		Back
	Unrounded	*Rounded*	
High	iː / ɪ	yː / ʏ	uː / ʊ
Mid	eː / ɛ	øː / œ	oː / ɔ
Low		aː / a	

2.4.5 CONCLUSION

Beyond these disputes about the appropriate phonological and phonetic characterization of the distinction between 'long' and 'short' vowels there is also the more fundamental question of the validity of the paradigmatic interpretation of length itself. We saw earlier (2.2) that the length of individual segments may often not be independent of the structural context in which they occur, and in particular, as in the case of Latin, may depend on the following consonants, but the paradigmatic approach assumes that the categories of sounds are mutually substitutable, and therefore takes no account of this dimension at all. It also naturally excludes any reference to such prosodic factors as syllable length and rhythm. In order to do justice to these wider implications of length we must therefore broaden our perspective to embrace the segmental and prosodic context. This involves, as an initial step, the *syntagmatic* interpretation of length.

2.5 The Syntagmatic Interpretation of Length

2.5.1 INTRODUCTION

In attempting to overcome some of the weaknesses of the paradigmatic approach to length outlined in 2.4, we may examine a somewhat different approach, which analyses length in terms not of oppositions but rather of combinations of sounds

---

[31] There is, in fact, only one stressed monophthong which falls outside this system, the vowel pronounced by some in *spät*, *sähe*, etc., which could be represented phonetically as [ɛː]. Since this is qualitatively closer to /ɛ/ than /eː/ is, it poses a problem for the quantitative analysis which pairs /eː/ with /ɛ/. However, this vowel is very marginal for many speakers, who use /eː/ in such words. A further detail which supports the quantitative analysis here is that the vowels /aː/ and /a/ are qualitatively indistinguishable for many Standard German speakers, length being the only distinctive feature. The different symbols for 'long' and 'short' here are therefore misleading.

[32] In spite of this assertion, a qualitative transcription is used in the present author's book on German (Fox, 1990), which follows the practice of MacCarthy (1975).

and their distribution. In essence, this involves regarding the distinction between 'short' and 'long' sounds as one of *structural complexity* rather than of a difference in the attributes of the individual sounds. 'Short' sounds, in other words, are *simple*, while 'long' sounds are *complex*, in the sense of consisting of more than one element. In practical terms this means that, phonologically speaking, 'long' sounds are regarded as a succession of (usually two) 'short' ones. Since in this approach the burden of contrast is shifted away from differences between segments themselves onto differences of *structure*, the emphasis here is *syntagmatic* rather than paradigmatic.

The main claim made in favour of such an approach is that it is *simpler* and therefore more *economical*. Since on the face of it the analysis of a long vowel as *two* segments would appear to be more complex than treating it as a unitary segment, this claim is not self-evidently justified, and needs to be substantiated. The principal argument here is that the bipartite analysis potentially uses fewer symbols *overall* and therefore implies a simpler system. That depends, however, on being able to identify the parts of a 'long' sound with existing segments, which occur independently elsewhere. Thus, if a 'short' vowel is analysed as a simple vocalic segment V, then we may regard a 'long' vowel as V+X, where X is an additional structural element. The V element of a 'long' vowel is, of course, to be identified wherever possible with an existing 'short' vowel of similar quality, but the identification of the X element is somewhat more flexible, and various alternative proposals have been made which we shall explore in the following discussion.

2.5.2 'ANALYTIC LENGTH'

In 2.4 we considered the contribution of Prague School linguists to the paradigmatic interpretation of length. The exploration of paradigmatic oppositions was undoubtedly the main focus of Prague School theory, but we nevertheless noted that one of the possible analyses of length advocated by Jakobson and Trubetzkoy allows a syntagmatic interpretation of the phenomenon in the form of *analytic length*. Here, the length of a 'long' vowel is considered to have the function of indicating a two-part structure. This interpretation depends on the possibility of regarding a long vowel as 'polyphonematic' (consisting of more than one phoneme), an analysis which is justifiable, according to Trubetzkoy (1939: 170–3), under certain specified conditions, as follows:

(a) the vowel contains a morphological boundary
(b) it is equivalent to a polyphonematic diphthong
(c) it behaves like two short vowels with regard to accent rules
(d) it has different tonal features at the beginning and the end
(e) it contains a glottal stop

Thus, in case (a), the long vowel may simply be the result of the juxtaposition of two identical short vowels in a morphological or syntactic construction. In Finnish, the partitive is marked by the suffix -a, and if this is added to a stem ending in -a, such as *kukka* (flower), then the result will be a long vowel: *kukkaa*. But we are not justified, according to Trubetzkoy's criterion, in recognizing a single long vowel phoneme here, even though the [-aa] constitutes a single syllable, since the vowel spans a morpheme boundary; the interpretation is polyphonematic, as a *geminate* (double) vowel forming a single syllable peak. Case (b) covers instances where a diphthong is appropriately analysed as a sequence of two phonemes, and the long vowel is treated analogously. Such a case is found in Slovak, where *both* long vowels *and* diphthongs are shortened after a syllable containing *either* a long vowel *or* a diphthong. In other words, long vowels and diphthongs are treated in exactly the same way, and the former should again be considered geminate.[33]

The Latin accent is an instance of case (c), since the accent falls on the antepenultimate syllable if the vowel of the penultimate syllable is short, but on the penultimate syllable if this is long (cf. 2.2.1). That is, we find 'V̆ V̆ V (*'dŏmĭnus*) but V 'V̄ V (*a'māre*), and the combination V̆ V̆ is therefore equivalent to V̄ for the purposes of the accent rules. A bipartite analysis of V̄ is therefore justifiable. This is also true if there are two different accentual types within the language, where the accent may fall on either the beginning or the end of the long vowel (Jakobson, 1931). This is usually manifested particularly in the pitch contour, since it will determine the point at which intonational features associated with the accent are likely to occur, and this comes under case (d). Examples are found in the different 'intonations' of Lithuanian, Slovenian or Ancient Greek.[34] In Lithuanian we may distinguish 'falling' and 'rising' intonations, depending on whether the first or second part of the vowel is prominent. Naturally, the two types of accent in these cases can only occur on a long vowel; on short vowels only one accent type will be possible.[35] Another manifestation of a two-part structure is found in the Danish *stød*, and a similar phenomenon in Latvian, which constitute case (e) (Jakobson, 1931). Here, glottalization breaks the vowel into two, justifying a bipartite analysis. Again such glottalization can occur only with long vowels, or with combinations of short vowels and sonorant conso-

---

[33] Jakobson (1937, pp. 32–3) is prepared to go further and accept a polyphonematic analysis of long vowels in *all* cases where there are polyphonematic diphthongs, even if the two are not treated equivalently. Trubetzkoy (1939: 173) rejects this.

[34] For discussion of this phenomenon from a different perspective see 4.7.3.

[35] For this reason, Trubetzkoy is able to establish a universal principle, according to which 'polytonic' languages (i.e. languages with different types of accent) must also have a 'quantity correlation' (cf. Jakobson, 1931). According to Jakobson (1937), such a universal is actually tautological, since the existence of bipartite vowels is contained in the definition of 'polytonic'. Jakobson's own principle, that free quantity and free 'monotonic' (dynamic) accent are incompatible in the same system, he also regards as tautological, since if a language has free quantity and a movable accent, the accent could fall on the beginning or the end of a long vowel just as well as on one of two short vowels, which would therefore make the language polytonic.

nants. In Danish we find glottalization at several points, for example, *pæn* [pʰɛʔn] ('nice') and *pen* [pʰɛnʔ] ('pen'), where [ʔ] represents the *stød*.[36]

In all these cases, therefore, it is justifiable to regard a long vowel as having two parts, so that the function of vowel length is here additional to the functions discussed in 2.4.6 above: to distinguish between a single and a two-part structure. This role is not obligatory, however, since these other features (accent type, pitch pattern, *stød*, etc.) may also be present, and additional length may therefore be functionally redundant. The same bipartite interpretation can therefore be given to cases in some African languages, such as Efik, where two tones occur on a *short* vowel. In Efik (Westermann and Ward, 1933: 149) vowel elision occurs, leaving the original tones intact and resulting in two tones on one syllable. Thus Efik *ké ùbóm* ('in the canoe'), with a high tone on the first syllable and a low tone on the second, is pronounced *kûbóm*, with a falling tone on the first syllable, combining the original high and low tones. Here, therefore, length is not involved. However, such cases are unusual, and length is likely to be a concomitant of the two-part structure.[37]

2.5.3 THE DISTRIBUTIONAL ANALYSIS OF LENGTH

Though provision was made by Prague School linguists for the syntagmatic analysis of length, this approach was initially associated primarily with linguists in the American structuralist tradition, who developed it in the particular methodological form characteristic of this school. However, the approach has much wider appeal than this; indeed, its fundamental principles have remained as the basis of much modern work on this topic, though cast in different theoretical moulds, as we shall see below. Initially, however, we shall consider the analysis of length in the distributional framework of American structuralist phonology.

2.5.3.1 The 'Glide' Solution

A fairly radical proposal for the distributional analysis of length is found in early work by the Bloomfieldian linguists Bloch and Trager (1942). They present an analysis of length in American English vowels, for example in words such as *calm* and *law* (which they represent phonetically as [aː] and [oː]), where the 'long' vowels have an additional 'lengthening element' which is a 'separate phonemic unit, which calls for a special allophone of the preceding vowel

---

[36] These examples are from Árnason (1980: 77), who writes: 'The *stød* could be seen as the surface realisation of underlying length in the vowels, and perhaps in the consonants too', and further remarks that *stød*-less dialects have long vowels, while *stød* dialects do not. This would indicate that vowel length is an underlying feature which is in some dialects realised as *stød*, in others as actual length. However, this does not quite square with Trubetzkoy's view that the *stød* occurs only with long vowels or their equivalent; it rather suggests that the *stød* is a *substitute* for vowel length.

[37] Van Wijk (1940) imposes a further restriction here: the presence of two tones on one vowel is to be regarded as evidence of bipartite structure only if there are also diphthongs which have such tones.

phoneme—longer and qualitatively different from the allophones in other positions' (p. 50). The 'X' element of the V+X formula is thus identified here with a 'lengthening element' which is able to account simultaneously for the greater length of the 'long' vowel and its different quality. Bloch and Trager note that this element is 'a voiced continuation of the preceding vowel', and it is therefore precisely the converse of [h], which is a 'partial or complete voiceless anticipation of the following voiced sound' (p. 51). And since the two sounds share an important property—that of borrowing their phonetic characteristics from the neighbouring vowel—and are in complementary distribution with regard to position, the lengthening element is identified with /h/, and the vowels [aː] and [oː] are interpreted phonemically as /ah/ and /oh/, respectively.

This conclusion is reached not on the basis of any 'opposition' between a long and a short vowel as such, but rather by a consideration of the distribution of length in relation to other features—here the occurrence of [h]—together with other factors such as the overall simplicity of the resulting pattern and questions of phonetic similarity. The gain in simplicity of the pattern is not immediately evident, but it becomes clear when we look at the overall distribution of the so-called *glides*, which include not only /h/ but also /w/ and /y/ (IPA /j/). English vowels may be preceded by one of these 'glides', as in /wiː/ 'we', /yuː/ (/juː/) 'you', and /hiː/ 'he', but the analysis of vowel length in the above terms allows such glides to occur *after* vowels as well as *before* them, since, in addition to the analysis of [aː] and [oː] as /ah/ and /oh/, [iː] and [uː] can also be analysed phonemically as /iy/ and /uw/. The net result is not only a smaller phoneme system (since the long vowels are eliminated) but also a more regular distribution of the glides, which can now occur both before and after vowel phonemes.[38]

It is interesting to note that a further effect of this analysis, as in the case of the paradigmatic approach discussed earlier, is to eliminate length from phonological significance, at least in English. But whereas in the latter approach this was concluded on the grounds that length could not be phonologically relevant in oppositions, here the conclusion is reached entirely on distributional grounds: the continuation of a sound can be identified with another sound that occurs in a different context. Thus, though the theoretical framework, the methodology, and the criteria are quite different, one final effect—the elimination of length as a phonologically significant feature—is the same.

For this solution to be satisfactory it must provide the desired economies, i.e. it must be possible to equate both parts of our V+X formula with other phonemes of the language. While the equation of V with existing 'short' vowels is usually possible, the 'glide' solution encounters the difficulty that the 'glides' may not be present in the system of the language concerned. German, for exam-

---

[38] It will be noted that this provides a further notation for the English vowels to supplement that presented in 2.4.8 above. For criticism, indeed rejection, of the category of 'glide', see Lass and Anderson (1975: 3–12).

ple, which, as we have seen, has a 'long'/'short' distinction comparable to that of English, has no initial /w/, which makes the analysis of [u:] as /uw/ problematic; Italian has no /h/, so that the analysis of [a:], [o:] and [e:] as /ah/, /oh/ and /eh/ would hardly be justifiable.

Hockett (1955: 76 ff.)[39] considers these matters in comparable terms, and offers a similar analysis of length in the American Indian language Fox, where the short vowels [ɪ, ɛ, ʌ, ʊ] are paralleled by the long vowels [iˑ, æˑ, aˑ, oˑ]. Like Bloch and Trager, he provides a 'glide' interpretation of length, regarding the lengthening element, here represented as [ˑ], as a 'covowel', which is given independent phonemic status as /ˑ/. He distinguishes a 'covowel' from a 'semivowel' and a 'semiconsonant', primarily on distributional grounds: given three structural positions in the syllable, 'peak', 'satellite' and 'margin' (where the 'satellite' is more closely associated with the 'peak' than the 'margin' is), a 'semivowel' may occur as peak or satellite, a 'semiconsonant' as margin or satellite, and a 'covowel' only as part of a complex peak. Thus in English /y/ (/j/), /h/ and /w/ are semiconsonants, occurring as both margin ('you', 'he', 'we') and as satellite ('boy' (/oy/), 'father' (/ah/), 'go' (/ow/)). German has a similar system, but here only the first two are semiconsonants, and /w/ is classed as a covowel, because it does not occur in the syllable margin (i.e. it is not a consonant) or as a satellite, but can be regarded as occurring as part of a complex peak in such words as *Haus* (/haws/).

Another example of this approach is Menomini, which, according to Hockett (1955: 79), has the phonetically simple peaks [i i ɛ ʌ ʊ u] and the phonetically complex peaks [iˑ eˑ æˑ aˑ oˑ uˑ iə uə]. These can be associated phonemically with one another as in Fig. 2.7. The symbol /ˑ/ represents 'a covowel with two allophones: a *scalar lengthener* (neither raising nor lowering) after /i u/, and a *lowering lengthener* with the other four', thus accounting for the differences of phonetic quality. /ə/ is 'a covowel which appears only as a centering glide'. The second allophone of /ˑ/ (the 'lowering lengthener') could also be grouped with /ə/.

Fig. 2.7 Simple   Complex
       [i] /i/   [iˑ] /iˑ/   [iə] /iə/
       [i] /e/   [eˑ] /eˑ/
       [ɛ] /ɛ/   [æˑ] /ɛˑ/
       [ʌ] /a/   [aˑ] /aˑ/
       [ʊ] /o/   [oˑ] /oˑ/
       [u] /u/   [uˑ] /uˑ/   [uə] /uə/

2.5.3.2 The Geminate Solution

If the 'glide' solution is potentially more economical than the establishment of distinct long phonemes, then a further possibility is still more economical: to

---

[39] For critical discussion of Hockett's approach, see Lass (1984: 136–8).

regard the X element as identical to the short vowel that it accompanies, so that V+X = V+V. This does not require us to identify the X element with existing glides, and therefore offers a solution in those cases where the language does not possess such glides. Under this analysis, long vowels are then double or *geminate*; [i:] = /ii/, [a:] = /aa/, and so on.

Within the American camp, Pike incorporates the geminate solution into his authoritative manual of phonemic practice. The relevant procedure is as follows:

When a long vowel is phonemically in contrast to a short vowel and is structurally analogous to clusters of diverse vowels, the long vowel must be considered as a sequence of two short identical vowel phonemes (Pike, 1947: 138–9).

Again the crucial criterion for a geminate interpretation in these procedures is the structural role of the sounds in question: only if the long sounds are *structurally analogous* to clusters of different sounds are they to be interpreted as geminates; otherwise they are single (long) phonemes. Further criteria are provided by Pike, according to the behaviour of the sounds in relation to prosodic features such as tone and stress:

If every short vowel has one toneme and one toneme only, but every long vowel has two tonemes, the investigator should conclude that the long vowels are sequences of two identical vowel phonemes rather than constituting single long phonemes with a complex tone. Similarly, contrasting stress on each of the long vowels (i.e. ['aˑ] and [aˑˈ]) tends to show that they are a sequence of phonemes (i.e. /ˈaa/ and /aˈa/) (Pike, 1947: 139).

These criteria recall strongly those of the Prague School for 'analytic length'.

Hockett (1955: 76–7) also considers the geminate approach to length, offering it as an alternative analysis of Fox long vowels (see above), so that [iˑ] is phonemically /ii/. Incidentally, there are no diphthongs in Fox, so that these geminate vowels are the only vowel clusters allowed, in violation of Pike's criterion, and this fact weakens this analysis. Hockett is unable to decide in such a case whether this or the earlier 'covowel' approach is the more satisfactory. With the Menomini case, too (p. 79), he considers treating the complex peaks as geminates: /ii ee ɛɛ aa oo uu/, with [iə] and [uə] analysed as /ia/ and /ua/. This has the virtue of greater economy, since we do not then need distinct glide phonemes, but Hockett is inclined to reject it because it gives undue special status to /a/.

It is not without significance, however, that both Pike and Hockett are still prepared to allow single long vowel phonemes in appropriate cases. Pike considers the geminate solution to be appropriate only in those cases where the 'long' sound is structurally analogous to a cluster, otherwise the sound is a single phoneme:

If long vowels are phonemically in contrast with short vowels but fill the same structural position as is filled by single short vowels, the investigator may conclude that the long vowels represent single long vowel phonemes (1947: 138).

Similarly, in the case of Fox, Hockett is unable to decide if either the glide or the geminate approach is actually preferable to having 'short' and 'long' vowels as distinct phonemes.

Discussion of the appropriateness of the 'geminate' or the 'long' interpretation of vowels is also found in other theoretical frameworks. We have already observed (2.4.3.2, above) that the preference in classical generative phonology is for a paradigmatic interpretation, with the feature [±tense]. The geminate possibility is also recognized, however. Schane (1973: 15), for example, observes that 'at times it may be useful to analyze a phonetically long segment as a sequence of two identical short ones, which are then called a *geminate*'.

An interesting case here is Lithuanian. Hjelmslev (1937) had already recognized that it is possible to simplify the analysis of Lithuanian vowels by treating 'long' vowels as complex versions of 'short' ones, forming a 'groupe d'identité', and the same conclusion is reached by Kenstowicz (1970). As in the case of Praguian 'analytic length', he distinguishes the two different accentual features of Lithuanian (the 'acute' and 'circumflex' accents) in terms of the part of the vowel on which the high pitch falls. This is clearest with diphthongs (including combinations of a vowel and a nasal or other consonant, which count as 'diphthongs' in Lithuanian), but the same principle applies with monophthongs (see Fig. 2.8). Various prosodic processes, including vowel shortening, likewise suggest that 'long' vowels are best regarded as geminates in Lithuanian.

Fig. 2.8 *káimas* /káimas/
      vaĩkas /vaíkas/
      ántis /ántis/
      añtis /añtis/
      matýti /matíiti/
      matýs /matiís/

On the other hand, there are also segmental processes in Lithuanian which appear to treat long vowels as single entities, including some which apply to all vowels regardless of length. In this case there is no justification at all for treating these vowels as geminates; a single segment with the feature [+long] is more appropriate here. This leads Kenstowicz to accept that *both* notations are necessary in Lithuanian, and that at some point in the grammar geminates are converted into long vowels. Thus, the prosodic rules requiring geminates will apply *before* the conversion into long vowels; the segmental rules requiring single [+long] segments will apply after it (cf. also Pyle, 1970, on a similar case in West Greenlandic Eskimo).

The evidence for the 'geminate' or the 'long vowel' approach is thus rather complex. The consensus is probably that stated by Anderson:

It is clear . . . that we need a feature which specifies purely phonetic length, and which is distinct from gemination. This feature does not ever, as far as we know, have distinctive values in underlying representations, however, since underlying length contrasts seem always to be representable in terms of clusters versus single elements (Anderson, 1974: 275).

2.5.3.3 Consonant Length

Comparable problems, and solutions, arise with the analysis of consonant length. This again was the subject of early Bloomfieldian work. Swadesh (1937) notes that long consonants can be analysed in three different ways: as allophonic variants, as separate phonemes, or as sequences of identical phonemes (geminates).

We may ignore the first case, where consonant length is of no phonological significance, and look at the last two, which provide similar possibilities to those available for the vowels, with the exception that a 'glide' interpretation is clearly inappropriate here. Swadesh suggests regarding long consonants as geminate clusters provided that certain conditions—analogous to those established by Prague linguists for a polyphonematic interpretation—are met. Thus, there must be a contrast between long and short consonants in some position in order to validate the phonemic status; the cluster must be comparable to other clusters in some respects; and there must be no conflict with other kinds of geminate clusters. On the other hand, if the long consonant behaves in its distribution like a single consonant, we will need to treat it as a single 'long' phoneme, distinct from the 'short' one. In practice, perhaps following Trubetzkoy, Swadesh asserts that length is never the *only* distinguishing feature of such consonants, and it could, therefore, again be excluded from phonological relevance.

These requirements for the geminate treatment of 'long' consonants are analogous to those for the interpretation of vowels, and Pike provides a parallel procedure:

Long consonants are analyzed in a manner similar to the analysis of long vowels. When long consonants are phonemically in contrast to short consonants and are structurally analogous to clusters of diverse consonants, the long consonants constitute sequences of identical short consonants. It would appear that long consonants are usually sequences of short phonemes, and only rarely single long phonemes (Pike, 1947: 139).

The analysis of long consonants as (phonologically) geminate clusters is also found in the framework of Firthian 'Prosodic Analysis'. A geminate solution is adopted for long consonants, in an unusual display of theoretical consensus, by Carnochan (1957) for Hausa, Mitchell (1957) for Arabic, and Palmer (1957) for Tigrinya. All point out that the difference between 'geminate' and 'long' is not a phonetic one, and that the adoption of one solution or the other is a purely phonological decision. The usual procedure is to recognize a 'prosody' of gemination, which has some function (mostly of a morphological kind) and to identify its 'exponents', i.e. its phonetic correlates. Palmer (1957: 141), for example, identifies the following as exponents of consonant gemination in certain Tigrinya plural forms:

(i)   consonantal duration, e.g. kɛnɛffər (ff = [fː]) vs. kɛnafər (f = [f]) ('lips')
(ii) tenseness of articulation (plosion as opposed to friction), e.g. mɛnɛbbər (bb = [b]) vs. mɛnabər (b = [ß]) ('seats')
(iii) position of articulation, e.g. mɛnɛddəq (dd = [ḍ]) vs. mɛnadəq (d = [d̪]) ('walls').

Similarly, Carnochan (1957: 165)[40] establishes an element g (for 'gemination') and an element $\bar{g}$ ('non-gemination') in Hausa, which are 'terms' in the junction system of infix and stem. In one dialect, the former occurs in singular forms, the latter in plural forms. In structures consisting of -$C_1V_1C_2V_2C_3\partial$-, e.g. -*nik kama*-, g includes among its exponents:

(i)   the short duration of the exponent of V_1
(ii) the long duration and tense articulation of the exponent of C_2.

In the plural forms, however, such as -*munka kama*-, both vowel and consonant are short, and the prosody is $\bar{g}$. Thus, the prosodies are intended to account simultaneously for both vowel and consonant length in a syllable with and without a 'long' consonant. In a similar vein, Mitchell (1957) sets up the prosodies *gc* (for 'geminate cluster') and *ḡc̄* ('non-geminate cluster') and *c̄* ('non-cluster') to account for the forms of Bedouin Arabic. Thus, words such as *ijjmaal* ('the camels') and *isstar* ('the jackets'), which have geminate clusters, are assigned the prosody *gc*, among whose exponents are 'C_1: sameness of phonetic feature in relation to C_2,' while *ilbayal* ('the mules'), with no geminate, has the prosody *ḡc̄*, with the exponent 'C_1: difference of phonetic feature in relation to C_2.'

The phonological characteristics of geminate consonants have been much debated (e.g. Hegedüs, 1959; Lehiste, 1970; Kenstowicz and Pyle, 1973, among others). The geminate interpretation is generally favoured over the feature [±long], but some doubt remains. In classical generative phonology, as we have seen, there is some ambivalence; Harms (1968) uses the feature [±tense] for long consonants as well as long vowels, and he asserts that 'the traditional contrast between long consonants and geminate clusters is probably unrealistic' (p. 36).

Sampson (1973) points out that the geminate analysis does not work for Biblical Hebrew, since the second part of 'long' plosives does not behave in the same way as the second element of a cluster. In certain contexts the latter change to fricatives, but 'long' consonants are not affected. Sampson concludes that such consonants must therefore be treated as single [+long] elements. However, Barkaï (1974) shows that in some cases long consonants in Hebrew do indeed behave like clusters rather than as single units, justifying the geminate interpretation. Again, therefore, it appears that the geminate interpretation remains the preferred option, but the possibility of single 'long' consonants must be kept open.

2.5.3.4 Multiple Systems

As a further illustration of the distributional approach to the analysis of length consider the case of multiple length systems, i.e. systems which have, from a paradigmatic perspective, more than one degree of distinctive length. Such systems are reported for a number of languages, including Estonian, Hopi, and

---

[40] For a comparable 'prosodic' approach to vowel length in Hausa see Carnochan (1951).

several others. Since a three-way length contrast is at odds with what many linguists believe to be the fundamental binarism of linguistic systems, there is pressure to reinterpret these systems as combinations of two-way contrasts. This can be done paradigmatically; Trubetzkoy (1939: 177–9) dismisses assertions of three- or four-way contrasts as 'misunderstandings',[41] and regards all such systems as combinations of two oppositions, in which length is combined with another feature, such as an accentual contrast (Estonian), 'contact' (Hopi), or tone (Croatian). However, as the following examples show, a syntagmatic reinterpretation is also possible.

Mixe

We may consider first the Coatlán dialect of the Mexican language Mixe, as described by Hoogshagen (1959). The data of Fig. 2.9 show a three-way distinction of vowel length where the differences cannot be attributed to conditioning factors. One possibility in such cases would be to invoke a difference in the number of syllables, so that the longest vowel is disyllabic: po·ʃ vs. po·-oʃ. However, distributional criteria rule this out, since in this language all syllables must otherwise begin with a consonant. Nevertheless, a closer examination of the sounds in this language allows a simpler solution with only two degrees of length.

Fig. 2.9   poʃ 'a guava'   pet 'a climb'
           po·ʃ 'a spider'   pe·t 'a broom'
           po:ʃ 'a knot'   pe:t 'Peter'

Hoogshagen observes that syllable nuclei can be of a number of types, in which not only length but also glottalization and aspiration are involved, giving the six types of Fig. 2.10. These can be related pairwise, so that V contrasts with V·, and Vʔ contrasts with VʔV, with a simpler sound opposed to a more complex cluster in each case. Vh and V: can be taken to be related in a similar way, allowing us to regard [V:] as phonemically /V·h/ and avoiding setting up a new phoneme. The three degrees of length are then phonemically /o/, /o·/ and /o·h/, and /e/, /e·/ and /e·h/. Another dialect in fact has [Vʔ] rather than [V:], suggesting that Coatlán has dropped a final glottal consonant and lengthened the vowel by way of compensation.

Fig. 2.10   V, Vʔ,   Vh
            V·, VʔV, V:

This solution does, of course, require a rather remote relationship between the sounds and the string of phonemes, but this is considered justifiable if it simplifies the pattern (the formal mechanisms for dealing with such remote relationships became commonplace within the framework of Generative Phonology in

[41] *Somit erweisen sich alle Fälle, wo angeblich bei den Silbenträgern drei oder mehr Quantitätsstufen auseinandergehalten werden, als Mißverständnisse.*

the form of phonological rules). It can be seen that the pursuit of this 'simplicity of the pattern', characteristic of the distributional model, is able to eliminate such three-way contrasts as that found in Coatlán.

Estonian

A further example is provided by Estonian, one of the most thoroughly described (though not, perhaps, the most thoroughly understood) of languages with multiple length systems. We may repeat here as Fig. 2.11 the examples given as Fig. 2.2 to illustrate the three-way contrasts of both vowel and consonant length (Ariste, 1939). These three lengths are often referred to as Q1 ('short'), Q2 ('long'), and Q3 ('overlong'). It will be noted that vowels in quantities 2 and 3 are not distinguished orthographically.

Fig. 2.11 sada *sada* ('100')   vs. sa·da *saada* ('send') vs. saːda *saada* ('to get')
          kapi *kabi* ('hoof') vs. kap·i *kapi*   vs. kapːi *kappi* ('wardrobe',
                                    ('wardrobe')   partitive singular)

Again there are distributional facts which may have a bearing on the interpretation of the contrasts: the three-way distinction is restricted to stressed syllables, since Q3 cannot occur elsewhere; all stressed monosyllables *must* contain at least one sound in Q3; and there is apparently a correlation between the occurrence of Q3 in the first syllable of a two-syllable word and the occurrence of a short vowel in the second syllable. There are, furthermore, relationships with other features; several observers note that there is a pitch difference between syllables with Q2 and those with Q3, and the vowel system likewise differs with the different quantities.

In order to clarify the issues here, a brief explanation of the origin of these contrasts is in order (cf. Comrie, 1981: 113–17). As far as the consonants are concerned, the contrasts are the result of the system of 'gradation' which characterizes most of the Balto–Finnic and Lapp languages. Historically, a consonant was 'weakened' at the beginning of a closed syllable: geminate consonants were simplified, voiceless plosives became voiced, voiced plosives became fricatives or disappeared, and a variety of other weakening or shortening processes occurred. Since the last syllable of a root ending in a consonant would be variously open or closed according to the affix which followed, the same word acquired different consonant 'grades' in different forms. Subsequent phonological changes have interfered with this pattern, though Finnish has retained the basic principle. In Estonian, on the other hand, although the consonant alternations have been retained, loss of final vowels and other changes have made the system rather arbitrary, with little relationship between the alternations and their original motivation in open and closed syllables. For example, *sõda* ('war') and *jalga* ('foot') —these are the nominative forms—originally had a genitive in -*n*, which, since it closed the final syllable, induced the weak grade of the consonant; but the -*n* was subsequently lost in Estonian, leaving the weak grade in an open syllable in the genitive forms: *sõja, jala* (*j* and *l* here being the weak grades of *d* and *lg*, respectively). Thus the alternation has acquired morphological significance as the only difference between the nominative and the genitive.

The final stage in this process is the analogical extension of these gradations to forms where they did not originally occur, to give systematic alternations of both consonant and vowel length in certain morphological forms. This included the creation of 'overlong' forms as the lengthened counterparts of 'long' vowels and consonants, as in Fig. 2.12. Although this gives only a two-way contrast within the paradigm itself, a third contrasting length is provided by other words not belonging to the same paradigm: [koli] (*koli* 'rubbish'), and [lina] (*lina* 'flax'), with a short vowel and a short consonant, respectively. On the whole, neither the 'short' vowels and consonants (Q1) nor their relationship to their 'long' counterparts (Q2) present any difficulty; it is the contrast between 'long' and 'overlong' sounds (quantities 2 and 3) that is problematical.

Fig. 2.12 nominative genitive   illative
        kool [ko:l]   *kooli* [ko'li] *kooli* [ko:li] 'school'
        linn [lin:]   *linna* [lin'a] *linna* [lin:a] 'town'

In the light of this complexity, it is not surprising that it has proved difficult to reach a consensus on the phonological properties of Estonian quantity. From a paradigmatic perspective, Trubetzkoy eliminates the distinction between quantities 2 and 3 by regarding the pitch difference as the distinctive property, with length as a mere concomitant of pitch (cf. also Durand, 1939). However, other linguists who have written on the subject (e.g. Must, 1959; Liiv, 1962; Tauli, 1966) have rejected this, arguing that the pitch difference depends on the length, rather than the other way round, and that Trubetzkoy's analysis is 'based on erroneous information and is entirely incorrect' (Must, 1959). In a similar vein, differences of stress have been held responsible for the difference, e.g. by Harms (1962) and Tauli (1966). The former associates Q3 with 'postposed stress'; the latter postulates different stress 'weights' as a means of distinguishing the two quantities, where Q3 is associated with 'heavy' stress and Q2 with 'light' stress.

Most scholars, however, seek a syntagmatic solution to the problem, which relies on the distribution of the different quantities. One aspect of this is the relationship between the quantities of vowels and those of consonants. Lehiste (1966), for example, notes that there is an interplay between vowel and consonant length in determining the overall length of the syllable:

'If the vowel is in quantity 1, the consonant in quantity 3 carries the whole burden in determining the syllabic quantity. If the vowel or diphthong is in quantity 3, the quantity of the consonant terminating the syllable is redundant as far as manifesting the syllabic quantity is concerned, but the quantity of the consonant remains contrastive on the segmental level. Under these circumstances, however, only a two-way contrast is possible; after a vowel in quantity 3, a consonant may occur either in quantity 1 or in a non-contrastively long quantity'.

She also observes (1965) that a vowel in Q2 cannot be followed by a consonant in Q3 and vice versa, i.e. we get V3 + C1 or V3 + C3 but *not* V3 + C2, and V2 + C1 or V2 + C2 but *not* V2 + C3 (cf. also Prince, 1980).

Another approach to the problem looks at the distribution of quantity in successive syllables. It has been argued that the occurrence of Q3 in the first syllable of a word depends on the presence of a *short* sound (Q1) in the second syllable (cf. Posti, 1950; Ravila, 1962; Lehiste, 1960, 1970); for Lehiste (1965), the occurrence of Q3 depends on whether the syllable is odd-numbered or even-numbered in the sequence.

None of these approaches appears to solve the problem of multiple quantities in Estonian, but the general drift is clear: the apparent 3-way contrast is resolved into a 2-way contrast, where the third quantity is seen as the result of distributional factors both within syllables (vowel and consonant quantities complement one another) and between syllables (syllables with 'overlong' sounds complement those without). However, the nature of the complementation of sounds and syllables is evidently complex. These matters will be taken up again below (2.9.4).

2.5.4 THE MORA (1)

One of the most important concepts that recurs in discussions of length within a variety of different theoretical frameworks is that of the *mora*. A precise definition of this term is difficult to come by, but we may take it to be a unit or measure of length, such that 'short' syllables can be said to constitute one mora, and 'long' syllables two moras. However, there are different interpretations here, and different writers appear to define the mora in ways which suit their own theoretical or descriptive principles.

Both the concept and the term 'mora' derive from the theory of verse, as applied to the classical languages, Greek and Latin. Verse in these languages is described as quantitative, since the feet of a line of verse are constructed not on the basis of the alternation of strong and weak syllables, as in English, but according to the 'quantities' of the syllables (Allen, 1964). The Greek or Latin hexameter, for example, has six feet, each foot having either two long syllables (a *spondee*) or one long and two short syllables (a *dactyl*). Metrically, therefore, a long syllable is equivalent to two short ones. Greek metricians use the term χρόνος πρῶτος (*chrónos prôtos* = 'primary measure') to refer to the minimum unit of length, so that a short syllable is considered to have one such measure and a long syllable two; the term *mora*—which is not itself of ancient provenance, but a product of later classical scholarship[42]—was introduced as a Latin equivalent of the 'primary measure'.

[42] According to Allen (1987: 112), *mora* (Latin = 'delay, space of time') was first used in this sense by the German classicist Gottfried Hermann (1772–1848).

The mora was incorporated into the phonological frameworks of a number of structuralist schools, and Prague School linguists, notably Jakobson and Trubetzkoy, adopted it as an important criterion for phonological typology. As we have seen (2.4.2.1), Trubetzkoy attempts to eliminate length as a phonologically distinctive feature, and reinterprets it in other terms. In the case of analytic length (2.5.2), where the length of a long vowel is considered to have the function of indicating a two-part structure, the long vowel is said to contain two moras. Trubetzkoy also uses the mora in cases which go beyond single syllables. If a short syllable counts as one mora and a long syllable counts as two, then the Latin accent rule, which places the accent on the antepenultimate syllable of a word if the penultimate syllable is short, but on the penultimate syllable itself if this is long, can be more efficiently stated in terms of moras: the accent falls on the syllable containing the penultimate mora before the final syllable. Other languages to which, according to Trubetzkoy (1939: 171), the mora can profitably be applied include Polabian, where the accent falls on the syllable containing the penultimate mora of the word (which will coincide with the first mora of the final syllable in the case of a long vowel and the penultimate syllable if the final syllable is short), Southern Paiute, where the accent falls on the second mora of the word, and Tübatulabal, where it falls on the last mora. Languages in which such phenomena are found are called 'mora-counting languages' (Trubetzkoy, 1939: 174); they are also said to have 'arithmetical quantity'.

The mora is also found in some American structuralist treatments of length. Sapir (1931) uses it extensively in his description of the Liberian language Gweabo,[43] but Bloomfield (1935: 110) gives it only a brief mention: 'in dealing with matters of quantity, it is often convenient to set up an arbitrary unit of relative duration, the *mora*. Thus, if we say that a short vowel lasts one mora, we may describe the long vowels of the same language as lasting, say, one and one-half morae or two morae.'[44] This usage raises some interesting questions about the nature of the mora; for Bloomfield, evidently, the mora is not a *unit* as such, but rather a *measure* of the length of a unit. This distinction can be explained analogically in terms of the length of, say, an object such as a chain. We might say that a chain is, for example, ten links long, or that it is ten centimetres long. In the first case, the chain *consists* of ten links; in the latter case, it clearly does not *consist* of ten centimetres, but *measures* ten centimetres. A link is a *part* of a chain; a centimetre is merely a measure of its length. Bloomfield's use of *mora* is evidently analogous to the centimetre rather than the link, hence he is able to envisage fractions of a mora. For other linguists, how-

---

[43] Sapir's analysis serves as the basis for Herzog's description of drum-signalling in this language, which he calls Jabo (Herzog, 1934). Herzog observes not only that the drum-patterns reflect the tones of the language but also that each drum-beat corresponds to a mora.

[44] Bloomfield's use of the Latin plural of 'mora' is not followed by the majority of writers, who prefer the anglicized plural 'moras'. The latter usage is followed in this book.

ever, the mora is comparable to the link; for them a syllable must consist of an integral number of moras.

Pike (1947: 242) defines the mora briefly, along similar lines to Bloomfield, as 'a unit of timing, usually equivalent to a short vowel or half a long vowel', but makes no specific use of it; Hockett (1955: 61) also has relatively little to say about the mora, reserving it for cases where the syllable and the mora are distinct, a situation which seems to prevail in the Apachean language Chiricahua, where 'a syllable containing two vocoids lasts about twice as long as a syllable containing one. We may therefore introduce the term *mora*: a syllable contains one or two moras. There is no need for this term (in addition to "syllable"), save when a language shows both types of unit, as Chiricahua seems to.' Under this interpretation, then, a mora is *part* of a syllable, rather than a measure of its length.

As a further example of the use of the mora in a basically distributional framework, we may take the studies of Stevick (1965, 1969b) on the African tone languages Yoruba and Ganda. In the former case there are problems in determining the number of tones, which seem to be bound up with duration. Though there are normally only three distinct tones (High, Mid, and Low), more occur with long vowels. Stevick solves the problems of tonal combinations by assuming that vowels can have one or two moras, and that the first mora can have more than one tone. In the latter case, he extends the use of the mora to consonants. In Ganda, all vowels and most consonants can be double, but there can only be one double consonant per syllable, and a vowel must be single before a double consonant. Stevick thus suggests that vowels and consonants have a value as moras:

a single consonant = 0 mora
a double consonant or a single vowel = 1 mora
a double vowel = 2 moras.

The distributional facts can then be accounted for by the simple principle that no syllable can have more than two moras. Here, then, the mora is the measure of the length of a phoneme or phoneme cluster, and only indirectly a measure of syllable length, since syllables are made up of segments or segment clusters of different mora-counts.

In spite of these apparently useful applications of the mora, it was from the start compromised by uncertainty as to its nature and status. One major difficulty, that was inherent in the concept from the first and continues to affect its more recent phonological applications, is that it is unclear whether it is a measure of the length of the *vowel* or that of the *syllable*. The Greeks themselves were divided on this question; the *rhythmikoí* took the former view, the *grammatikoí* the latter (Allen, 1968: 99–100). Defining the mora in terms of the vowel alone encounters the problem that a Greek or Latin syllable is metrically long not only if it contains a long vowel (when it is said to be long 'by nature') but also if it contains a short vowel in a closed syllable (when it is said to be long 'by position'). On the other hand, if the mora is defined in terms of the length of the syllable as a whole, we have to account for the fact that initial consonants, and some final ones, are ignored in counting moras.

Trubetzkoy makes no claim that his view of the mora is the same as that of the classical grammarians, and in fact he explicitly warns against equating them, but his theory encounters very similar problems. In particular, although prosodic features are for him in principle properties of the syllable as a whole,[45] in practice they are confined to the syllable nucleus ('Silbenträger'), which is in almost all cases the vowel; consonants are admitted to the nucleus only in exceptional cases, since in the majority of instances they are 'prosodically irrelevant'. It is not at all clear, therefore, how Trubetzkoy can employ the mora where syllables can be long 'by position', as in the case of the Latin stress rule.

There are similar ambiguities with the American structuralist position. For Sapir (1931) the mora characterizes the *syllable*, while for Bloomfield (1935: 110) it is unequivocally a measure of the length of the *vowel*. Hockett (1955: 61) is more ambivalent; he states that 'a *syllable* contains one or two moras' (emphasis added), but in fact in his analysis of Chiricahua the number of moras appears to depend solely on the length of the *vowel*, and he does not consider the role of possible coda consonants.

There are some difficulties in delimiting the mora from other units. In Trubetzkoy's analysis, regarding long vowels as having two moras implies a polyphonematic analysis, i.e. an analysis into a sequence of phonemes. If long sounds are divided into separate phonemes, and also are divided into moras, what is the difference between the phoneme and the mora, and is the latter not redundant? This is evidently not Trubetzkoy's intention. He cites (1939: 172) some Chinese dialects with short diphthongs; in his view they have two phonemes (because they are diphthongs) but only one mora (because they are short). But such cases are clearly exceptional, and in the majority of languages moras are likely to correspond to phonemes. Nevertheless they remain distinct, as the mora is the bearer of prosodic features, while the phoneme is the bearer of segmental features. But though in theory this may be clear, in practice it is not, and not all Prague School phonologists have followed Jakobson and Trubetzkoy in this distinction. Van Wijk (1940), for example, prefers to allow some prosodic properties to be associated with specific vowel phonemes rather than moras.

But if it is difficult in Trubetzkoy's theory to distinguish the mora from the phoneme, there are cases, notably that of Japanese, where the mora has been equated with the *syllable*. Bloch (1950), for example, analyses Japanese in terms of equal-length fractions, which he describes as syllables, but he goes on to

---

[45] *Die prosodischen Eigenschaften kommen nicht den Vokalen als solchen, sondern den* Silben *zu* (1939: 166).

define the syllable in terms of duration rather than structure, and to identify it with the mora. However, the majority of scholars (e.g. Jakobson, 1931; McCawley, 1968; Shibatani, 1990: 158) regard the syllable and the mora as distinct in Japanese. In his description of the language in terms of classical generative phonology, McCawley (1968) makes use of the mora as the basic 'unit of distance' in the language. The mora is the bearer of the pitch features which constitute the pitch–accent of the language, but there is nevertheless a place for the syllable, since if we analyse a long vowel as constituting a single syllable but consisting of two moras, the pitch–accent cannot fall on the second mora of the syllable. Thus, in conflict with Trubetzkoy's classification, Japanese is a syllable language, but one which counts moras.

In summarizing the discussion of the mora in earlier theory it is difficult not to conclude that the concept is somewhat ill-defined. Though ostensibly a measure of *syllable* length, it is in practice mostly applied to the length of the *vowel*; in some cases it is difficult to justify its separate existence from the *phoneme*, and in others it is indistinguishable from the *syllable*. Furthermore, as we have seen, it is a matter of dispute whether the mora is a *unit* or merely a *measure of length*. It is not surprising, therefore, that some linguists have found the mora less than helpful. Martinet (1949: 16–18) regards the mora as a purely 'operative concept' of limited theoretical value, and contends that there are only three kinds of languages:

(i)   those where the mora concept is useful
(ii) those where we can do without it
(iii) those where it would complicate the picture.

We shall examine the mora again below.

2.5.5 CONCLUSION

The approach to the specification of length considered in 2.5 shows that some degree of economy can be achieved by breaking down 'long' segments into sequences of 'short' ones. By the elimination of 'long' sounds, we reduce the number of distinct phonological items in the system, and the system itself becomes more homogeneous. The 'cost' here is that the complexity of syllable structure is increased (syllables with 'long' sounds require an additional structural element in the syllable nucleus), but this is not regarded as a serious weakness.

We may ask, however, to what extent this approach solves the problems identified above in relation to the paradigmatic approach, i.e. the neglect of the context in which the sound occurs. In fact, despite the splitting up of long sounds into sequences and the examination of the distribution of the parts, this approach still treats the length of segments in relative isolation from the wider context. The more complex structures for 'long' sounds which result from this are not related in any way to the structure of the syllables in which they occur. We shall need, therefore, to explore such relationships more explicitly.

2.6 Length and the Syllable

2.6.1 LENGTH AND SYLLABLE STRUCTURE

Although the syllable has been referred to informally in our discussion so far, we have not yet considered its role explicitly. The *definition* of the syllable is, however, a matter which is beyond the scope of the present chapter; for our present purposes it is sufficient to recognize that the syllable has a certain *structure* in the sense that it consists of an ordered arrangement of sounds. Typically, though not exclusively, it has at its centre or nucleus a vocalic element (which we may represent as V), flanked by consonantal elements (here C). Syllables need not contain a vowel, of course, as the syllabic nasal and lateral of such English words as *button* [bʌtn̩] and *bottle* [bɒtl̩] demonstrate, and in some languages, such as Czech, such syllabic consonants are especially numerous. For the sake of simplicity, however, we shall ignore these cases here, or else assume that V includes any syllabic element, whether phonetically vocalic or consonantal.[46]

Our discussion of the classical tradition of phonological description in 2.2.1, above, has already noted the close relationship between vowel length and syllable structure. In particular, we saw that Latin syllables (or sometimes, erroneously, the vowels themselves), are considered long 'by position' when a 'short' vowel is followed by more than one consonant. Since the same length is assigned to a syllable containing a 'long' vowel, with or without following consonants, it appears that VCC is equivalent to V̄.

Some refinements are required here, however. First, the role of the consonant or consonants following the vowel depends on where the syllable-division falls. An intervocalic consonant is generally assumed to belong to the following syllable, so that the syllabification of the sequence CVCV will usually be CV·CV (the dot represents the syllable division). Intervocalic consonant clusters may, depending on the consonant types, be split between syllables, so that CVCCV is likely to be CVC·CV, though some combinations may be assigned wholly to the following syllable. Thus, though Latin *arbor* ('tree') is syllabified as VC·CVC, *libri* ('books') is syllabified as CV·CCV. The principle—we are here talking not about spelling conventions concerning line-breaks but about phonological

---

[46] Trubetzkoy (1935, 1939) refers to the nucleus of the syllable as the *Silbenträger* ('syllable bearer'), which covers both vocalic and non-vocalic elements. However, he explicitly excludes cases such as the syllabic consonants of English and German, since these can be regarded phonologically as variants of ə+consonant. Pike (1943) makes a useful distinction between *vocoid* and *contoid*, as articulatory and acoustic terms, and *vowel* and *consonant*, as phonological terms denoting the role of the sound in the syllable. Thus, vocoids and contoids are only vowels and consonants when functioning as 'syllable crests' and 'nonsyllabics' respectively.

syllable-division—appears to be that consonants are assigned as far as possible to the following syllable (the principle of 'maximal onsets'), limited only by the proviso that the resulting syllable-initial consonant cluster must be a possible word-initial cluster in the language in question. According to this principle, the English word *petrol* would be syllabified as *pe·trol*, since *tr-* is a possible initial cluster in English; *pelting*, however, would be syllabified as *pel·ting*, since *lt-* is not a possible initial cluster. Other factors might include the morphological structure; *toe-strap* and *toast-rack* (Jones, 1956: 327), or *nitrate* and *night-rate* (Trager and Smith, 1951: 38) may be differently syllabified (-·*str*- vs. -*st·r*- and -·*tr*- vs. -*t·r*-).[47]

The significance of this is that the rule for syllable length in Latin and many other languages is best stated in terms not of sequences of consonants and vowels but rather of syllable structure. If a single intervocalic consonant belongs to the following syllable and a -CC- cluster may be divided between two syllables, then the familiar Latin rule that a syllable is long 'by position' if it contains a short vowel followed by more than one consonant is in effect simply a matter of whether it is 'closed' or 'open' (whether it has a final consonant or not). The sequence -VCV- (with a single consonant following the vowel) is syllabified as -V·CV-, giving an open syllable, while -VCCV- (with two consonants following the vowel) is generally syllabified as -VC·CV-, giving a closed syllable. Thus, although it is stated that a syllable is long 'by position' if the vowel itself is 'long' or if it is 'short' but followed by more than one consonant, implying an equivalence of V̄ and VCC, in fact the equivalence is between V̄ and VC, while VCC is equivalent to V̆C.

Syllabification is, however, a controversial issue; some scholars regard intervocalic consonants as *ambisyllabic*, i.e. they belong to *both* syllables. Hockett (1955: 52), for example, recognizes an *interlude*, a consonant or group of consonants that belongs to *both* the coda of the first syllable *and* the onset of the second, so that for him the difference between *nitrate* and *night-rate* or *syntax* and *tin-tax*, is that the cluster -*tr*- or -*nt*- is an interlude in the first word and a coda + onset in the second (in the latter case the two consonants are said to be separated by an 'internal open juncture'). Later phonologists, such as Kahn (1976) and Leben (1977), have adopted the same principle, dividing long intervocalic consonants between both preceding and following syllables. In a framework which permits such an analysis, the syllable division is in principle indeterminate, and syllable structure is less easily used in discussions of length.

A further point to be noted is that initial consonants do not contribute to the length of a syllable at all, so that 'short' syllables in English may be V̆ ('*arrow*'),

---

[47] These are the places where classical Bloomfieldian structuralist phonology would insert a 'juncture' phoneme, a non-pronounced phoneme which is the phonological equivalent of a morphosyntactic boundary. Thus, Trager and Smith (1951: 38) transcribe *nitrate* and *night-rate* as /náytrèyt/ and /náyt+rèyt/, respectively, where /+/ is a 'plus-juncture'. In practice, many of these theoretical distinctions are obliterated in actual speech; the possibility of consistently distinguishing between such pairs as *nitrate* and *night-rate*, *a name* and *an aim*, etc. in normal speech is rather remote.

CV̌ ('*bi*tter'), CCV̌ ('*pla*tter'), or even CCCV̌ ('*stra*pping'). Nor do final consonants increase the length of 'long' syllables which contain a 'long' vowel: V̄C ('art'), V̄CC ('aunt') and V̄CCC ('aunts') are all equally 'long', and no 'longer' than V̄ 'are'), even though they contain *both* a 'long' vowel *and* the requisite number of consonants.[48] In this case the syllables are said to be *hypercharacterized*.

In the light of this discussion, it is clear that the relationship between vowel length, syllable structure, and syllable length is not a simple one. Nevertheless, it may be said that the basic finding here, that V̄ is in some sense equivalent to V̌C, appears to justify the interpretation of length in syntagmatic terms: in some languages, at least, the 'X' of the V+X formula for long vowels is equivalent in its structural role to a consonant. However, this does not necessarily mean that, phonologically speaking, it *is* a consonant, but merely that it is *structurally equivalent* to one. It is also clear that vowel length is not completely accounted for in terms of syllable structure. Although V̄ may be equivalent to VC, the existence of hypercharacterized syllables, in which V̄ is also followed by consonants but the syllable length is not increased further, as well as the exclusion of initial consonants from the equation, means that vowel length and syllable structure are not wholly interdependent, and that the length of a syllable is not the arithmetic sum of its segmental parts.

2.6.2 SYLLABLE WEIGHT

On the basis of our conclusions regarding the relationships between long vowels and short vowel + consonant combinations, we may deduce, with Kuryłowicz (1948), that length is not an exclusively segmental matter: it can also be regarded as a property of the syllable as a whole, or at least of the syllable *minus* its initial consonants. Syllables containing a short vowel followed by not more than one consonant (or, more accurately, short vowels in open syllables)—let us provisionally call them Type A syllables—evidently differ from those with a long vowel or with a short vowel followed by more than one consonant (i.e. short vowels in closed syllables)—let us call them Type B syllables.

The terminology here is potentially confusing, however. As we saw in 2.2.1, above, in the quantitative metre of classical verse, two syllables of Type A are equivalent to one syllable of Type B, so that a dactyl (¯ ˘ ˘) is equivalent to a spondee (¯ ¯) in certain positions in the line. Hence we may regard type A syllables as *short* and type B syllables as *long*. The fact that both syllables and vowels can be 'long' or 'short' naturally invites mistakes of the sort discussed in 2.2.1, above. Allen (1973) points out that the Sanskrit grammarians avoided this problem by referring to syllable *weight* rather than length, which provides us with the adjectives 'heavy' and 'light', and allows the terms 'long' and 'short' to be restricted to segments.

48 A British RP pronunciation is assumed here: [ɑːt], [ɑːnt], [ɑːnts], and [ɑː].

In a classic discussion, Newman (1973) gives many examples from different languages of the significance of syllable weight in the languages of the world.[49] He demonstrates that in languages as diverse as Latin, Classical Greek, Finnish, Estonian, Classical Arabic, Gothic, and the Chadic languages of West Africa, a variety of phonological processes depend on the weight of syllables. For example, in the Chadic language Bolanci, the tone pattern of one class of verbs (those ending in -*u*) depends on the weight of the first syllable, heavy syllables having a low tone (marked `) and light syllables a high tone (marked ´) (Fig. 2.13).

Fig. 2.13 *Heavy*   *Light*

ràamú	'repair'	tónú	'sharpen'
sòorú	'fall'	shírú	'steal'
mòyyú	'wait for'	móyú	'see'
ɓòltú	'break' (intrans.)	ɓólú	'break' (intrans.)[50]

Furthermore, in the subjunctive of these verbs, where the tone pattern is fixed, the quality of the final vowel also depends on the weight of the first syllable. If this is heavy, the vowel is -*e*; if it is light the vowel is -*i* (Fig. 2.14):

Fig. 2.14 sòoré   'fall' (subj.)
    yòrí (<yórú) 'stay' (subj.)

Similarly, in another Chadic language, Kanakuru, derived nominals with -*ək* have the tone pattern High–High if the first syllable is light, but High–Low if the first syllable is heavy (Fig. 2.15).

Fig. 2.15 mòné > mónək 'forget'
    pàaré > páarək 'exchange'

Such phenomena are widespread in the languages of the world. However, the specific structures which count as heavy or light are subject to some variation. Though syllables of the type (C)V̆ (the number of initial consonants is irrelevant as they do not contribute to syllable weight—see above) will always be light, and syllables of the type (C)V̄(C) will always be heavy, syllables of the structure (C)V̆C are variable, depending on the language (cf. Hyman, 1985: 5–6; McCarthy and Prince, 1986: 32–4; Hayes, 1989: 255–6; Tranel, 1991).

It is important to note, however, that length cannot be totally equated with or accounted for by weight, since, as Newman points out, although weight may in part be dependent on vowel length, weight differences cannot necessarily be analysed in terms of units of duration or correlated with actual time-length

---

[49] Newman builds on the work of Kuryłowicz (1948), who makes two essential points about syllable weight: (1) given onset, peak and coda, the peak and coda group together as one constituent, the *core*, as opposed to the onset; (2) syllable weight exists only in languages with phonemic vowel length.

[50] Note that, as this example shows, it is the syllable weight in the actual verb stem, not in the underlying root, that is crucial here.

differences. There is nevertheless an evident connection between weight and prosodic features, including length, and Newman concludes (1973: 320) that 'it seems natural to find that syllable weight as a distinctive variable functions most often in the realm of tonal, accentual, and rhythmic phenomena'.

2.6.3 THE SYLLABLE AS A UNIT OF LENGTH

Our discussion so far has made it clear that there is an intimate relationship between segment length and syllable structure, where the length of specific segments combines with structural patterns in determining the weight of syllables. However, it is also possible that syllable weight is not merely determined by segments and their length; the length of segments may itself be determined by the syllable structure and syllable weight. If this is so, then the syllable itself is to be interpreted not merely as a structure whose quantity is determined by that of its segments, but also as a *unit of length* in its own right.

2.6.3.1 Historical Evidence: The Development of Quantity Systems

Evidence for such an interpretation is provided in part by a number of historical processes involving length. These processes, lengthening and shortening changes in different phonological environments, are well documented, though the historical and phonological interpretations put on them vary.

The classical languages, Greek and Latin, in common with other ancient Indo–European languages, are assumed to have had a pitch–accent system and were (in Praguian terms) 'mora-counting' (cf. the discussion of Latin in 2.5.4). However, in Latin this system seems to have broken down with the development of a stress-based accentual system, and, according to some authorities, the subordination of quantity contrasts to the stress system. In effect this means that the quantity (or weight) of a syllable became determined by whether it was stressed or not rather than by a mora-count dependent on its structure (Sommerfelt, 1951; Weinrich, 1958; Spence, 1965).[51]

Subsequent developments follow from this uniform stressed syllable quantity, affecting the occurrence of different segmental lengths. According to Weinrich (1958), Latin of the classical period had the four types of syllable structure given in Fig. 2.16 ($\bar{V}$ = long vowel or diphthong; $\bar{C}$= double consonant or consonant cluster).

Fig. 2.16   (i) $\check{V} + \bar{C}$
        (ii) $\check{V} + \bar{C}$
       (iii) $\bar{V} + \bar{C}$
      (iv) $\bar{V} + \bar{C}$

In terms of our previous discussion, type (i) is light, types (ii) and (iii) are

---

[51] For more detailed discussion of accentual phenomena see Ch. 3.

heavy, and type (iv) is hypercharacterized. But a uniform syllable weight in stressed syllables would exclude the co-occurrence of all of these. Type (iv) disappeared early, followed by type (i), so that ultimately the quantities of vowel and consonant became mutually dependent, a situation which, roughly speaking, prevails in modern Italian, with oppositions such as *fatto* ([fat:o] = 'fact') vs. *fato* ([fa:to] = 'fate'). Note that the quantity system is not thereby destroyed but reconstituted following the collapse of the classical system; length is therefore still distinctive in Italian but its independence is limited, firstly by accent (distinctions only apply in stressed syllables) and secondly by the interdependence of vowel and consonant length. The first stage of this process, the loss of the classical system, also entailed the shift from quantitative pairing of vowels to a qualitative one, with a number of different results in different parts of the Romance-speaking area.

Similar developments took place in other European languages, particularly the Germanic languages, during the mediaeval period.[52] Early Germanic may have had a quantitative system similar to that of Latin, but later developments suggest a strong stress on the root and quantity distinctions restricted to stressed syllables. But in Middle English, Middle High German, Low German, and later the Scandinavian languages, lengthening and shortening processes analogous to those described for late Latin took place, to varying extents and at different times. The actual processes, and their timing and motivation, have been discussed in detail by many scholars; here only some of the more salient and secure findings will be singled out, in so far as they are relevant to our present discussion.

As evidence for a 'mora-counting' system in Old English we may cite the various alternations between monosyllabic and disyllabic forms in certain noun classes (Lass, 1984: 251–4), for example the nominative plural of a-stem neuter nouns, which is disyllabic if the stem is light (*fætu* 'vessels', *hofu* 'dwellings') but monosyllabic if the stem is heavy (*wīf* 'women', *word* 'words'). If light syllables have one mora and heavy syllables have two, then this rule ensures that the plurals have two moras overall. The same is true of the nominative singular of u-stem masculine nouns, which are disyllabic if the first syllable is light (*sunu* 'son', *lagu* 'sea') and monosyllabic if it is heavy (*gār* 'spear', *feld* 'field').

In Middle English various lengthening and shortening processes took place, which went hand in hand with the restriction of quantity distinctions to stressed syllables and the equalization of weight in these syllables. Various interpretations have been put upon these processes. Vachek (1959), adopting a classical Praguian stance, considers that the breakdown of the older 'mora-counting' system, with 'polyphonematic' long vowels, involved a change to the 'monophonematic' interpretation of long vowels, and the development of 'contact' as the distinguishing feature of 'long' vs. 'short' pairs in English. An alternative view, however, is that

---

[52] Sommerfelt (1951) links the Latin and Germanic developments, assuming Latin influence on Germanic.

new quantity relationships were created by means of resyllabification due to the loss of a final vowel (Dobson, 1962). For example, a word such as *name* ('name') was pronounced /nă·mə/, the first syllable having the structure CV. The equalization of length in stressed syllables resulted in the lengthening of the vowel to give /nā·mə/, with the structure C̄V·CV, while the subsequent loss of the final vowel closed the initial syllable to give /nām/, with the structure C̄VC, contrasting with CV̆C, and creating a quantity distinction in the vowels. In a more recent interpretation, Minkova (1982) shows that this lengthening appears to take place almost exclusively in cases where the word-final schwa is dropped; her analysis will be considered below.

Whatever the interpretation, all of these developments illustrate the crucial role of the syllable (and in many cases the *accented* syllable) in the rise and fall of quantity systems, with the equalization of syllable weight through lengthening and shortening processes. The lengths of individual vowels are adjusted to preserve the appropriate syllable weight, thus making the segment length dependent on the syllable weight, rather than the reverse.

2.6.3.2 Scandinavian Systems

Developments of the sort just described, leading to a changed quantity system largely restricted to accented syllables, produce, in one group of languages, a specific set of quantity relationships in such syllables. The languages concerned are those of Scandinavia, including Iceland, though two qualifications must be made here: first that the Scandinavian system is merely the end-point of a set of developments to have embraced all the Germanic languages to different extents and at different times (as discussed above), and second that, of the Scandinavian languages, Danish stands somewhat apart, and does not have the system typical of the other Germanic languages.

As a typical example of the Scandinavian situation, consider the Icelandic words given in Fig. 2.17. In these examples, a long vowel is followed by a short consonant, and a short vowel by a long consonant, while words such as *man or *iːs:, with either a short vowel and a short consonant, or a long vowel and a long consonant, do not occur. There is thus complementarity of vowel and consonant length.[53]

Fig. 2.17	maːn	*man*	'slave'	man:	*mann*	'man' (acc.)
	huːs	*hús*	'house' (nom.)	hus:	*húss*	'house' (gen.)
	iːs	*ís*	'ice' (nom.)	is:	*íss*	'ice' (gen.)

Though there is no question that there is a phonological distinction between the members of each pair, there is less agreement about where to assign it. One

[53] From a phonetic point of view, this situation is not restricted to the Scandinavian languages; Sweet (1877) notes the complementarity of vowel and consonant length in English (cf. 2.2.2), and this is endorsed by Lehiste (1971). Unlike the Scandinavian case, however, this complementarity is of a purely phonetic nature, with no phonological implications.

solution, suggested by Malone (1953), is to regard length as distinctive in *both* the vowel *and* the consonant, so that [maːn] and [manː] are phonemically /maːn/ and /manː/, respectively. However, this seems uneconomical, and a number of scholars, such as Bergsveinsson (1941) and Garnes (1973), allocate the distinctiveness to the vowel, regarding the consonant length as allophonic and predictable. The opposite view is taken by Benediktsson (1963) and by Árnason (1980), who take the length of the consonants to be phonologically relevant, with vowel length as predictable from this.[54]

The arguments in favour of this latter view seem to be the more compelling. As Benediktsson and Árnason point out, this is morphologically the most satisfactory, since an analysis of the pair *hús* vs. *húss* as /hus/ and /husː/, especially if the latter is represented as /huss/, reflects the addition of a genitive suffix /-s/ to the latter, which is also found elsewhere, e.g. in *vors*, genitive of *vor* ('spring'). An analysis of the pair as /huːs/ vs. /hus/, with the length distinction ascribed to the vowel, would suggest that the genitive is formed by shortening the vowel in the case of *hús* but adding -s in the case of *vor*, whereas the process is the same in both cases. This solution, in which vowel length is predictable from the following consonants, also explains the presence of a short vowel before a consonant cluster in words such as *hestur* ('horse') (Árnason, 1980: 21). For Árnason, therefore, 'vowels are short before two or more consonants, but long otherwise' (p. 22).

Again, therefore, we may draw a general conclusion that the shape of the syllable *as a whole* may determine the quantity of individual sounds, and that the syllable itself is therefore a unit of quantity. We shall explore this principle further below.

2.7 The Non-linear Approach to Length

2.7.1 INTRODUCTION

Current phonological theory has largely abandoned the view of phonological structure as a string of segmental units—'beads on a string'—in which much of both structuralist and generative phonology was couched until the late 1970s. Instead, these structures, and the representation of them, are regarded in a more multi-dimensional way.

In the present context, the most relevant of such 'non-linear' approaches are Metrical Phonology and Autosegmental Phonology (there are other theories, but they are less significant for the description of length). In the former,[55] phonological representations are seen as hierarchical arrangements of binary-branching

---

[54] For full discussion, see Árnason (1980: 14–23). A further analysis, proposed by Malone (1953) and endorsed by Haugen (1958), is to regard the length difference as part of the 'accent' of the syllable.

[55] On Metrical Phonology see especially Liberman and Prince (1977); Hogg and McCully (1987); Goldsmith (1990).

nodes; in the latter,[56] multidimensionality takes the form of a representation which arranges different kinds of units and features on quasi-independent, parallel 'tiers', which are linked by principles of association, and the whole is thus rather like a musical score in which the independent staves are co-ordinated by the temporal or rhythmical organization. Though rather different, these two approaches have in common a complex, non-linear structure; since they are also not incompatible with each other, more eclectic scholars have been able to combine them in a number of useful ways.

The adoption of one or other of these frameworks forces us to reconsider and develop the notions of length presented so far. Since they provide more elaborate conceptions of timing and of syllable structure, they offer further possibilities for the interpretation and analysis of length in a wider context.

2.7.2 THE NON-LINEAR REPRESENTATION OF SYLLABLE STRUCTURE[57]

We have so far adopted a rather crude view of the syllable as a 'structured string' of segments (Lass, 1984), containing C and V elements in ordered patterns. Thus, the nucleus or peak of the syllable is assumed to be basically vocalic (V), optionally flanked by consonantal elements (C). In Metrical Phonology we need to approach the structure rather differently, as a hierarchically ordered arrangement of branching nodes, dominated by the syllable node itself.

The idea of a hierarchically organized branching structure in phonology can be traced back some way. An influential early application of this is the analysis of Mazateco syllable structure by Pike and Pike (1947), who give the tree diagram of Fig. 2.18 as a representation of the syllable /ncʔoai3–4/ (3–4 is the tone pattern).

Fig. 2.18

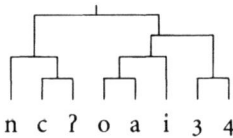

n c ʔ o a i 3 4

This is refined somewhat by Wells (1947), who applies the theory of Immediate Constituent Analysis (Bloomfield, 1935), to the description of phonological structure. Though the model was designed for syntax, Wells provides extensive discussion of its application to phonology.

Hockett (1955: 52) uses the labels *onset*, *peak*, and *coda* for the parts of the syllable: the 'peak' is the central vocalic element; the 'onset' is the preceding, and

[56] On Autosegmental Phonology see especially Goldsmith (1976, 1990).
[57] The very brief exposition given in this section of the basic principles of these varieties of non-linear phonology can be supplemented by the works referred to in notes 55 and 56, and current standard manuals of phonological theory, such as Durand (1990), Kenstowicz (1994), Roca (1994), Goldsmith (ed.) (1995), Spencer (1996), Gussenhoven and Jacobs (1998), and others.

the 'coda' the following, consonantal part. Each of these may be simple or complex. Unlike Pike and Pike, however, Hockett does not group any two of these more closely together, implying that the syllable is divided into three equal constituents. More recent developments, which incorporate some of Hockett's categories but provide rather more structure, include the approaches of Kahn (1976) and Selkirk (1978, 1980), which assume the binary-branching 'syllable template' of Fig. 2.19(a), and that of Levin (1985), who interprets this in terms of X-bar theory (Jackendoff, 1977), regarding the syllable as a 'projection' of the nucleus, as in Fig. 2.19(b).

Fig. 2.19 (a) 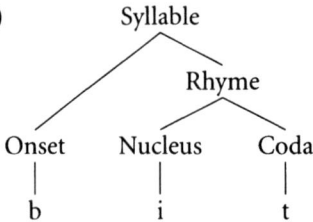   (b)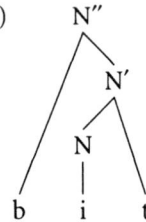

This representation (as opposed to a non-binary, three-fold division of Hockett) can be justified by an appeal to the internal relationships within the syllable. Since the initial consonant or consonant cluster plays no part in syllable weight, and the remaining two parts have a closer unity, we can justify an initial cut into 'onset' and 'rhyme'; the latter divides into 'nucleus' ('peak'), and 'coda'. There can be further constituents in those cases where there are consonant or vowel clusters. Exactly how the trees should be drawn is open to discussion, but if we assume binary-branching and right-branching structures we obtain representations such as those of Fig. 2.20 (σ = syllable node). In Fig. 2.20(a) there is a branching nucleus, in Fig. 2.20(b) a branching onset, and in Fig. 2.20(c) a branching coda.

Fig. 2.20 (a) 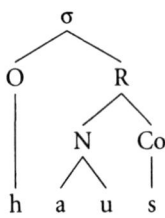   (b) 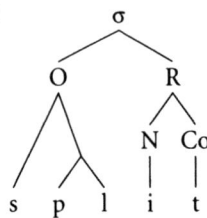   (c)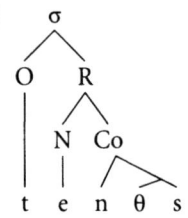

('house')   ('split')   ('tenths')

In Metrical Phonology the nodes of metrical trees are labelled 'strong' or 'weak', thus ranking the syllables according to relative prominence.[58] For exam-

---

[58] For discussion of the Metrical approach to the specification of accent see 3.5.3.

ple, Fig. 2.21(a) shows a possible tree for *elephant*. This form of representation can be extended to the structural parts of the syllable, as in Fig. 2.21(b), and ultimately to the segments themselves (Fig. 2.21(c)).

Fig. 2.21 (a)   (b)   (c)

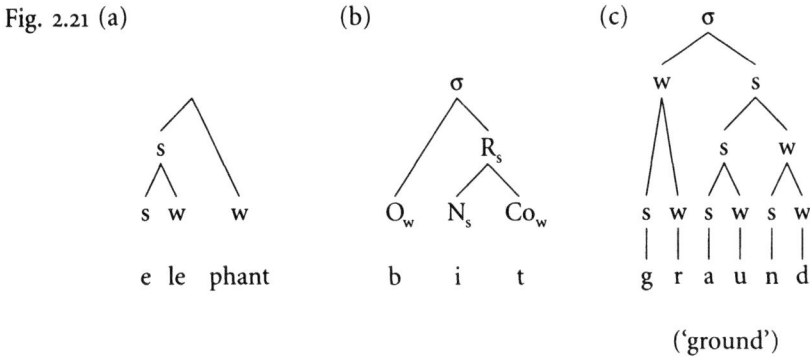

('ground')

As the theory has developed, however, such labelling of nodes as 'strong' and 'weak' has been less used, and for our present purposes we can dispense with it. The structural labels (Onset, Rhyme, Nucleus, and Coda) can, however, be supplemented by the labels C and V for consonantal and vocalic (or [−syllabic] and [+syllabic]) segments, respectively.[59] A typical representation of 'ground' would thus be as in Fig. 2.22(a). As we shall see, the C and V labels have been dispensed with in some versions of this approach (Levin, 1985; Lowenstamm and Kaye, 1986), since the role of a segment as C or V may be predictable from the configuration of the tree, and therefore redundant. All that we need, therefore is an indication of each segmental position, as in Fig. 2.22(b), which consequently can be labelled 'X', further specification being recoverable from the tree. However, we shall retain C and V for clarity in the following discussion.

Fig. 2.22 (a)   (b)

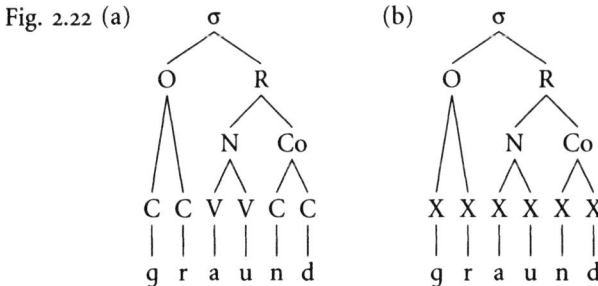

[59] The establishment of a 'CV tier', on which the segmental positions and their role as [+syllabic] or [−syllabic] are represented, was proposed by McCarthy (1979), and developed and codified by Clements and Keyser (1983) in their 'CV phonology'.

A different, and in some ways complementary, approach to the representation of syllable structure has been adopted in Autosegmental Phonology. Initially a theory of tone, this model recognizes separate *tiers* for prosodic features such as tone, which are independent of the segments as such, but linked to them in an appropriate way. This captures the relative independence of tonal and segmental features in many languages, especially the African languages to which the theory was first applied. Thus, for example, in Mende (Leben, 1973a), tone patterns such as High + Low and Low + High are applied to words regardless of the number of syllables they contain, so that the same pattern is differently linked to the segmental material in each case (Fig. 2.23). Further 'tiers' have been accommodated within the model as its scope has been extended to other features, such as nasality, backness, rounding, etc.

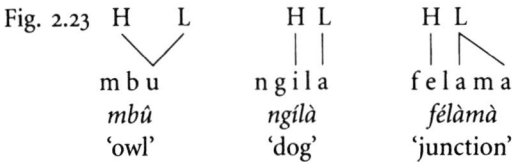

Fig. 2.23
```
     H    L          H L          H L
      \  /           | |          | \
      m b u          n g i l a    f e l a m a
      mbû            ngílà        félàmà
      'owl'          'dog'        'junction'
```

In this approach the interest is clearly not in the complexities of segmental syllable structure as such (which is by some scholars reduced to a non-hierarchical string of C and V segments), but rather in how this structure relates to phonetic features. The C and V (or X) positions thus constitute a framework, a *skeleton*, or *root tier*, which accounts for the distribution of these features. The linking of the features to the skeleton is achieved by the application of the *Wellformedness Condition*, initially devised by Goldsmith (1976: 27) for tone (cf. 4.4.3.2), though easily generalized to other features:

(1) All vowels are associated with at least one tone.
(2) All tones are associated with at least one vowel.
(3) Association lines do not cross.

However, these do not provide a unique way of linking the tiers, and further principles must be applied, some of them language specific. Since the association is also subject to modification by phonological processes (both synchronically during a derivation and diachronically through time), rules for *linking* (the initial association), *delinking* (the severing of links, which may leave certain segments or tones unassociated), and *relinking* (the re-establishment of links between the two) are required. In some cases further segments or tones, etc., may be deleted; in others they may be inserted. More will be said about some of these processes below, though clearly not all are relevant for our present discussion.

This brief explanation of the framework and the linking mechanisms will serve as a background for our discussion of the role of length in non-linear theories, to which we shall proceed directly.

2.7.3 THE NON-LINEAR REPRESENTATION OF LENGTH

Different phonological models may require a different interpretation—or at least a different representation—of phonological features, structures, and processes, and this is true of the application of non-linear phonology to length. In 2.6 we considered the role of length in terms of syllable structure, and the non-linear view of this structure just outlined imposes a similarly non-linear view of length.

From a Metrical perspective, 'long' vowels and consonants can be interpreted as geminates (Kenstowicz and Pyle, 1973; Guerssel, 1977), occupying two positions in the metrical 'tree'. Thus, a 'long' vowel could take the form of Fig. 2.24(a), and a 'long' consonant the form of Fig. 2.24(b) ($ = syllable node; the subscript co-indices identify the segments as geminates).

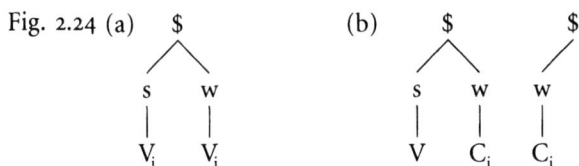

Fig. 2.24 (a)

```
        $
       / \
      s   w
      |   |
      Vᵢ  Vᵢ
```

(b)

```
     $        $
    / \      /
   s   w    w
   |   |    |
   V   Cᵢ   Cᵢ
```

Under this interpretation, geminate vowels are dominated by the same syllable node, while geminate consonants are assumed to be intervocalic and are therefore split between two syllables. We can accommodate syllable initial (Fig. 2.25(a)) or syllable final (Fig. 2.25(b)) geminate consonants with slightly more elaborate 'trees'.

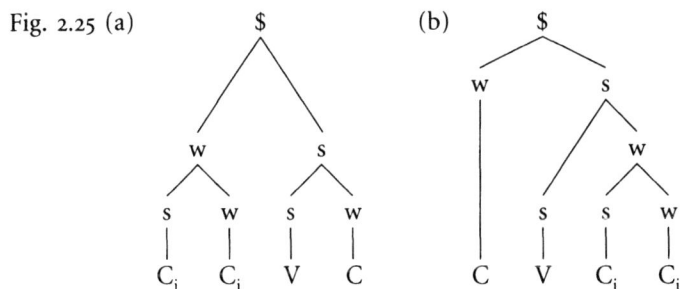

Fig. 2.25 (a)

```
              $
            /   \
          w       s
         / \     / \
        s   w   s   w
        |   |   |   |
        Cᵢ  Cᵢ  V   C
```

(b)

```
            $
          /   \
        w       s
        |      / \
        |     s   w
        |    / \  |
        C   V Cᵢ  Cᵢ
```

With the elimination of 'strong' and 'weak' nodes in the Metrical representation of syllable structure, and the use of labels for structural parts, the trees become more complex but rather clearer. Thus a geminate interpretation of a 'long' vowel can be represented as a branching nucleus; a 'long' consonant as a branching onset or coda. Syllables such as [bit], [biːt] and [bitː] may thus be represented as in Fig. 2.26.

Fig. 2.26 (a) 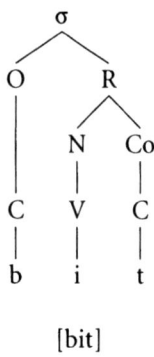   (b) 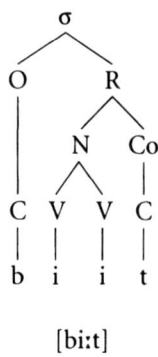   (c)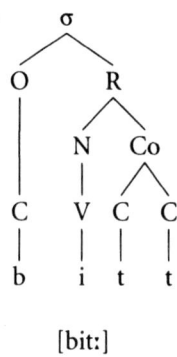

[bit]   [biːt]   [bitː]

This representation also makes transparent the nature of syllable weight. If a 'light' syllable has a short vowel with no coda, and a 'heavy' syllable has either a long vowel or a short vowel with a coda, then the respective representations are as in Fig. 2.27.

Fig. 2.27 (a) 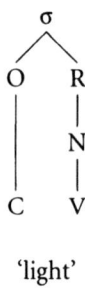   (b) 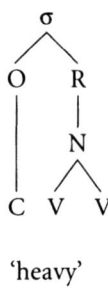   (c)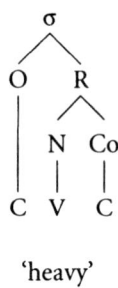

'light'   'heavy'   'heavy'

The definition of a 'heavy' syllable in these terms is therefore simply that it has a branching rhyme, though the branching is at different levels—the nucleus or the rhyme itself—according to whether the weight is the result of vowel length or of the presence of a final consonant. 'Hypercharacterized' syllables, with *both* a long vowel *and* a following consonant (e.g. [biːt]) will naturally have branching at the level of *both* the nucleus *and* the rhyme, as in Fig. 2.28.

Fig. 2.28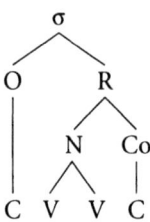

In an Autosegmental framework the interpretation of length is somewhat

different. As we have noted, C and V elements are here seen as segmental positions to which the phonetic material is associated. These two parts of the representation—the C and V slots and the vocalic or consonantal material—belong
to different tiers; if 'long' segments are seen as geminates, then the same material
extends over two such slots. A 'long' vowel is therefore represented not as
Fig. 2.29(a) (as in Metrical theory) but as Fig. 2.29(b) (cf. van der Hulst and
Smith, 1982; Vago, 1985; Clements, 1986).

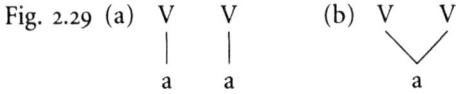

Fig. 2.29 (a) V   V   (b) V   V
              | | \ /
              a   a   a

In an early application of these principles to length in Hausa, which is cast
largely in the Metrical mould, Leben (1977, 1980) represents the words *damoo*
and *gammoo* as in Fig. 2.30.

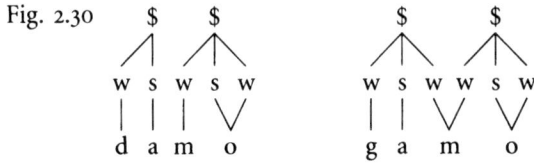

Fig. 2.30

It can be seen that Leben adopts the metrical analysis of 'strong' and 'weak'
nodes, but does not subscribe to the binary view of their relationships. The approach is similar to the Metrical analysis given above, but the major difference
is that 'long' segments are associated to two positions within the syllable, rather
than having a double representation with co-indexed vowels or consonants.
Thus, 'long' vowels are associated to both a 'strong' and a 'weak' position, while
'long' consonants are treated as 'ambisyllabic': the consonant is associated to the
final 'weak' position of the first syllable and the initial 'weak' position of the
second.

As it stands, this analysis caters only for intervocalic long consonants, and not
for initial or final ones; it also only accommodates long vowels in open syllables.
Ingria (1980) includes these by adopting the more orthodox binary-branching
analysis, and by allowing a long consonant in initial or final position also to be
associated with strong+weak nodes (Fig. 2.31(a)), while a long vowel in a closed
syllable can be strong+strong (Fig. 2.31(b)).

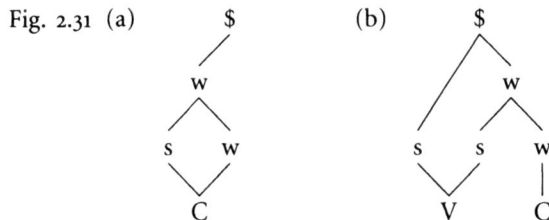

Fig. 2.31 (a) $ (b) $

Again with the elimination of the 'strong' and 'weak' nodes, and the incorporation of structural labels, the structures of Figs. 2.26(b) and 2.26(c) can be represented as in Fig. 2.32.

Fig. 2.32

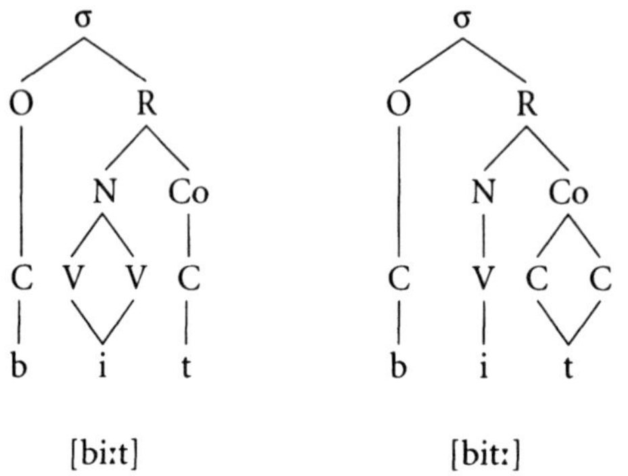

[biːt]   [bitː]

It should be noted that a representation with two contiguous identical segments—as in Fig. 2.26(b)—is in principle excluded in Autosegmental Phonology
because of the 'Obligatory Contour Principle', which rules out a sequence of
identical elements on a specific tier, unless these belong to different morphemes
(Goldsmith, 1976). We can therefore in principle distinguish between geminates
'proper' and sequences of identical segments, where the latter will belong to
different morphemes (cf. McCarthy, 1986; Lowenstamm and Kaye, 1986; Schein
and Steriade, 1986; Goldsmith, 1990). For example, a syllable final geminate [tt]
would have the representation of Fig. 2.33(a), a non-geminate sequence, consisting of a syllable final [t] and a syllable initial [t], that of Fig. 2.33(b).

Fig. 2.33 (a)   R   (b)   R

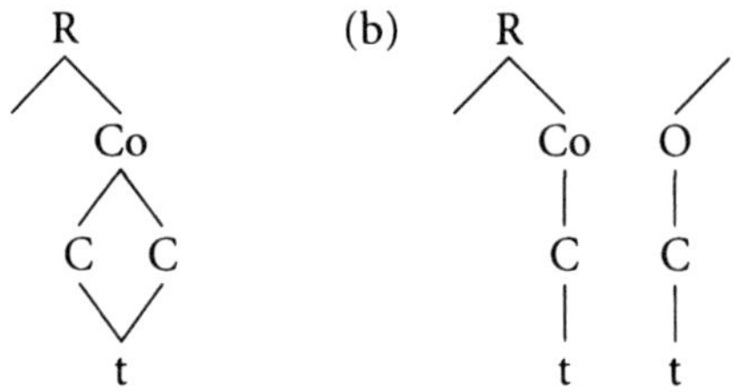

In sum, therefore, an Autosegmental approach to length involves separating
the actual segmental material—the qualitative features of the vowels and consonants—from the structural positions within the syllable where these occur, and
associating these two according to a variety of principles. The C and V (or alternatively X) elements which represent these structural positions are construed not
merely as structural slots but also as units of *timing*. The length of individual
segments is therefore the result of their being associated with different numbers
of such slots.

It may be asked whether the non-linear approach to length presented here actually involves a different interpretation of the phenomenon itself, or is merely a different way of representing it. In so far as non-linear phonology recognizes an elaborate syllable structure with different structural positions, and regards 'long' segments as occupying two such positions, it is comparable to the syllable-based approaches outlined in 2.6, though providing a more graphic representation of this structure. However, Autosegmental Phonology goes somewhat further, by representing this double nature on a separate tier from the phonetic quality of the sound itself. The fact that there is a *single* representation on the segmental tier could in itself be said to involve recognition that 'long' sounds also constitute in some sense a single element, and the approach thus achieves a useful conceptual ambiguity—useful, that is, in that it is able to reconcile the apparent dual status of geminates as *simultaneously* double units and single units. In this sense, therefore, the Autosegmental representation of length could be said to constitute an advance on approaches which are forced to choose between the double and the single nature of 'long' sounds.

2.7.4 LENGTHENING PROCESSES

In order to illustrate the application of non-linear—principally Autosegmental —theory to questions of length, and to evaluate its claim to provide new insights into the phenomenon, we may examine a number of phonological processes from the perspective of this approach. These processes, which can be interpreted either historically or as part of synchronic grammars, involve lengthening (and, to some extent, shortening) in specific contexts. We shall see that Autosegmental theory provides a way of describing these processes in terms of the relationship between a segmental 'tier' and a structural 'tier' (or CV tier), as discussed above.

2.7.4.1 Open Syllable Lengthening

A widely attested process in the history of many languages is Open Syllable Lengthening, which involves the lengthening of short vowels in syllables where there is no final consonant. Such a process occurred in Middle English during the thirteenth century, and has been the subject of much scholarly work (Jones, 1989: 98–127; Lass, 1992: 47–8, 73–6); comparable processes also took place in Middle High German and Dutch. This process was referred to briefly in 2.6.3.1, in connection with the equalization of length in stressed syllables.

Further examples are given in Fig. 2.34, which presents Old English and Middle English versions of a number of words. Apart from the change of vowel

Fig. 2.34	*Old English*		*Middle English*		
	faran	/faran/	*fare*	/faːrə/	'to go'
	wudu	/wudu/	*wode*	/woːdə/	'wood'
	beran	/beran/	*bere*	/bɛːrə/	'to bear'

quality (which we ignore here), it will be observed that there has been a change in vowel length from Old to Middle English. This change took place in open syllables, i.e. in syllables with no consonantal coda. In the examples of Fig. 2.34, the syllabification is assumed to be /fa·ran/, etc., so that the first syllable is open.

Exactly what mechanism led to this development has been the subject of much debate, the details of which are beyond the scope of the present discussion. One significant factor is assumed to be the strong stress on the first syllable, which may have led to the equalization of length in stressed syllables (see 2.6.3.1 above). But whatever the origin and cause of the change, the fact that it affects *short* vowels in *open* syllables suggests that *light* stressed syllables (with a short vowel and no coda) became *heavy*.

We have seen that, in terms of Autosegmental representations, 'heavy' syllables have a branching rhyme; 'light' syllables do not. Open Syllable Lengthening can therefore be seen as the creation of a branching rhyme. A further timing slot is produced, and the lengthening processes can be interpreted as the automatic spreading of the vowel to this additional slot. These processes are depicted in Fig. 2.35, where (a) shows the original situation: a short vowel in an open syllable. Creation of a branching nucleus gives the structure of (b), with an empty V slot; this is filled by being linked to the existing vowel, as in (c).

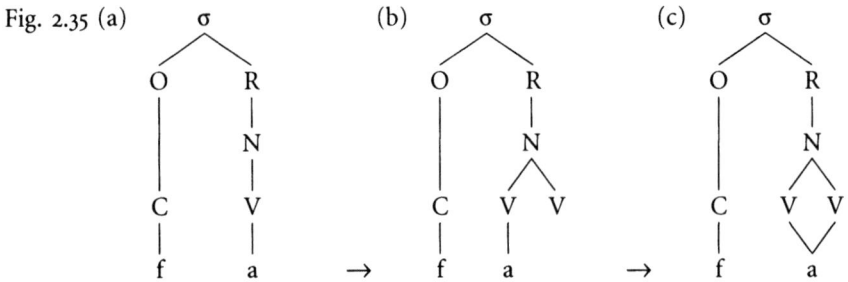

Fig. 2.35 (a)

```
          σ                        (b)        σ                      (c)        σ
         / \                                 / \                              / \
        O   R                               O   R                            O   R
        |   |                               |   |                            |   |
        |   N                               |   N                            |   N
        |   |                               |  / \                           |  / \
        C   V                               C V   V                          C V   V
        |   |                               | |                              | |  /
        f   a        →                      f a          →                   f a
```

The crux of the problem is, of course, the process represented in Fig. 2.35(b) which, unlike that of (c), which is automatic, appears unmotivated. Referring back to our discussion in 2.6.3.1 of the equalization of length in stressed syllables, we may hypothesize that the intolerance of light stressed syllables led to the automatic generation of an additional slot in the rhyme. Why this should be a slot in the nucleus of the syllable as opposed to the rhyme itself (which would generate a coda) remains unclear, however (see below, 2.7.4.2).

The same principles underlie a complementary process in Middle English: the *shortening* of vowels in *closed* syllables. Thus, the long vowels in the initial syllables of Old English *wīsdōm* ('wisdom'), *cēpte* ('kept'), had by the thirteenth century become short: Middle English *wisdome* /wisdəm/, *kepte* /kɛptə/ (Jones, 1989: 105; Lass, 1992: 72). The internal consonant clusters here are such that the first consonant of the cluster must belong to the first syllable, which is consequently closed. The assumption here is that a long vowel *and* a coda, which forms a hypercharacterized syllable, is reduced to a simple *heavy* syllable. The outcome is therefore the same as Open Syllable Lengthening, resulting in the equalization of stressed syllables, but the process itself is the reverse of lengthening, and can be represented as in Fig. 2.36. Here, the nucleus loses its branching structure, leaving the vowel attached to only a single vowel slot, and thus short. Again, the motivation for this development—the loss of the vowel slot—is, of course, not contained in this representation, which displays only the *result* of this loss.

Fig. 2.36

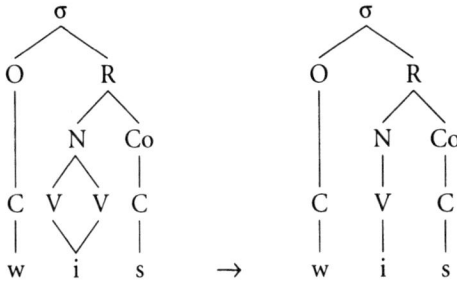

There are other kinds of lengthening processes in open syllables. Consider, for example, the Old English forms given in Fig. 2.37 (De Chene and Anderson, 1979; Hogg, 1992: 173).

Fig. 2.37 *nominative   genitive*

holh	hōles	'hole'
feorh	fēores	'life'
wealh	wēales	'foreigner'

The short vowel of the stem has been lengthened in the genitive with the loss of stem-final -*h*. This can be explained by assuming that loss of the *h* in the genitive form (/holhəs/ > /holəs/) left a single intervocalic consonant, which was reassigned to the following syllable (/hol·əs/ > /ho·ləs/), and the first vowel was lengthened as a result (/ho·ləs/ > /hō·ləs/.[60] In Autosegmental terms, the process can be described as in Fig. 2.38. Fig. 2.38(a) represents the original state of affairs, with a short vowel followed by a consonant cluster /lh/; loss of the /h/ leaves an empty slot in the syllable onset position, as in (b). Realignment according to the principle of maximal onsets (as many intervocalic consonants as possible are assigned to the onset of the following syllable) results in the delinking of the /l/ from the coda position of the first syllable (indicated by the cancelling of the association line) and relinking to the vacant onset position of

[60] Though this process is treated here as an instance of Open Syllable Lengthening (De Chene and Anderson, 1979), it is usually regarded as a form of 'Compensatory Lengthening' (e.g. by Hogg, 1992). An interpretation in terms of the latter will be presented below.

the second (Fig. 2.38(c)), leaving a vacant coda position at the end of the first syllable which is pruned from the tree (Fig. 2.38(d)). Open Syllable Lengthening can proceed as before, generating a V slot (Fig. 2.38(e)) and linking it to the preceding vowel (Fig. 2.38(f)), which thus becomes long.

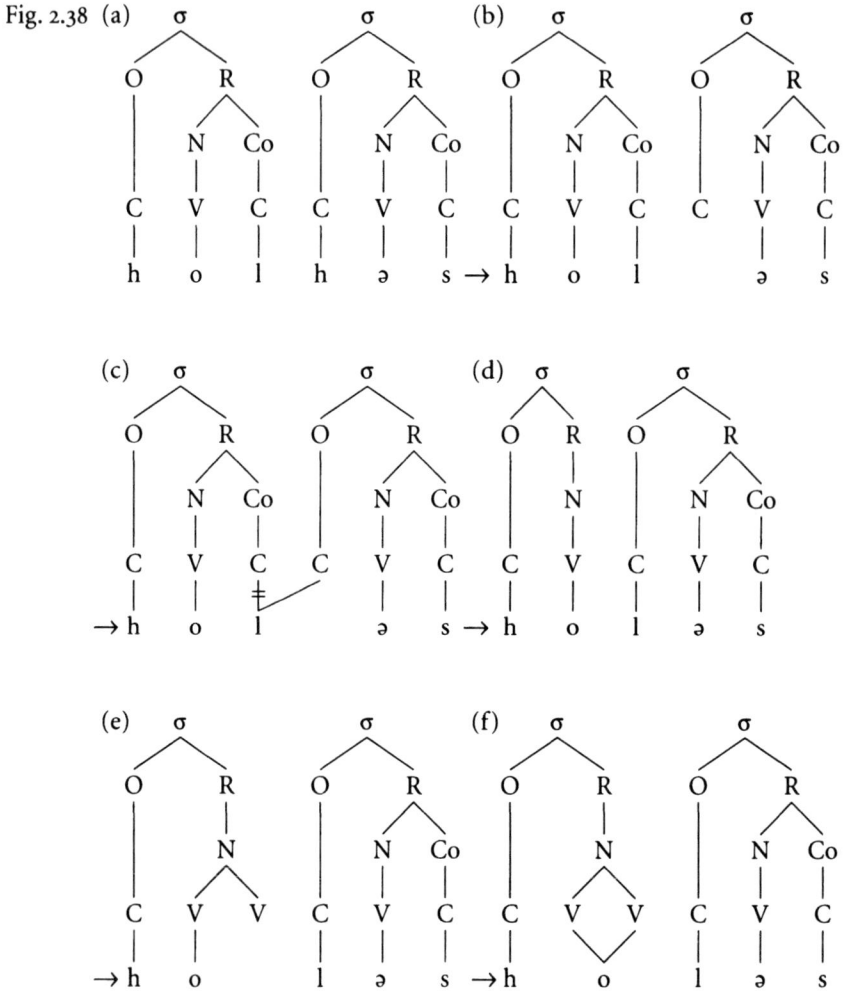

Fig. 2.38 (a)

```
        σ                    σ          (b)    σ                    σ
      /   \                /   \              /   \                /   \
     O     R              O     R            O     R              O     R
     |    / \             |    / \           |    / \             |    / \
     |   N   Co           |   N   Co         |   N   Co           |   N   Co
     |   |   |            |   |   |          |   |   |            |   |   |
     C   V   C            C   V   C          C   V   C            C   V   C
     |   |   |            |   |   |          |   |   |            |   |   |
     h   o   l            h   ə   s    →     h   o   l            ə       s
```

```
   (c)  σ                    σ          (d)  σ                    σ
      /   \                /   \              /   \                /   \
     O     R              O     R            O     R              O     R
     |    / \             |    / \           |    |               |    / \
     |   N   Co           |   N   Co         |    N               |   N   Co
     |   |   |            |   |   |          |    |               |   |   |
     C   V   C            C   V   C          C    V    C          C   V   C
     |   |   ‡            |   |   |          |    |               |   |   |
   → h   o   l            ə       s    →     h    o    l          ə       s
```

```
   (e)  σ                    σ          (f)  σ                    σ
      /   \                /   \              /   \                /   \
     O     R              O     R            O     R              O     R
     |     |              |    / \           |     |              |    / \
     |     N              |   N   Co         |     N              |   N   Co
     |    / \             |   |   |          |    /\              |   |   |
     C   V  V             C   V   C          C   V  V             C   V   C
     |   |                |   |   |          |   \/               |   |   |
   → h   o                l   ə   s    →     h   o                l   ə   s
```

There is a serious weakness in this presentation of the process, however, since the lengthening here is not, as in the case of Middle English Open Syllable Lengthening, taken to be an independent development, but is assumed to arise directly from the loss of the /h/ and the subsequent resyllabification. The causal link between these processes is not expressed in Fig. 2.38, which treats the creation of a heavy syllable (Fig. 2.38(e)) as unmotivated. We shall take up this question in 2.7.4.2, providing a better interpretation of this process.

It can be seen, nevertheless, that Autosegmental Phonology provides a graphic notation for the mechanisms involved in lengthening and shortening. In the case of the processes described here, the developments are attributed to the increase or decrease in the number of structural slots in the syllable, thus affecting the availability of such slots for association with the segmental material. In this way, the lengthening and shortening of vowels is seen as a reflection of changes to the structural characteristics of the syllable as a whole.

2.7.4.2 Compensatory Lengthening

The term 'compensatory lengthening' is usually applied to the process in which segments—usually 'weak' ones such as nasals and 'liquids'—are lost, and the accompanying vowel is apparently lengthened to 'compensate' for its loss. Well attested examples are found in the development of Latin, where, in the accusative plural, an original *-ons became Classical Latin -ōs, or in the Germanic languages, where Proto-Germanic *gans ('goose') and *finf ('five') became Old English gōs and fīf. In each case a structure containing a short vowel and two consonants became one with a long vowel and a single consonant, i.e. V̆CC became V̄C. The process is assumed to have involved the loss of the first C, followed by the lengthening of the vowel by way of 'compensation'. Similar processes, some involving different kinds of loss of phonological material, are postulated in the synchronic phonology of a number of languages. This confirms that a long vowel is in some way equivalent to a combination of short vowel and following consonant. Compensatory lengthening also provides evidence for the role of the syllable in determining the length of sounds, since in this case the vowel is lengthened in order to maintain the original syllable weight after the loss of the consonant. Non-linear representations of syllable structure, in which the basic syllable template remains constant, in spite of the apparent loss of segments, can be used to support such a principle.

The process of Compensatory Lengthening is, however, a controversial one, not least because it requires the *simultaneous* application of two independent processes: the loss of one segment and the lengthening of another. Such simultaneity is rare in historical terms, and demands that we establish a close causal connection between the two processes. Not all scholars are willing to admit such a connection; De Chene and Anderson (1979), for example, are reluctant to admit that compensatory lengthening exists at all: 'There is no such distinct phonetic process as compensatory lengthening, and accordingly no unified phonetic explanation (such as 'preservation of syllable weight' or the like) should be sought' (p.507). Their preferred explanation is that the consonant whose loss is supposed to trigger the process in fact becomes a glide, resulting in the formation of a diphthong, which is subsequently monophthongized to form the long vowel. That is, VCC > VGC > V̄C, where G is a glide. An example of such glide formation is found in Old English thegn > thēn ('thane'). Furthermore, there are many cases of consonant loss which do not result in 'compensatory lengthening'. According to De Chene and Anderson, such lengthening will only occur if there is already a length distinction in the phonological system of the language; 'compensatory lengthening' does not create such a distinction. An example of this is French where, according to De Chene and Anderson, consonant loss before AD 850 did not result in lengthening, but consonant loss after AD c. 1100 did, a circumstance that they attribute to the lack of a length distinction in French before the earlier date, and the presence of one after the later date.

Though De Chene and Anderson are dismissive of compensatory lengthening, and hence of any role for the overall structure of the syllable in determining the length of sounds, most other phonologists are prepared to accept it as a legitimate process. This approach has been enhanced by the introduction of the more elaborate notational devices of the non-linear framework, presented in 2.7.2 and 2.7.3. Ingria (1980), for example, describes compensatory lengthening in Metrical terms, proposing that the process 'should not be treated as a purely segmental phenomenon, but should rather be viewed as the result of the interaction of changes on the segmental level with well-formedness conditions on the syllabic level . . . Since length, within the framework to be outlined here, is treated as an aspect of syllabic structure, rather than as a segmental feature, changes on the syllabic level can, in turn, affect the length of segments. It is this latter series of changes that constitutes compensatory lengthening proper' (p. 465).

Consider, for example, the loss of *s* in pre-consonantal position in pre-classical Latin, and the corresponding lengthening of the preceding vowel, e.g. *sisdo: > si:do: ('sit'), *pesdo > pe:do: ('furnish with feet') (Ingria, 1980). This process is assumed to have involved voicing of [s] to [z], followed by the loss of the [z], but for simplicity we shall collapse this into a single process of s-loss. Given a metrical representation of *sisdo:, as in Fig. 2.39(a), the loss of the *s* will result in an 'empty' slot (marked here by 'Ø'), as in Fig. 2.39(b). However, this loss is compensated for by doubling the vowel [i], giving the representation of Fig. 2.39(c). This has the effect of adjusting the segmental representation to match the metrical tree; the latter remains unaffected by the changes, and the syllable weight is preserved. There is, however, a weakness here, since Metrical Phonology does not provide any principle which requires the vowel to be doubled following the loss of the following consonant; there is thus no real link between the two processes, and no reason for regarding the lengthening as 'compensatory'.

Fig. 2.39 (a)

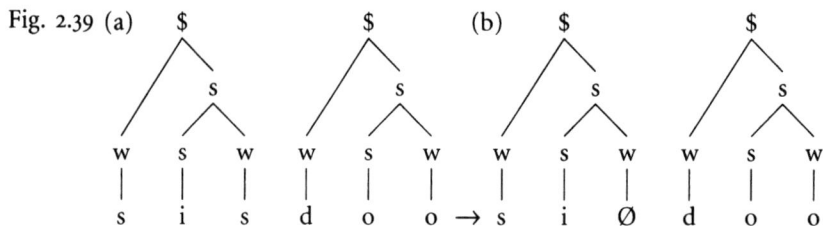

Fig. 2.39 (c)

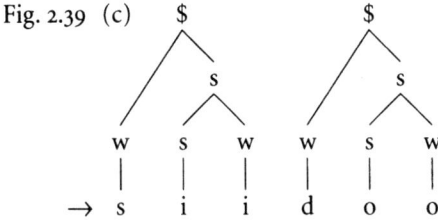

This process can also be accounted for under an Autosegmental interpretation. Here, as we have seen, long segments can be represented by a single element on the segmental tier, linked to two positions in the skeleton. The result is similar to the metrical approach, though converting the metrical tree to an Autosegmental tree (Fig. 2.40) reveals some differences, and an anomaly. First, unlike the Metrical interpretation, the Autosegmental approach does provide a motivation for the lengthening of the vowel; if we assume that the coda slot occupied by [s] in Fig. 2.40(a) is not deleted following the loss of the consonant, but retained on the CV tier, then the relinking of this slot to the preceding vowel (Fig. 2.40(c)) is an automatic process which follows from the Wellformedness Conditions: an unassociated slot is not permitted.

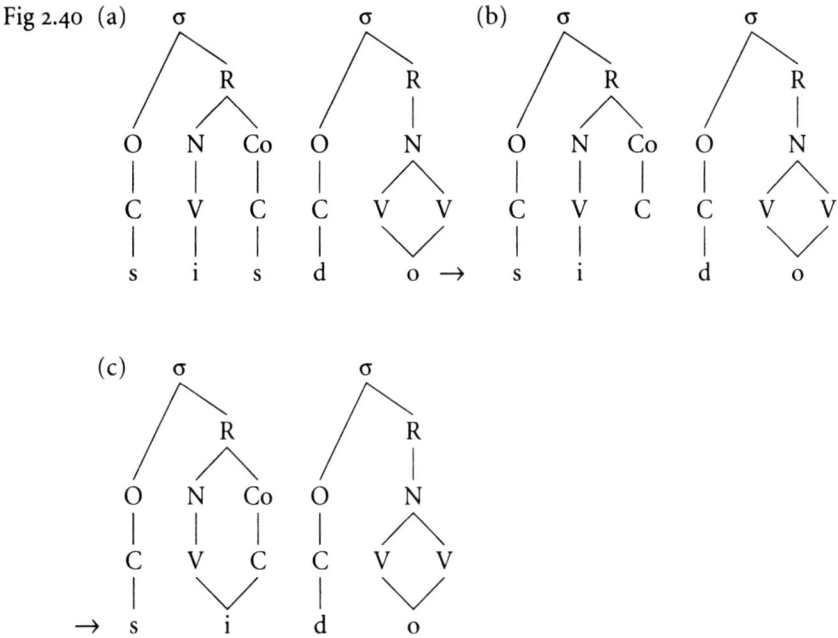

Fig 2.40 (a)   (b)

(c)

It will be observed, however, that the *vowel* ([i]) is associated to a [−syllabic] slot (C), which is hardly satisfactory; we would expect a vowel to associate to a

[+syllabic] slot (V). In fact, the version of this process given by Lass (1984: 260) (which does not adopt the Autosegmental representation of long vowels as doubly linked), is formalized in a way which avoids this anomaly. The change from Proto-West-Germanic *finf* to Old English *fīf* is presented in Fig. 2.41. Here, the lengthening process is construed as the creation of an additional V slot in the nucleus, to replace the C slot in the rhyme. This avoids the domination of a vowel by a C slot, but of course it forfeits the causal link between the consonant loss and the vowel lengthening; the latter cannot be seen as compensatory.

Fig. 2.41

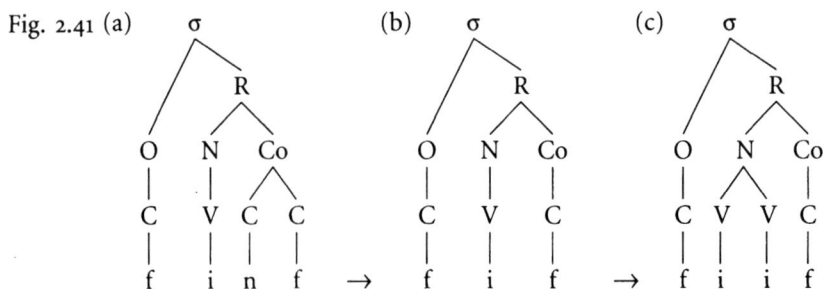

This is exactly the problem that was encountered in 2.7.4.1 in connection with lengthening in the Old English form *hōles* (see Fig. 2.38). The lengthening in that process was seen as the result of consonant loss and resyllabification, but again the lengthening was in the *vowel*, though the loss was of a *consonant*, and consequently of a C slot, and hence no direct link could be established between the two. That process, too, can be described more neatly by not deleting the C slot and relinking it to the vowel, as in Fig. 2.42. Fig. 2.42(a) is identical to Fig. 2.38(c), while Fig. 2.42(b) replaces all of Fig. 2.38(d) to Fig. 2.38(f). Again the motivation for the lengthening can be found in the Wellformedness Conditions which rule out an empty slot. Preservation of the syllable structure on loss of the consonant thus automatically results in a long vowel, though it requires us to link the vowel to a consonant position.

Fig. 2.42

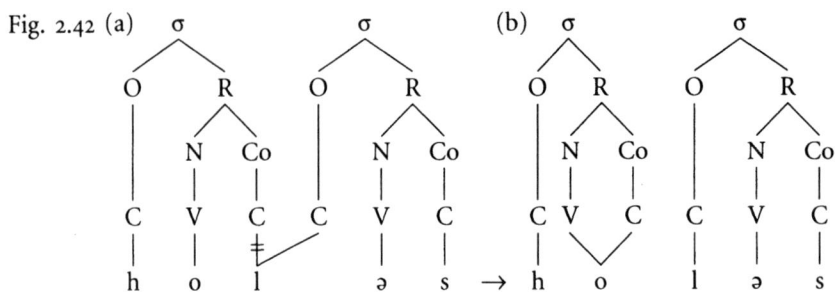

In defence of this approach, it may be said that this solution reflects the equivalence of VC and V: in the structure of the syllable: the latter replaces the former and has the same structure.[61] However, it would make a long vowel which results from compensatory lengthening structurally different from one which does not, unless, of course, we were to represent *all* long vowels in this way, and thus eliminate all branching in the nucleus. Apart from this, there are a number of other solutions to the problem. Lass (1984: 260) appears happy to accept the replacement of branching in the rhyme by branching in the nucleus because there is 'a structural distinction between syllables-as-units and simple linear strings of Vs and Cs. . . . Syllables, then, are *hierarchical* structures, and (apparently) "branching" is a structural primitive.' Thus, compensatory lengthening preserves syllable weight by preserving *branching* (which, as we have seen, is the defining characteristic of heavy syllables), even if the branching is in a different place.

In the approach of Clements and Keyser (1983), the syllable is represented simultaneously on a number of separate 'planes', including the 'segmental display', the 'syllable display' and the 'nucleus display'. The word *stout*, for example, has the 'segmental display' of Fig. 2.43(a), the 'syllable display' of Fig. 2.43(b), and the 'nucleus display' of Fig. 2.43(c).

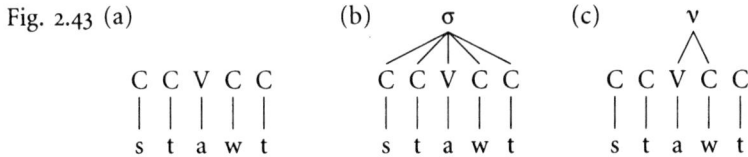

Fig. 2.43 (a)   (b)   σ   (c)   v

C C V C C   C C V C C   C C V C C
| | | | | | | | | | | | | | |
s t a w t   s t a w t   s t a w t

Clements and Keyser reject the hierarchical view of the syllable, so that the syllable display has no intermediate branches; the nucleus (v) consists of 'any tautosyllabic sequences of the form V(X), where X ranges over single occurrences of C and V' (p. 13), i.e. it consists of the vocalic element and one following element, be it vowel or consonant. Since no hierarchical structure is recognized, they avoid the difficulties which arise in cases of compensatory lengthening, when branching in one part of the structure is replaced by branching in another, or when a vocalic element comes to be dominated by a consonantal node.

By way of illustration, consider their treatment of another case of compensatory lengthening, 'preaspiration' in Icelandic (Thráinsson, 1978). When, in Icelandic, two identical voiceless aspirated stops are juxtaposed, the first is replaced by *h*; this process can be regarded as the deletion of the supralaryngeal features of the consonant and the compensatory extension of the corresponding features

---

[61] Vago (1987) adduces evidence from Hungarian which supports the view that long vowels can be equivalent to VC. In this language, the final *-j* of imperatives causes palatalization of a preceding *t*, e.g. *nevet+j* → *neveʃʃ* ('laugh'), but the *t* becomes *č* if it is preceded by *either* VC or V:, as in *költ* → *kölčč*, *dü:t* → *düčč* ('turn over'). The palatalization rule thus requires V: to be equivalent to VC.

of the preceding vowel to the now vacant consonant slot. This happens, for example, with the addition of the past tense suffix *t* to a stem with a final *t*, for example in [maihtı] < [mait - tı] ('met') or [veihtı] < [veit - tı] ('granted'). For the change *att* > *aht*, the process can be presented as in Fig. 2.44, where there is a 'laryngeal tier', with *h* representing [+spread glottis], a CV tier, and a 'supralarygeal tier' for the segmental features.

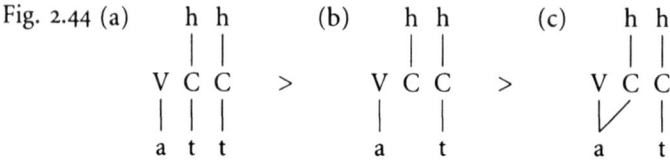

Fig. 2.44 (a)
$$
\begin{array}{cccccc}
\text{h} & \text{h} & \quad(\text{b}) & \text{h} & \text{h} & \quad(\text{c}) \quad \text{h} \quad \text{h} \\
| & | & & | & | & \quad\quad | \quad\ \ | \\
\text{V} \ \ \text{C} & \text{C} & > & \text{V} \ \ \text{C} & \text{C} & > \quad \text{V} \ \ \text{C} \ \ \text{C} \\
| \ \ | & | & & | & | & \quad\quad \diagdown \ \ | \\
\text{a} \ \ \text{t} & \text{t} & & \text{a} & \text{t} & \quad\quad \text{a} \quad\quad \text{t}
\end{array}
$$

The first of the *t* segments of Fig. 2.44(a) is deleted to give Fig. 2.44(b), but the C slot is preserved, and is filled by the spreading of the supralarygeal features of the vowel *a*, to give Fig. 2.44(c). The features of the laryngeal tier are unaffected. Since the nucleus tier can embrace both vowel and consonant slots, no structural adjustment is required as part of the compensation.

Again, however, there is a difficulty here. In the case of Icelandic preaspiration the *h* is arguably still consonantal, since it preserves the laryngeal feature of the original consonant, and it therefore appropriately occupies a C slot, but if we apply this approach to cases of *total* replacement of a consonant by a vowel, as discussed above, we will still find a vowel attached to a C slot, and a change of category (though not of structure) will be necessary. An alternative solution would be to adopt the X slot theory in preference to the CV theory, in which case the anomaly of having a vowel in a consonant slot is resolved: the slots themselves are not categorized as C or V. However, this does not really solve the problem; in most theories it still leaves the vowel attached to an X slot under the coda node (Co) instead of under the nucleus node (N), where it belongs. The non-hierarchical CV theory of Clements and Keyser is incompatible with the X theory, since the necessary structural information must be represented somewhere if phonological processes are to be adequately specified. The CV theory can only dispense with the hierarchical representation of syllable structure because the information is represented in the C and V classification; the X theory can only dispense with the C and V classification because the information is contained in the hierarchical tree. Clearly, we need one or the other.

2.7.4.3 Conclusion

The application of non-linear—and specifically Autosegmental—phonology to these processes of lengthening and shortening thus appears to offer a formal means of representing the role of syllable weight in determining such processes. In all these interpretations, it is assumed that the segmental processes—the lengthening and shortening of the vowels—follow either from changes at the level of syllable structure (as with Open Syllable Lengthening) or from the attempt to maintain the existing syllable weight following the loss of the consonant (as with compensatory lengthening). The claim is that a non-linear representation of syllable structure, where syllable weight is reflected in the configuration of the tree and is represented separately from the vowel and consonant features themselves, is able to account for these process automatically, in terms of general conditions on phonological representations.

Nevertheless, it is evident that there are also some difficulties here, particularly in cases of compensatory lengthening, since, in the majority of cases, the compensation involves the lengthening of a *vowel* in order to replace a *consonant*. The theory, as presented so far, is not quite able to accommodate this in a natural manner.

2.8 Length as a Prosodic Feature

2.8.1 INTRODUCTION

We have so far considered length in terms of progressively wider and more inclusive contexts. Implicit within some of these approaches is the view that length is not only to be seen *in relation to* its context, but that some, perhaps all, of the durational properties of individual segments should be *derived from* this context. Length, in other words, is primarily a property of more inclusive, or 'higher', units of speech, above all of the syllable, and is only secondarily to be attributed to individual sounds. Such an approach can be called 'prosodic', in the sense that length is regarded as distinct from the segments themselves.

The classical non-linear view described in 2.7 adopts this assumption in placing segments on a different 'tier' from the timing slots associated with particular structural positions. However, although this separates the segments from the structure, this structure is still described in terms of a linear sequence of slots. Length is therefore still a property of the slots, and therefore, in a sense, still linearly specified. We therefore need to consider more genuinely prosodic views which regard length as distinct from both the segments and the structural positions (timing slots).

2.8.2 'CHRONEMES'

The treatment of the length of segments separately from the segments themselves is not new; an approach of this kind is suggested by Jones (1944, 1967: ch. XXIII) and endorsed by Abercrombie (1964: 28–9). This approach consists in regarding 'long' and 'short' vowels as identical, and treating the length difference as a separate feature (a 'chroneme') which is independent of the vowels themselves. This solution relates to the quantity/quality problem considered in 2.4.4, since it provides a motivation for the 'quantitative' conception of vowel distinctions, with the additional principle that the differences of quantity are abstracted out.

Unlike the quantitative and qualitative approaches discussed in 2.4.4, therefore, this approach does not treat length paradigmatically but prosodically.

The idea here is that a pair of corresponding 'short' and 'long' phonemes can be regarded as the same phoneme in different conditions of length. Abercrombie (1964: 28) illustrates this as follows. Given, say, the words *bit* and *beat*, the vowels in each case would appear to be in the same environment, *b . . t*, and therefore in contrast with each other. However, according to Abercrombie 'the environments are in fact different from each other in one very important respect: the *b* and *t* are more widely separated from each other in the second word than in the first, and the vowel in the second word therefore has a bigger gap to fill' (p. 28). Thus the two environments are, in fact, *b . . t* and *b . . . t*, respectively. This means that the difference between the two vowels is ascribed to the context, and the vowels themselves can be interpreted as phonologically the same.

The difference in the environment is described by Jones (1967: ch. XXIII) in terms of 'chronemes'. If we regard any different duration as a 'chrone', then a set of non-distinctive chrones can be grouped together into a 'chroneme' in the same way that sounds can be grouped into phonemes. The different lengths of the vowels of *see*, *seed*, and *seat* thus constitute a single chroneme, as do the lengths of the vowels of *sin*, *sit*, and *sitting*, but the first group constitute a different chroneme from the second. These chronemes are, however, separated from the vowel itself, which is the same phoneme in all six words.

It may be helpful to compare this approach to the way in which tone is treated in tone-languages (see Ch. 4, below). In a language such as Mandarin Chinese we may distinguish words such as *bā*, *bá*, *bǎ*, *bà*, where the accent marks indicate the four different tones of this language. We would not normally say that there are four different *vowel* phonemes here, but rather that there is a single vowel appearing with four different tones. Jones is effectively using 'chroneme' in the same way (he uses the term 'toneme' for what has here been called 'tone'): in *sit* and *seat* we have the same vowel appearing with two different chronemes.

A problem here, however, is the lack of formal explicitness; neither Jones nor Abercrombie makes clear *how* or *where* the different chronemes are to be accommodated, nor whether they are to be associated with the vowel position in the syllable or with the syllable as a whole. As a result, although this theory is suggestive of an interesting approach to the problem of length, it remains unsatisfactory, or at least incomplete.[62]

---

[62] A similar approach is adopted by Trager (1940) in relation to Serbo–Croat, who concludes that, although there is distinctive vowel length in this language, short and long vowels should not be treated as separate phonemes. Instead, length should be considered separately. 'The proper statement is that there are a number of vowel phonemes, each of which may be accompanied by either short quantity or long quantity, these being prosodic phonemes.' Another approach, which likewise regards prosodic features such as length as separate from segmental phonemes, is that of Haugen (1949), who labels such features 'prosodemes'. Again, however, no formal apparatus is provided which would allow us to incorporate such prosodemes satisfactorily.

2.8.3 THE MORA (2)

The mora was introduced in 2.5.4 within a structuralist framework as a measure of syllable length: 'short' syllables consist of one mora, and 'long' syllables of two. As we saw, there is some ambivalence about its nature and role, since it can be construed either as a *constituent* of the syllable or as a *measure* of its length. Further, it can be regarded simply as a function of the number of segments in the syllable or as an independent feature of the syllable.

The mora was rarely invoked in early generative discussions, with the exception of some descriptions of languages such as Japanese where it has traditionally been considered appropriate (e.g. McCawley, 1968), though with no formal means of incorporating it into the theoretical framework. The concept has been revived in more recent non-linear approaches, however, in which the necessary formal means are available. Prince (1980), for example, resumes the discussion of length in Estonian (see above, 2.5.3.4) within a metrical framework, and is able to restate the problems in terms of moras. He starts from the rather inexplicit standard view of the mora ('a mora, James McCawley has somewhere written,[63] is *one* of what heavy syllables have *two* of' (pp. 525–6)), and observes that moras cannot simply be equated with segments or segmental positions. We cannot simply say that 'long' syllables have more moras because they have more segments, since hypercharacterized syllables, with either VVC or VCC rhymes, are still only bimoraic, and not trimoraic. However, if we adopt the hierarchical view of syllable structure typical of metrical phonology, with binary-branching, then the mora can be incorporated into the tree at a higher level than the individual segment, and defined as an 'immediate constituent of the rime'. For example, a syllable with the segments CCVVC can be represented as in Fig. 2.45. Additional coda consonants will be accommodated *under* the second mora, and will therefore not increase the mora count.

Fig. 2.45

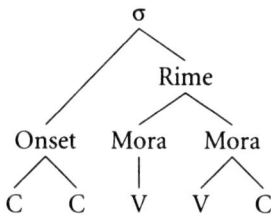

Clements and Keyser (1983: 79–80) adopt a similar approach, but they define the mora in a slightly different way. As we have seen (2.7.4.2), the 'nucleus display' in their theory consists of the vowel and a following vowel or consonant belonging to the same syllable. Given this approach, they are able to define the mora as 'any element of the CV tier dominated by the node "Nucleus" in the Nucleus display'. In the case of *stout* (cf. Fig. 2.43), with the structure CC[VC]C

[63] The reference sought by Prince is, in fact, to McCawley (1968).

(the nucleus is enclosed in brackets), there are two such elements, *a* and *w*, and hence the syllable is bimoraic. It will be evident that, since the nucleus excludes not only the onset but also any further coda consonants, 'heavy' syllables, whether their weight is the result of a 'long' vowel or of a following consonant, will always have two (and no more than two) moras, as will hypercharacterized syllables.

A further illustration of this approach is found in the treatment of the Danish *stød* (cf. above, 2.5.2). The glottal constriction of the *stød* may occur in stressed syllables either on the second part of a long vowel, as in [hu:ˀs] ('house'), or, if the vowel is short, on the following consonant, as in [manˀ] ('man'). Clements and Keyser (1983: 84) assume, as in the case of Icelandic, a laryngeal tier for the *stød*; given the representation of Fig. 2.46(a), the glottalization is automatically associated with the *second mora*, as in Fig. 2.46(b), accounting for both of these cases (note that both a long vowel and a short vowel followed by a consonant are represented as VC).

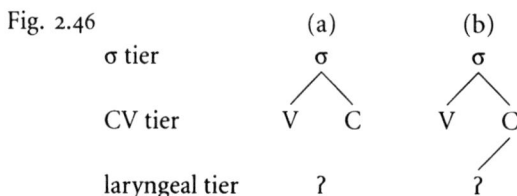

Fig. 2.46   (a)   (b)

σ tier   σ   σ

CV tier   V   C   V   C

laryngeal tier   ʔ   ʔ

The purpose of all this is to demonstrate that the mora is not to be equated with timing slots *as such*; only certain kinds of slots contribute to the mora count. Nevertheless, it will be clear that the mora is still considered segmentally, in the sense that it is defined in terms of the presence of segments in certain structural positions. A truly *prosodic* view of length is only possible if it is treated as completely separate from the segmental positions.

2.8.4 THE 'WEIGHT TIER' AND MORAIC PHONOLOGY

In our discussion so far, the mora has generally appeared in a rather informal guise, the only formal representation of it being in the work of Prince (1980), who includes moras as constituents of the rhyme, dominating nucleus and coda slots. A number of scholars have followed Prince's lead in explicitly including moras, or their equivalent, in phonological representations, though in a number of different ways. While Prince adopts a metrical view, and regards the mora as part of the metrical structure of the syllable, other scholars have incorporated the mora into Autosegmental representations.

Hyman (1985) argues for the replacement of the CV tier with a *weight tier* on which the syllable weight is represented directly, rather than being derived from the syllable structure. The CV tier itself, according to Hyman, is incorporated to provide information of three kinds:

(a) to provide the value of syllabicity, since C = [–syll] and V = [+syll]
(b) to provide a measure of the number of units
(c) to provide a core through which Autosegmental and prosodic tiers connect.

Hyman suggests that the CV tier can be dispensed with, and the information provided in different ways. We have already noted that an alternative to C and V slots is the X slot theory, in which syllabicity is derived from the branching structure itself, and the X is simply interpreted as [+segment]. Hyman proposes interpreting the X differently: not as [+segment] but as a *weight unit*, where each such unit represents a potential 'beat'. Since these units are (in terms of the original Autosegmental theory) also 'tone-bearing units', they can also be interpreted as potential moras.

The word 'potential' is important here, since clearly not every segment corresponds to a mora. At the very least, onset consonants must be eliminated as weight units, since they do not contribute to syllable weight. Hyman therefore introduces an Onset Creation Rule which deletes the weight of a [+cons] segment followed by a [–cons] segment (i.e. an onset consonant followed by a vowel), and attaches it to the latter to form a single weight unit. This will have the effect of producing structures such as those given in Fig. 2.47.

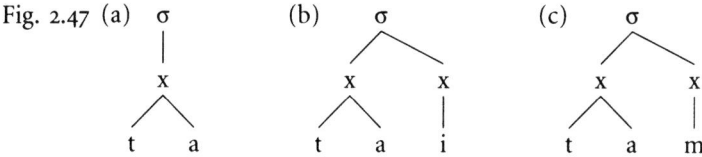

Fig. 2.47 (a) σ   (b) σ   (c) σ

In all these examples each segment is initially associated with a weight unit (x) on the weight tier, but the onset consonant loses its weight and is attached to the x of the following vowel. The result is a single unit for a light syllable (Fig. 2.47(a)), but two units for a heavy syllable (Figs. 2.47(b) and 2.47(c)). Since languages differ in what they consider to be a light syllable, some language-specific principles must be provided; a CVC syllable with a final non-sonorant consonant might, for example, constitute only a single weight unit, as in Fig. 2.48. Here a further rule (the Margin Creation Rule), attaching a coda consonant to the preceding vowel, is required.

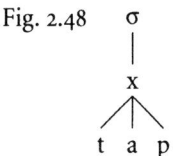

Fig. 2.48   σ

It will be evident that the 'weight unit' postulated here is, in fact, equivalent to the mora, and is explicitly identified with it, and although it is still ultimately linked to the occurrence of specific segments it disregards syllable structure as such. In fact, Hyman's approach is clearly incompatible with branching metrical structure within the syllable. This naturally provides a rather drastic solution to the problems discussed above in relation to lengthening processes and compensatory lengthening, where the structure of a heavy syllable with a long vowel is different from that of a heavy syllable with a coda consonant. If no such structures are postulated, then no such problems arise.

This theoretical approach to syllable weight has been explored under the heading of *Moraic Phonology*. Following on from work by Hock (1986), and McCarthy and Prince (1986), Hayes (1989) develops a theory in which the mora has a still more prominent place. Instead of X slots the mora is represented directly (as μ), so that light and heavy syllables take the form of Fig. 2.49. Note that onset consonants are here attached directly to the syllable node rather than grouped with the first mora, though coda consonants are grouped under the final mora. The latter case involves language specific rules for 'weight by position', whereby closed syllables may become heavy by the addition of an extra mora.

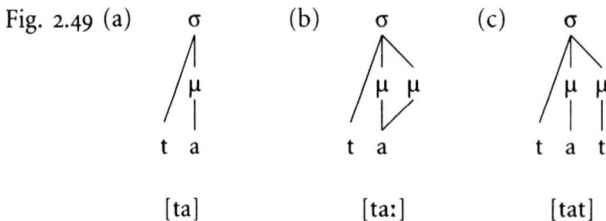

Fig. 2.49 (a)   σ   (b)   σ   (c)   σ

[ta]   [taː]   [tat]

To illustrate these points, we may consider the derivations given in Fig. 2.50. The underlying forms (Fig. 2.50(i)) give representations of the mora-count for each of these forms—two in the case of [ata] and [apta], three for the other two—and the vowels, together with their onset consonants, are assigned to syllables as in Fig. 2.50(ii) and Fig. 2.50(iii). In languages where a coda consonant contributes to the weight of the syllable, a new mora is created, to which the consonant is assigned, as in Fig. 2.50(iv), and the remaining links are assigned as in Fig. 2.50(v). It will be noted that in the case of [aːpta] the coda consonant does not contribute to the weight of the syllable (which is hypercharacterized), and hence does not receive an additional mora. The peculiar treatment of the geminate consonant of [atta] reflects an assumption that such consonants are moraic (hence they have an underlying mora in Fig. 2.50(i), and are doubly linked, as an onset of the following syllable (hence linked in Fig. 2.50(iii)) and a coda of the preceding one (hence ultimately linked in Fig. 2.50(v)).

Fig. 2.50   [ata]   [apta]   [aːpta]   [atta]

(i) underlying forms:

(ii) σ-assignment:

(iii) adjunction:
prevocalic
consonants:

(iv) adjunction:
weight by
position:

(v) adjunction:
remaining
segments:

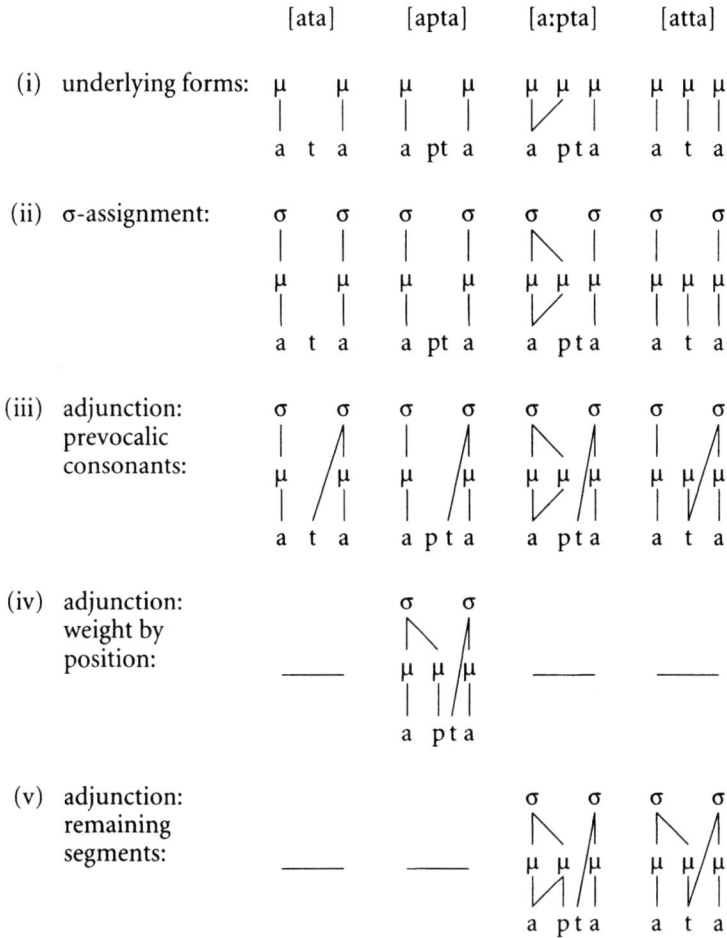

This elaborate procedure is intended to demonstrate that it is possible to derive structures of this kind from underlying forms which include a direct representation of moras. Vowel and consonant segments are associated with moras according to general principles (with a language specific principle in the case of 'weight by position'). Onset consonants are independent of the moras; coda consonants are not. According to Hayes (1989: 260), 'the representations that result appear to be adequate for the two tasks that moraic theory must carry out: representation of segment length and of syllable weight'. Segment length is here specified by the association of segments to moras: 'long' segments are associated to two moras; syllable weight is specified by the association of moras to syllables: 'heavy' syllables are likewise linked to two moras.

The direct representation of moras (rather than C and V or X slots) is claimed to offer advantages in the specification of processes such as compensatory lengthening (cf. 2.7.4.2, above). This process has been extensively discussed,[64] and since a commonly accepted motive is the preservation of length, the mora has been invoked here as an explanatory factor: compensatory lengthening is assumed to work by maintaining the mora count (Hayes, 1989; Bickmore, 1995b).

Consider once again the case of Latin *sisdo: > si:do: ('sit') discussed in 2.7.4.2 (Ingria, 1980). One of the difficulties encountered in metrical and Autosegmental treatments was shown to be the fact that the loss of a *consonant* is compensated for by the addition of a *vowel* slot, so that although the number of slots is preserved, the structure is affected. Alternatively, the vowel must be associated with a C slot or placed under the coda node. Expressing this process in terms of moraic theory, however, no such anomalies arise. Fig. 2.51(a) shows the original state of affairs; loss of the consonant (Fig. 2.51(b)) is followed by re-attachment of the vowel to the stranded mora (Fig. 2.51(c)).

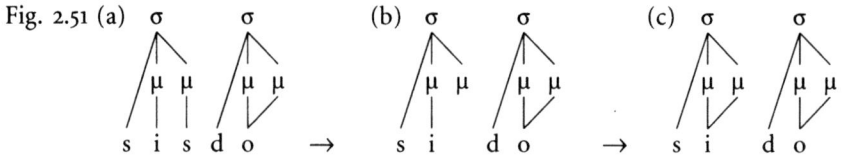

Fig. 2.51 (a) σ   σ   (b) σ   σ   (c) σ   σ

A somewhat different case, but leading to the same kind of result, is that of the 'Double Flop', in which compensatory lengthening is preceded by resyllabification. For example, the development of Greek *odwos to o:dos (Steriade, 1982; Wetzels, 1986; Hayes, 1989) can be accounted for by the processes given in Fig. 2.52. This interpretation assumes loss of the post-consonantal [w], resyllabification by the association of the [d] to the following syllable, and the lengthening of the first vowel by association to the vacated mora (Hayes, 1989: 266).

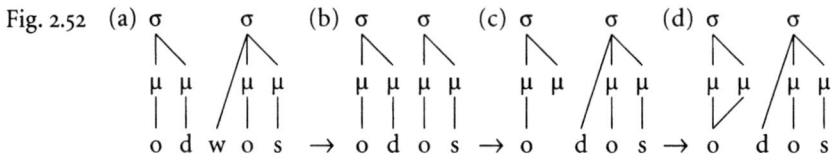

Fig. 2.52 (a) σ   σ   (b) σ   σ   (c) σ   σ   (d) σ   σ

Consider, however, the change from Proto-West-Germanic *finf to Old English *fīf*, which was presented in Fig. 2.41 in a metrical framework, using C and V slots. The loss of the nasal consonant is here compensated for by the lengthening of the vowel, the motive apparently being the preservation of the

---

[64] See, for example, Grundt, 1976; De Chene and Anderson, 1979; Ingria, 1980; Clements and Keyser, 1983; Lass, 1984; Wetzels and Sezer (eds.), 1986; Hock, 1986; Hayes, 1989; Bickmore, 1995b, among others.

timing slot. In the moraic framework there are no CV slots, so that this motive is unavailable, and we must assume that it is *moras* that are to be preserved. But in a normal interpretation of this case, where light syllables have one mora and heavy syllables have two, the mora count is unaffected by the consonant loss; both **finf* and **fif* (the latter resulting from the loss of the nasal) are heavy and therefore bimoraic, and there is no motivation for vowel lengthening to preserve the mora count. The solution, suggested by Hayes (1989), is to regard words such as **finf* as *trimoraic*, as in Fig. 2.53. As before, the loss of the nasal (Fig. 2.53(a)) leaves a stranded mora (Fig. 2.53(b)) to which the preceding vowel is attached (Fig. 2.53(c)), giving a long vowel. Since there is otherwise no reason to assume that syllables with final consonant clusters were 'overlong', it might well be asked whether this is not merely equivalent to the reintroduction of a C slot or X slot.

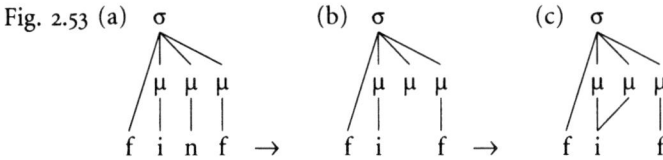

Fig. 2.53 (a) σ   (b) σ   (c) σ

μ μ μ   μ μ μ   μ μ μ

f i n f →   f i   f →   f i   f

2.9 Length and Prosodic Structure

2.9.1 INTRODUCTION: SYLLABLE QUANTITY

We have now discussed length in the broader context of the syllable as a whole, either as a reflection of syllable structure or as an independent feature of the syllable, represented by the mora. We cannot stop here, however; the next stage is to consider the length of the syllable itself. We cannot assume that the latter is fixed and constant; on the contrary, it is often quite variable. It will be recalled (2.2.2) that early phoneticians, such as Jespersen, drew attention to the different lengths of syllables, for example in words such as *gloom*, *gloomy*, and *gloomily*, where each word takes approximately the same amount of time to pronounce, and as a consequence the initial syllable becomes progressively shorter. We must therefore consider the various factors that determine syllable length.

We have already encountered one such factor: syllable *weight*. Weight is, as we have noted, primarily a matter of structure: a closed syllable, or an open syllable containing a long vowel, is regarded in many languages as *heavy*; an open syllable with a short vowel is *light*. But the additional vowel length or more complex structure may often entail greater length for the syllable as a whole; a heavy syllable is therefore likely to be *long*, and a light syllable *short*. For this reason, too, heavy syllables are equivalent to more than one light syllable, for example in classical quantitative verse, but also more generally, for example in accentuation rules such as the rule for Latin discussed in 2.2.1. This difference of length is captured by assigning a single mora to a light syllable and more than one to a heavy syllable. However, syllable length is not necessarily to be equated with weight,[65] first because in some cases heavy syllables are not long (cf. 2.6.2), and, second, because other factors are involved in determining the length of syllables.

One of these factors is *accent* (stress).[66] The relationship between segment length and accent has been noted at several points in the discussion in this chapter; Prague School theory generalized the notion of 'extendibility' with that of stress, under a single heading of 'intensity', with the further proviso that stress and length cannot both have independent functions within the same system. Further links between the two are found in cases where length distinctions are restricted to accented syllables; it is in such languages that, according to Jakobson (1937), the 'contact' feature is relevant. We have also observed (2.6.3) that, in the historical development of length systems in a number of European languages, such principles as the 'equalization of length' are confined to accented syllables. These cases suggest that the relationship between segment length and accent is more than just the interaction of two independent features; it is a rather more intimate interdependence. Furthermore, accent is not merely relevant for the length of segments; since it is a property of syllables, it is closely bound up with syllable quantity, too. However, though it is clear that syllable quantity and accent are, in many languages, closely related, the nature of this relationship is a matter of some dispute. One key to this relationship, mediating between them, is *rhythm*.

2.9.2 RHYTHM

Rhythm[67] is a fundamental component of much human activity, including speech. There is, however, considerable disagreement about its linguistic role, and it is rarely taken into account in a formal way in phonological theory and description. Rhythm is a matter of timing, but it is more than this; it involves *regularity*, such that there is a pattern of recurrence of some particular event. In speech, this 'event' may be identified with some particular salient point in utterances, especially accent, but it may also be interpreted as coinciding with the

---

[65] It will be recalled that the terminological separation of segment length and syllable weight was found in the writings of the Sanskrit grammarians, whereas grammarians of Greece and Rome made no such distinction.

[66] The relationship between 'accent' and 'stress', and their phonological nature, will be considered in Ch. 3. In the present context the two terms will be used interchangeably.

[67] On rhythm in general, see, for example, Fraisse (1956, 1963). Discussions of rhythm in a linguistic context include those of Pike (1945: 34 ff., 1947: 13), Shen and Peterson (1962), Abercrombie, (1967: 96–8), Uldall (1971), W. S. Allen (1973), G. D. Allen (1975), Catford (1977: 85–8), Lehiste (1977), Roach (1982), Wenk and Wioland (1982), Buxton (1983), Dauer (1983), Jassem, Hill and Witten (1984), Scott et al. (1985), Levelt (1989: 392–8), Beckmann (1992), Laver (1994: 523–33), and others.

beginning of a speech unit, such as a syllable. There is thus a certain ambivalence as to what is recurrent in speech rhythm, *events* or *units*, though the two may perhaps be regarded as interchangeable if units are defined in terms of events or vice versa: the occurrence of accent defines a 'stress unit', while a syllable is defined by its 'onset'. The 'stress unit' (or *foot*) and the syllable are the two main candidates for the unit of rhythm in different languages, with the potential addition of the *mora* as a third possibility. In each case it is assumed that the unit in question is a *measure of timing*, and successive units are, in these terms, approximately the same length. Thus, languages may have a different rhythmical organization, according to the unit that is used, but governed by the same rhythmical principle.

A basic typology of languages on this basis is put forward by Pike (1945: 35), who categorizes languages into *stress-timed* (for example, English) and *syllable-timed* (for example, French), according to whether it is stresses or syllables that occur at equal intervals of time. Abercrombie (1967: 96–8) endorses this categorization, claiming that 'as far as is known, every language in the world is spoken with one kind of rhythm or with the other' (p. 97). Examples of 'stress-timed' languages given by Abercrombie include English, Russian and Arabic; examples of 'syllable-timed' languages include French, Telegu, and Yoruba. However, another category, *mora-timed* languages, has also been recognized, though in practice the only language which has been consistently assigned to this category is Japanese.

The rhythmical principles involved in this categorization are clearly of considerable importance for the understanding of length, since they determine the timing, and therefore the relative lengths, of parts of the utterance. However, there is much controversy here, particularly with regard to 'stress-timing', and we must therefore examine some of these questions in more detail.

2.9.3 TIMING

2.9.3.1 Stress-timing and Isochrony

The basis of 'stress-timing' is that, in languages which have it, stressed syllables occur at approximately equal intervals of time. This is the principle of *isochrony* (or *isochronicity*).[68] In English, for example, the theory claims that the utterance 'four large black dogs',[69] in which every syllable would normally be stressed, is spaced out so that each of these syllables is of approximately equal length, as in Fig. 2.54(a) (the vertical lines are intended to indicate equal intervals of time). The same is true for utterances where each word contains more than one sylla-

---

[68] The term could in principle be applied equally to other forms of timing, but it is generally only discussed in relation to stress-timing.
[69] The example is taken from Abercrombie (1964: 217).

ble, only one of which is stressed, for example 'seventy terrible menacing elephants', in Fig. 2.54(b). Thus far the equal spacing could be attributed to the equal number of syllables in the words of each utterance, but the principle of isochrony is illustrated when we combine words with different numbers of syllables, as in 'seventy large menacing dogs' (Fig. 2.54(c)) or 'four terrible black elephants' (Fig. 2.54(d)). The speaker has the impression that the words are still of equal length, and that the stressed syllables are still evenly spaced, despite the different numbers of unstressed syllables between them. That this is not a matter of equal length *words*, however, is clear from utterances such as 'four unfortunate deceased dogs', given in Fig. 2.54(e), or 'seventy unsuccessful old administrators', given in Fig. 2.54(f), where it is the stressed syllables that are felt to be aligned with the regular rhythmical 'beat', regardless of which word they occur in.

Fig. 2.54	(a)		four			large		black		dogs	
	(b)		seventy			terrible		menacing		elephants	
	(c)		seventy			large		menacing		dogs	
	(d)		four			terrible		black		elephants	
	(e)		four	un-	fortunate	de-	ceased		dogs	
	(f)		seventy	unsuc-	cessful		old	ad-	ministrators	

In these terms, the occurrence of the stressed syllable could be regarded as defining a stress unit, the *foot*; each foot having a single stress. Furthermore, it is clear from Fig. 2.54 that the foot is seen as *beginning* with the stressed syllable. This is the normal assumption, though some scholars assume *final* stress within the foot.[70] Either of these will ensure that feet are of equal length; to allow the stressed syllable to occur elsewhere in the foot would forfeit this equality.

There have been numerous experimental studies designed to test the phonetic reality of isochrony.[71] Almost without exception, their results fail to confirm the principle; the time intervals between successive stressed syllables in languages for which a 'stress-timed' rhythm is assumed are found to be very variable. As a result, some linguists have felt it necessary to abandon the concept of isochrony, at least in its strong form. Levelt (1989: 392) asserts that 'stress-timing would imply that feet tend to be equally long. This notion of the foot as a prosodically relevant entity has been largely abandoned in linguistics, and I see no role for it in a theory of language production either.' Others (Dauer, 1983; Laver, 1994: 527–32) have taken the view that, although there may be some perceptual basis

---

[70] A distinction has been made between 'leader-timing' and 'trailer-timing', the former having units commencing with an accent, the latter having an accent at the end of the unit (Wenk and Wioland, 1982). This might be related to the traditional distinction in verse metrics between feet with a *trochaic* rhythm (´ ∪) and those with an *iambic* rhythm (∪ ´), where ´ indicates the stressed 'ictus' and ∪ the unstressed 'remiss'). The assumption of 'leader-timing' in speech implies that all (two-syllable) feet are trochaic.

[71] E.g. Lehiste (1977), Cutler (1980), Cutler and Isard (1980), Nakatani, O'Connor and Aston (1981), Dauer (1983), Jassem, Hill and Witten (1984), Cooper and Eady (1986), Kelly and Bock (1988), Levelt (1989: 392–8).

for rhythm, this perception may be the result of other features of utterances, including syllable structure, vowel quality, and syllable weight. On this view, the apparent difference between 'stress-timing' and 'syllable-timing' is the result of a combination of such factors, rather than of timing itself; the latter is at best subordinate, and probably irrelevant.

Another approach which ascribes the spacing of syllables to other factors is that of Bolinger (1981) and Dasher and Bolinger (1982). Like Levelt, they reject the principle of isochronous feet, but they seek to explain the more or less equal spacing of stresses by other principles. In comparing the utterances 'Money makes the mare to go' and 'Money makes the mare go', they note that 'mare' is longer in the second utterance than in the first. Instead, however, of attributing this to isochronous stressed syllables, and the need to accommodate different numbers of syllables between them, they advance the hypothesis that 'a syllable containing a full vowel will be longer when followed (in the same phrase or breath group) by another syllable containing a full vowel than when followed by a syllable containing a reduced vowel' (Dasher and Bolinger, 1982: 58–9). Hence 'mare' is longer in the second utterance, where it is followed by 'go', with a full vowel, than in the first, where it is followed by 'to', with a reduced vowel.

This approach effectively reverses cause and effect. While the majority of scholars have seen the shortening and reduction of vowels in unstressed syllables as the result of rhythmical factors and the lack of stress, Dasher and Bolinger (1982: 60) claim that the converse is true: stress and rhythm are the result of the presence of a reduced vowel, since 'vowel quality is a given and not a product of stressing rules or rhythm rules, and can be used to predict the possibility of accentuation' (Dasher and Bolinger, 1982: 60). This view naturally denies rhythm, and the principle of isochronous feet, a primary role in the determination of timing.

In spite of these alternatives, the concept of isochrony has persisted, even among those whose experimental results appear to contradict it (e.g. Dauer, 1983), and instead of abandoning the notion, many scholars have sought to find alternative formulations, or alternative explanations, of the principle. As Laver (1994: 524) puts it, 'the concept of an approximately isochronous rhythm in speech has been so tenacious in the history of phonology and phonetics that it seems unlikely that it is completely without foundation'. Thus, though completely rejecting the *phonetic* basis of isochrony, Levelt (1989: 392) accepts the foot as a legitimate *phonological* entity. Another approach is to regard isochrony as *subjective* rather than *objective* (Laver, 1994: 523–4). In this way, it is possible to reconcile the intuitive feel for regular rhythm in speech with the difficulty of detecting it experimentally.

The view taken here is that much of the temporal structure of English (and other comparable languages) is only explicable in terms of some form of isochrony, since the lengths of syllables must be determined at least in part in relation to the regular occurrence of stress. Thus, for example, the shortening of syllables in polysyllabic words (cf. Jespersen's examples), the occurrence of so-called 'silent stress' (cf. Abercrombie, 1971), and a variety of intonational phenomena, seem to require the existence of a prosodic unit defined in relation to the regular occurrence of an accentual 'beat'.

Bearing in mind the negative results obtained in experimental studies, however, it is necessary to interpret the principle of isochrony in an appropriate way, and to understand its nature. Many assumptions are made about isochrony which are clearly both unrealistic and untenable. The 'strong' form of the principle implies that stresses occur at measurably equal intervals of time throughout an utterance, but this is a priori very unlikely, as we would not demand such a degree of phonetic precision from any other feature of speech production. But in fact there is in any case no reason to require it, as rhythm is not defined by strict temporal regularity. A useful analogy is with musical rhythm: any musician knows that a natural rendering of most pieces of music, even fairly rhythmical ones, will require considerable deviation from the regularity of a metronome. Rubato, lengthening some notes at the expense of others, is fundamental to musical performance, as are adjustments of speed in response to musical phrasing. Speech, which shares with music some features of structure but lacks most of the constraints on its form, allows much more freedom of this kind. Significantly, however, this does not mean that either music or speech have no regularity of rhythm, since *rhythm is not a matter of absolute temporal equality*.

Consider, for example, the illustrations of Fig. 2.54. Even if we go out of our way to pronounce these as rhythmically as possible, there will inevitably be variations, many of them perceptible, in the lengths of the rhythmical feet, largely because there are different numbers of unstressed syllables to accommodate between the stressed ones. In the case of sentence (f), for example, absolute regularity demands that we fit the five syllables of the first foot into the same time as the two syllables of the second and third. A moment's self-observation shows that we do not do this: the foot with five syllables is noticeably longer that the ones with two (though not in the ratio of five to two); we apparently attempt to keep the feet more or less equal, but nevertheless adjust their lengths in order to accommodate all the syllables in a natural manner. This, of course, suggests that there is no regularity of rhythm, but this is not so. We still *feel* that we are maintaining a regular rhythm even though we can hear that the stresses are not equally spaced. In other words, rhythmical regularity, though having a close relationship to equal spacing of stresses, does not require it, and considerable latitude is allowed without destroying the sense of rhythm. The same is true, though not to the same extent, in music: it is possible to deviate from metronomic regularity without abandoning the rhythm; indeed, *not* to do so is often a sign of an unmusical performance.

What, then, is the role and status of isochrony? In one respect we could argue that it is merely subjective, since it is not borne out by 'objective' measurements. But this subjectivity should not be construed in a negative sense, as the speaker's *mistaken* impression of regularity; most phonological constructs—from the 'phoneme' onwards—are subjective in this sense, and we could therefore regard the failure to detect phonetic isochrony as equivalent to the failure to find consistent phonetic characteristics of a phoneme, an enterprise that has long been abandoned as it rests on a category mistake. Isochrony can therefore legitimately be seen as a *phonological* principle, in the sense on the one hand that it is mentally real for the speaker and on the other hand that it is a significant organizing principle of prosodic structure.

There are other methodological difficulties, too, which obscure the issues here. We might assume that isochrony is maintained throughout utterances, but there is considerable evidence that it is confined to relatively short stretches of speech, such as the 'intonational phrase', or 'tone-group' (see below, Ch. 5). The 'ideal' foot length appears to be reset for each such phrase. Averaging the lengths of feet over sentences or longer utterances is therefore likely to produce meaningless results. Furthermore, it is by no means clear where we should measure from; we could measure from the *onset* of the stressed syllable, from its *peak*, or from some perceptually significant point, such as the *P-centre* of Morton, Marcus and Frankish (1976) (cf. Buxton, 1983), the point at which speakers perceive the 'beat' to occur. Measuring from these different points will produce significantly different results. However, as we have noted, it is not necessary to 'prove' the phonetic existence of isochrony in order to accept it as a valid phonological concept.

2.9.3.2 Other Factors Affecting Foot Length

A tendency to isochrony is evidently only one of the factors determining the spacing of stresses and hence the length of feet. Other factors include the number of syllables to be accommodated between the stresses, and the place of the foot in a higher phonological unit. The former case, which was considered above (Fig. 2.54), illustrates a countervailing principle to that of isochrony: that each syllable tends to be given the same space. In the case of 'syllable-timed' languages (see 2.9.3 below) this is considered to be the basic principle of timing, but it appears to play some role in 'stress-timed' languages, too. However, the available experimental evidence (Levelt, 1989: 389 ff.) suggests that the ultimate spacing of stressed syllables represents a kind of compromise between these two principles, since although the length of a foot increases with the number of syllables, it does not increase proportionately, and the syllables within the foot are compressed in an attempt to maintain isochrony. An alternative strategy, noted by Levelt (1989: 392), is for speakers to 'shift accents to create a more even distribution of stressed syllables', rather than to 'stretch or compress syllable durations, depending on the number of syllables in a foot'.[72]

For some scholars, these results are interpreted differently: as evidence of the

---

[72] An example of this is to be found in so-called 'stress-clash' or 'iambic reversal', to be discussed in 3.5.3, below.

role of the *word* as a unit of rhythm. Lehiste (1970: 40 ff.) suggests that in some languages there is tendency for words to be of equal length, regardless of the number of syllables, though other experimenters provide evidence to the contrary.[73] Another domain of quantity put forward by Lehiste (1970: 42 ff.) is the disyllabic sequence, which she claims is relevant for Slovak and for Estonian; this is endorsed by Grundt (1976), who argues that a variety of developments in the Germanic languages were brought about by changes in vowel duration ratios in disyllabic words. Again the evidence is inconclusive.

Another factor which may contribute to determining the length of the foot, again modifying the basic isochrony of stresses, is its place in a still larger unit of speech. We have already noted that the intonation unit (the 'tone-group' of the British tradition) appears to constitute the domain of isochrony, but a number of deviations have been noted depending on where in the intonation unit the foot is located. One of these is the so-called 'final lengthening', according to which the final foot of an intonation unit is lengthened (cf. Beckmann and Edwards, 1990; Fowler, 1990; Cutler, 1990). Again, this has been interpreted in syntactic terms by some (e.g. Klatt, 1975), as the lengthening in *sentence*-final position, though a sentence-final foot will, of course, also be intonation-unit final.[74]

These various factors will inevitably affect the extent to which isochrony is measurable in speech, but, as noted above, they do not affect isochrony itself, seen as a phonological principle. Rather they are factors which determine the way in which isochrony is realized phonetically.

2.9.3.3 Syllable Quantity in Stress-timed Languages

According to the view adopted here, the length of syllables within the foot is dependent on the length of the foot as a whole, but also on *internal* factors which operate within the foot itself. Two major factors involved here are the nature of the syllable—specifically its weight—and syntactic factors which determine word groupings within the foot.

As far as the former is concerned, we have already observed (2.9.1) that syllable weight is a major factor in determining syllable quantity: heavy syllables are usually (though not necessarily) longer than light ones. However, this gives us a principle for relative length of different kinds of syllables, but does not determine the apportionment of length within the foot overall. This is in part because the heavy/light distinction, in a language which has stress, appears to be generally confined to stressed syllables. What, then, determines the quantity of unstressed syllables?

An attempt to provide an answer to this question is made by Abercrombie (1964), who asserts that 'there *are* consistent relations of quantity to be found

---

[73] Cf. Nakatani, O'Connor and Aston (1981), Levelt (1989: 387 ff.).

[74] Other discussions of the relationship between length and syntax include Kisseberth and Abasheikh (1974); Klatt (1976); Lehiste, Olive, and Streeter (1976).

between English syllables, and that these relations are quite important in the phonetics and phonology of English' (p. 216). He regards English disyllabic feet as being basically in triple time, though 'this is probably no more than a convenience, largely of notation' (p. 217), and recognizes three types of such feet, according to the quantity relations between their syllables. Type A feet have a short syllable followed by a long syllable; examples are the words |*shilling*|, |*never*|, |*atom*|, |*cuckoo*| (where '|' represents the foot boundary). Type B feet contain two syllables of equal length, as in |*greater*|, |*firmly*|, de|*cisive*|, |*matches*|. The final type, Type C, has a long syllable followed by a short syllable, as in |*tea for*| two, per|*haps I*|did. In addition to musical notation, Abercrombie devises a notation in traditional metrical terms, where ∪ = short, ∩ = medium, and — = long. The three types can then be represented as in Fig. 2.55.

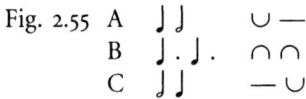

Fig. 2.55   A   ♩♩   ∪ —
             B   ♩.♩.   ∩ ∩
             C   ♩♩   — ∪

For the feet of types A and B, Abercrombie gives an explanation based on syllable weight. The first syllable in a type A foot (as the first syllable of the foot it is, of course, accented) is light; the first syllable of a type B foot is heavy. This evidently produces the different lengths of the first syllable, and the second, unaccented, syllable fills the remainder of the foot, regardless of its structure. In order to predict type C we must invoke factors of a morphosyntactic kind. In a disyllabic foot of this type, the two syllables are separated by a word-boundary. This provides an explanation of the difference noted by Scott (1940) between utterances such as *Take Grey to London* and *Take Greater London*. Under Abercrombie's analysis the difference is between | — ∪ | and | ∩ ∩ | for the sequence [greitə], with a word division in the former but none in the latter.

Abercrombie's principles can, as he points out, be extended to feet with more than two syllables, and he gives the examples of Fig. 2.56 of trisyllabic feet, where the different syllable weights of the stressed syllable and the different locations of word boundaries give a different apportionment of syllable quantity in each case (Abercrombie, 1964: 220). Abercrombie also observes that not all cases where there is a word division behave like type C; in a number of constructions the word division is ignored, and the words joined together as a single unit, so that the foot is treated like type A or type B, according to the weight of the first syllable. Words which are attached to the preceding word in this way are called *enclitics*. Examples include object pronouns, as in |*stop her*|

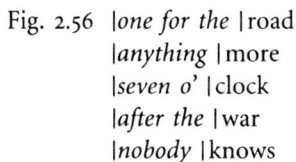

Fig. 2.56 |*one for the* |road
             |*anything* |more
             |*seven o'* |clock
             |*after the* |war
             |*nobody* |knows

(Type A) or |*take it*| (Type B), and some occurrences of prepositions (|*piece of*|).

The fact that word-division plays a part here allows us to reconcile, to some extent, the views of those who treat quantity as purely a matter of phonology and those who see a role for grammatical categories such as the word. In the interpretation given by Abercrombie, the foot is determined phonologically, but the apportionment of length within the foot depends partly on phonological characteristics of the syllables (weight) and partly on the word divisions.

The principles given by Abercrombie are not, of course, intended to be universal, but cover only certain accents of English, and he concedes that the principles operating in other languages—and other varieties of English pronunciation—may be different. In German, for example, the equivalent conditions for type A feet give a quantity distribution similar to the English type B (| ∩ ∩ |), for example in |*Mutter*| ('mother'), which has equal length syllables, while the conditions for type B give a distribution like the English type C (| — ∪ |), as in |*Vater*|, ('father'). A word division within a disyllabic foot gives a still longer initial syllable which has no equivalent in English, as in |*gut zu*| wissen ('good to know'). This last case could be thought of as being in quadruple rather than triple time, where the time pattern is | ♩ . ♩ | or | ♩ . ♪ |.

2.9.3.4 Syllable-timing

According to Pike's typology, in syllable-timed languages it is syllables rather than stresses that are considered to occur at equal intervals of time. In French, for example, the syllables of a phrase such as *Est-ce que'elle est ici?* ([es-kɛl-ɛt-i-si]) or *Je ne voulais pas vous le dire* ([ʒən-vu-lɛ-pɑ-vul-dir]) are claimed to occupy approximately the same time.[75] In Spanish, too, a sentence such as *Juan no sabe lo que dijo Pepe* is said to contain a sequence of ten equally spaced syllables.[76] Some syllables are stressed (*Juan, no, sa-, di-, Pe-* in this sentence), but the equal spacing of syllables means that the stresses cannot be isochronous. Since French has no word-stress as such,[77] stress-timing is in any case excluded for this language.

Experimental evidence is not so readily available for 'syllable-timed' languages, but, as in the case of stress-timing, what evidence there is offers no support to the hypothesis. From a strictly phonetic point of view, there can be no doubt

[75] The examples are from MacCarthy (1975: 13–14). Note that it is the *spoken* syllables that are equal, and these do not always correspond to the written ones. MacCarthy writes that 'continuous French spoken fluently by native speakers conveys the general auditory impression that syllables in each group . . . are being uttered at a very regular rate' (p. 6).

[76] The example is from MacPherson (1975: 34), who writes that 'the syllable is the basic rhythm unit of Spanish, and one of the most characteristic features of the spoken language is that all syllables in a rhythm group, whether stressed or unstressed, tend to follow each other at more or less evenly spaced intervals of time'.

[77] French is sometimes said to have word-final stress, but this is a misconception. It is the final syllable of a *phrase* that is prominent, and a word spoken in isolation constitutes a phrase and is therefore accented on the final syllable. But *within* the phrase there is no such accent.

that the syllables of French and Spanish, and of other languages of this type, are *not* of equal length in connected speech. As in the case of stress-timing, however, there are a number of pitfalls in the measurement of syllable length. In French, it again appears that the approximate equality of syllable length is restricted to relatively short accentual phrases such as those given above, and considerable divergences are found between such phrases; to measure the syllables across more than one accentual phrase will in many cases easily 'disprove' the hypothesis. More importantly, however, the principles applied above in relation to 'stress-timing' must be observed: objective instrumental measurements of the lengths of syllables do not necessarily 'disprove' the principle of syllable-timing, since equality of perceptual spacing does not depend on equality of physical spacing. It is sufficient to demonstrate that a perceptual approximation to equal-length syllables is the basis for the overall prosodic organization of utterances in the language concerned for the principle to be valid phonologically. In languages such as French and Spanish, such evidence is readily available.

Strong criticism of the principle of syllable-timing in French is made by Wenk and Wioland (1982). They utterly reject any principle of syllable-timing for the language,[78] and seek the rhythmical basis of the language in the accented syllables—the final syllables of each accentual phrase. For them, 'rhythms are *not* "successions" of like elements, but rather presuppose alternation between marked (accented) and unmarked (unaccented) elements' (p. 207). Hence speech rhythm depends on accentuation, and since such accents occur only phrase-finally in French, these phrases must be the basis of French rhythm.

The argument is, however, flawed on several counts. First, it is by no means certain that rhythm requires accentuation, and many languages appear to have no accentuation at all; second, if alternation of 'accented' and 'unaccented' elements is required for rhythm, it is perfectly possible to see each successive syllable peak as an 'accent' in this loose sense, separated by the (unaccented) syllable margins;[79] finally, rhythm requires regularity, but French phrase-final accents are far from regular, and thus cannot serve as the basis of rhythm. This approach also takes no account of the fact that isochrony of syllables (like that of stresses in 'stress-timed' languages) is limited to each accentual phrase; given this restriction, the principle of syllable-timing is not incompatible with the occurrence of the phrase-final accent of French.

Similar controversies are found with other assumed 'syllable-timed' languages. Pointon (1980) reports on experimental studies which fail to confirm the principle of equal-length syllables in Spanish, and he concludes that 'Spanish has no regular rhythm in the sense of an isochronous sequence of similar events, be

---

[78] Presumably in an attempt to discredit once and for all the 'syllable-timing' theory, Wenk and Wioland (ironically?) suggest that, since (i) all languages must have rhythm, (ii) rhythm must depend on accentuation, and (iii) the syllable-timing theory takes no account of accentuation, therefore (iv) the theory claims that French is not a language.

[79] See also the comments in 2.9.2 above on 'events' and 'units' in rhythm.

they syllables or stresses' (p. 302). Again, however, factors such as the limitation of syllable isochrony to the accentual phrase are ignored.[80] Balasumbramanian (1980) similarly finds no evidence for either stress-timing or syllable-timing in Tamil, but his measurements likewise take no account of phrasing.

In the light of our previous discussion of 'stress-timing', however, it will be clear that experimental evidence which fails to confirm the equal length of syllables cannot be considered as 'proof' of the absence of 'syllable-timing' as a phonological principle. Such a principle can still underlie the rhythm of a language even if it is not manifested phonetically in a consistent fashion. As with 'stress-timing', there are other factors at work in determining the length of syllables which may modify the principle without, however, destroying it or rendering it irrelevant. One such factor is the weight of the syllables. For Tamil, Balasumbramanian (1980) finds that the length of a syllable depends on its structure, so that he can group them into four types on the basis of their duration, as in Fig. 2.57. It can be seen that these categories reflect syllable weight. Similarly, Pointon (1980: 295) reports that in Spanish 'the more complex the syllable structure, the greater the duration of that syllable is likely to be'.

Fig. 2.57	V	lighter
	CV	light
	VC, CVC, $\bar{V}$, C$\bar{V}$	heavy
	$\bar{V}$C, C$\bar{V}$C	heavier

A further factor affecting the length of syllables is stress. Although MacPherson (1975: 34) writes that the five stressed syllables in the Spanish example given above 'are neither longer nor shorter in duration than the five unstressed syllables', the experimental studies reported on by Pointon (1980) all show a difference of duration in stressed and unstressed syllables in Spanish. In French, the *final* syllable of the phrase, which is accented, is also significantly longer than the other syllables (Wenk and Wioland, 1982: 210–11).

The syntactic structure of the utterance, identified by Abercrombie (1964) as a factor affecting syllable quantity in English, does not seem to be relevant in French in quite the same way. Whereas in English it affects the length distribution within the foot, in French it appears to have no effect within the accentual phrase itself, but may be relevant for the division of the utterance into such phrases, and will thus affect length indirectly, since the last syllable of the phrase is lengthened. Wenk and Wioland (1982: 195–6) find that listeners are able to disambiguate syntactically different sentences on this basis; the two utterances *ces deux, papa* ('these two, father') and *c'est de papa* ('it's from father'), which are both phonemically /sedøpapa/, can be distinguished as | sedø |papa | vs. | sedøpapa | respectively, where '|' represents the phrase boundary; in the former

---

[80] Pointon in fact criticizes one of his sources (Olsen) for 'limiting himself to sense groups and ignoring pauses between them' (p. 297).

case, but not the latter, the syllable /dø/ is lengthened, as it occurs at the end of the phrase. Other examples of such disambiguation include *la moustache tomba* ('the moustache fell off') vs. *la mousse tache ton bas* ('the foam stains your stocking'), and *j'ai vu des moines au couvent* ('I saw monks in the convent') vs. *j'ai vu des moineaux couvants* ('I saw some sparrows sitting on their eggs'), where appropriate phrasing induces phrase-final lengthening in different places.[81]

2.9.3.5 Mora-timing

The third category of timing that has been recognized is based on the *mora*. As in the case of 'stress-timing' and 'syllable-timing', the assumption is that the unit in question—here the mora—is of consistent length, thus providing a rhythmical basis for the utterance. As with the other forms of timing, mora-timing implies that segmental length is the result of distributing the available mora-length among the segments.

The language that is always cited in this connection is Japanese. Superficially, it resembles French in having no perceptible stress within the phrase, and an even succession of syllables. However, there are some differences; French has a phrase-final accent, whereas in Japanese there is a pitch–accent which may occur within the phrase without, however, disturbing the rhythm. But a further difference is that the 'syllables' of Japanese may include not only consonant-vowel sequences, e.g. to-ko-ro ('place'), but also the syllabic nasal, e.g. sa-n ('three'), the second part of long vowels, as in te-e-bu-ru ('table'), or the first part of geminate consonants, as in ta-t-ta ('stood'). The unit in question would thus appear to be not the syllable as such but the mora.

That these units are more or less equal in length has been remarked upon by many scholars. Bloch (1950) notes that 'the most striking general feature of Japanese pronunciation is its staccato rhythm. The auditory impression of any phrase is of a rapid pattering succession of more-or-less sharply defined fractions, all of about the same length'. Thus, 'two phrases containing the same number of fractions are heard as equal in duration'. Although Bloch states that 'all these fractions, of whatever type, will henceforth be called *syllables*', he also notes that such 'syllables' do not correspond to 'peaks of sonority' or 'chest pulses'; 'in short, the Japanese syllable is a unit of duration. Such a unit is often called a mora'.

Jakobson (1931) also recognizes that the basis of timing in Japanese is the mora. He suggests that Japanese is an example of a language with a two-mora accent which can fall either on the first part of a two-mora syllable, or on two short syllables, and where quantity serves to indicate whether the syllable nucleus is unitary or two-part. Many other scholars have gone further, and eliminated reference to the syllable altogether, so that the language is regarded simply as having a succession of moras.

---

[81] Length is, however, not the only indication of the end of the phrase; other features, such as intonation, are also involved.

Yoshiba (1981), for example, takes the mora to be the basic unit of Japanese phonology, since an utterance must consist of a chain of moras, and the mora is the traditional unit for the description of pitch–accent and verse metre. He describes a number of processes using the feature [±mora]. Kubozono (1989, 1995) provides further arguments for the mora, using evidence from speech errors and perception.

As might perhaps be anticipated from our experience of 'stress-timing' and 'syllable-timing', however, experimental studies have failed to confirm the temporal regularity of the mora. Beckman (1982) finds no evidence that moras are of equal length, and thus 'no convincing evidence for the phonetic reality of the mora'. She thus attributes the claims of native speakers about the reality of such a unit to the influence of the *kana* writing system, which assigns a symbol to each mora.

The arguments deployed earlier in defence of stress-timing and syllable-timing may be extended to mora-timing: the fact that such units of timing appear to have no consistent correlate in the physical lengths of the units concerned should not surprise us, since rhythm, as a phonological and mental phenomenon, does not require such phonetic precision. We would, of course, expect to find a loose connection between rhythmical units and the actual phonetic durations, and there is evidence that this is so; Hoequist (1983), for example, compares the durations of sounds in Spanish and Japanese, and concludes that while there is certainly no confirmation of strict isochrony with regard to syllables and moras, respectively, there is 'evidence fitting a less strict hypothesis of rhythm categories'. But we would not expect, or require, a stricter observance of isochrony than this, in order to confirm the basic hypothesis.

In our earlier discussion of the mora (2.5.4) we noted some inconsistency with its definition, since some scholars see it as a unit in itself, a part of the syllable, and others as a measure of syllable length. The view of Japanese as 'mora-timed', consisting of a string of moras, would tend to reinforce the former view, since the syllable does not appear to be relevant here. However, for a number of scholars, the syllable, as well as the mora, is a significant unit in Japanese, and this allows us to maintain the view that the mora is not a unit as such but rather a measure of the length of a syllable. We have seen that Jakobson (1931) uses both the syllable and the mora in describing Japanese, since a two-mora accent may fall either on a long syllable or upon a sequence of two short syllables. This view is reinforced, within a different theoretical framework, by McCawley (1968), who points out that, although the mora is a unit of timing in Japanese, the accent cannot fall on the second mora of a long vowel. In effect, therefore, the accent falls on the *syllable*, which consequently has an important place in the phonology of Japanese.[82] Shibatani (1990: 158) is thus able to con-

---

[82] The situation is complicated by the fact that the principles of accentuation vary from dialect to dialect. It has been claimed that different dialects also vary according to whether it is the syllable or the mora that is the relevant unit. Cf. Shibatani (1990: 160); Tsujimura (1996: 78–80).

clude that 'a word such as *sinbun* "newspaper" consists of two syllables *sin* and *bun*, but a Japanese speaker further subdivides the word into the four units *si*, *n*, *bu* and *n*.'[83]

Other prosodic units have also been claimed to be relevant for Japanese phonology. Jakobson's view that Japanese may have a two-mora accent which characterizes either a long syllable *or two short syllables*, suggests that the principles of length assignment may transcend the individual syllable. This is explicitly claimed by Poser (1990), who argues, largely on the basis of accentuation rules, for the existence of a 'bimoraic foot' in Japanese, which is comparable to the foot of stress-timed languages. But however relevant such a unit might be for the placing of the pitch–accent, there is no evidence that it actually determines timing in the language.

2.9.4 SEGMENT LENGTH IN A PROSODIC CONTEXT

We have concluded that segment length must be seen in the context of the syllable as a whole, and that syllable quantity must be seen in the context of larger prosodic units. There is therefore an inevitable relationship—albeit an indirect one—between segment length and the larger prosodic context, and it is possible to consider this relationship more directly. We shall examine some specific cases here where segment length can be shown to depend on this larger context.

Old English High Vowel Deletion

In 2.6.3.1 we considered the alternations between monosyllabic and disyllabic forms in some noun-classes of Old English, notably the plural of neuter a-stems, and the nominative singular of ō-stems, i-stems, and u-stems. In each case there are two different forms, depending on the weight of the initial syllable: if this is light, the form is disyllabic, but if it is heavy, the form is monosyllabic. Examples are given in Fig. 2.58.[84] Data of this kind were used in 2.6.3.1 to illustrate the significance of the mora, since the words in the two different columns all have two moras, but different numbers of syllables, as a heavy syllable counts as two moras and a light syllable as only one.

Fig. 2.58		*heavy*	*light*
	neuter a-stem	word ('words')	scipu ('ships')
	ō-stem	lāf ('remnant')	lufu ('love')
	i-stem	giest ('guest')	wine ('friend')
	u-stem	feld 'field'	sunu 'son'

[83] Yoshida (1990) argues, from the perspective of Government Phonology, that units such as these are actually syllables rather than moras. However, this seems to be based on the aprioristic assumption of this theory that final consonants are actually the onsets of further syllables, and therefore that even English words such as 'cat' are actually disyllabic. Whatever the theoretical motivations for such an assumption, it does not seem to have much relevance for the principles of timing.
[84] Data from Lass (1994: 129–33).

What was not considered earlier, however, is the fact that the length equivalence between the two sets of forms cannot be dealt with at the level of the syllable itself, but only in terms of the sequence of two syllables, and, since the first syllable is stressed in such words, this sequence is equivalent to the *foot*. It may be concluded, therefore, that the foot is relevant for length in Old English in so far as the foot length is kept constant (in terms of the number of moras). Historically, an original final high vowel was lost after heavy syllables, but *not* after light syllables, thus ensuring that all such forms have two moras.

Middle English Lengthening

The lengthening of open syllables in Middle English has already been considered above (cf. 2.6.3.1; 2.7.4.1). As we have seen, a standard interpretation of this phenomenon is in terms of stress or equalization of weight. However, Minkova (1982) shows that this lengthening takes place almost exclusively in cases where the word-final schwa is dropped—for example [talə] > [taːl] (Modern English 'tale')—and it can therefore with some justification be interpreted as a case of compensatory lengthening.

Hayes (1989: 266–9) uses this example to illustrate what he calls 'compensatory lengthening by vowel loss'. This process appears to be very similar to other kinds of compensatory lengthening that we have considered, with the loss of a segment and the preservation of its mora. After deletion of the second syllable node, together with its structure, the first vowel is automatically attached to the stranded mora, resulting in additional length, as in Fig. 2.59.

Fig. 2.59 (a) σ   σ   (b) σ   σ   (c) σ   (d) σ

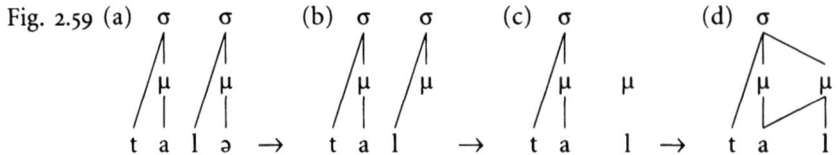

Although this case appears to be analogous to other instances of compensatory lengthening, in fact there are significant differences. First, the structure of the second syllable has to be entirely deleted in order to allow its onset consonant to become the coda consonant of the first syllable ('Parasitic Delinking'). Second, the vowel of the first syllable has to be linked to the stranded mora of the original second syllable. The first of these is a radical measure which is not required in most other processes of Compensatory Lengthening,[85] the second is unmotivated by the normal principles of the model, since, according to one view at least, the syllable would be perfectly well-formed without this linking; the final

---

[85] Hayes in fact uses it for two other processes of compensatory lengthening, those induced by Glide Formation and by 'Managerial Lengthening'. Both of these also involve vowel loss, since a vowel becomes non-syllabic.

mora would be linked to the final consonant and thus not left stranded. Hayes glosses over the difficulty here, and merely motivates this particular aspect of the process by an appeal to an external principle, taken from Îto (1986), that 'syllable structure (indeed, all prosodic structure) is created maximally'.

But the major difference between this case of vowel loss and other types of compensatory lengthening is that it involves the loss not merely of a segment but of a *syllable*, and this means that the motivation for the compensation must ultimately be different. In other cases, such as those exemplified in 3.7.4.2, the motivation can be seen as the maintenance of syllable weight, where this is represented in terms of the mora count, since the mora serves, in Hayes's terms (1989: 285), as 'the basic unit for syllable weight'. But in the case of Middle English Lengthening and similar cases of 'compensatory lengthening by vowel loss', maintenance of syllable weight clearly cannot be the motivation for the compensation, since here the weight of one syllable is increased and that of another is deleted altogether. What is maintained in such cases is, of course, not the weight of the syllable but rather the length of the whole word, or rather, since here the original form of the word consists phonologically of a disyllabic sequence of stressed and unstressed syllables, of the *foot*. This difference is significant, since it is clear that if the mora serves as 'the basic unit for syllable weight', then Hayes's principle of 'Moraic Conservation' is inappropriate where, as here, syllable weight is *not* maintained.

'Overlength' in Low German

Another case where length is related to a larger prosodic context is that of 'overlong' vowels in Low German. The phenomenon can be illustrated by pairs such as those given in Fig. 2.60, from a North Saxon dialect[86] (: = 'long'; :: = 'overlong'; the High German counterparts are given in brackets). Though the phonological interpretation is obscured by the fact that the vowel quality may vary, and that the following consonant has also been claimed to differ in 'tension' in the two cases,[87] the length difference is clear, and it provides a three-way contrast here: 'short', 'long' and 'overlong'.

Fig. 2.60

bru:t	(Braut)	'fiancée'	bru::t	(braut)	'brews'
stu:f	(stumpf)	'blunt'	stu::f	(Stube)	'parlour'
zi:t	(seit)	'since'	zi::t	(Seide)	'silk'
hu:s	(Haus)	'house' (nom.)	hu::s	(Haus(e))	'house' (dat.)
bre:f	(Brief)	'letter'	bre::f	(Briefe)	'letters'

The historical origin of these 'overlong' vowels is relatively transparent: they arose as a result of the loss of a following unstressed /ə/, either morpheme-

---

[86] Cf. Keller (1961: 343–4). A recent treatment, on which much of this discussion is based, is Chapman (1993).

[87] Keller (1961: 343).

finally or before a voiced consonant. Thus, the development is [bru: + ət] > [bru::t], [bre:v + ə] > [bre::f], and so on. This means that the 'overlong' vowels can again be seen as the result of compensatory lengthening, in which the loss of the [ə] is compensated for by the lengthening of the preceding vowel. It should also be pointed out that this phenomenon affects consonants, too, giving distinctions such as [kan] (*kann* = 'can' (verb)) vs. [kan:] (*Kanne* = 'can' (noun)) (Chapman, 1993), though here there is simply a two-way contrast between 'short' and 'long'.

From an Autosegmental perspective, this phenomenon poses certain additional problems in comparison with other cases of compensatory lengthening. In the first place, there is some indeterminacy about the appropriate representation of 'overlong' vowels. They appear to need a three-fold attachment to timing slots to differentiate them from 'short' and 'long' vowels, but this could be done in different ways, with either a multiply branching nucleus slot (see Fig. 2.61(a)) or with a shared coda, as in Fig. 2.61(b). This aside, the major difficulty is, as with Middle English Lengthening, that the segment which is lost and that which is lengthened belong to different syllables and are not contiguous; the process of compensation cannot therefore be dealt with satisfactorily in terms of redistribution within the syllable.

Fig. 2.61 (a)

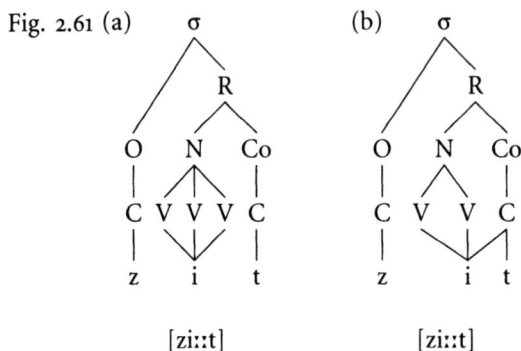

With a process such as [bre:və] > [bre::f], the first part—the loss of the [ə] and the attachment of the stranded onset to the preceding syllable—is straightforward, and is given in Figs. 2.62(a) and (b) (the devoicing of final [v] to [f] is taken for granted). However, this does not provide for the lengthening of the already long vowel, and the outcome—Fig. 2.62(c)—is incorrect and must be supplemented by the generation of an additional V slot under the nucleus node, as in Fig. 2.62(d). However, this last step is unrelated to the loss of the vowel, and the compensatory nature of the process is not captured.

Fig. 2.62 (a)

(b)

(c)

(d)

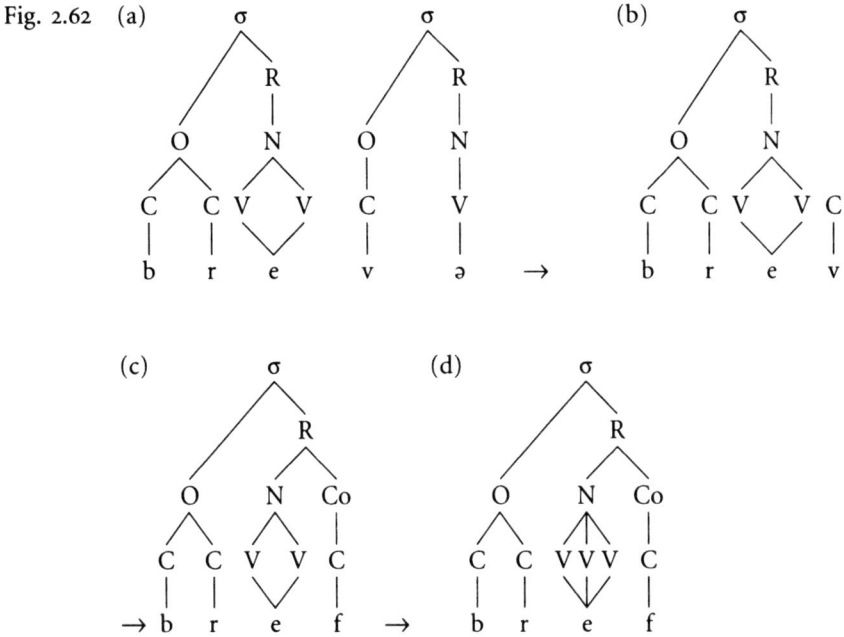

The situation can be restated in terms of moraic theory, as in Fig. 2.63. As-suming that the syllable with the overlong vowel is trimoraic, the problem is to get from the representation of Fig. 2.63(a) to that of Fig. 2.63(b). This cannot be achieved simply by deleting the second syllable node, attaching its mora to the first syllable node, and relinking the vowel to the mora, since the intervening consonant presents an insuperable barrier.

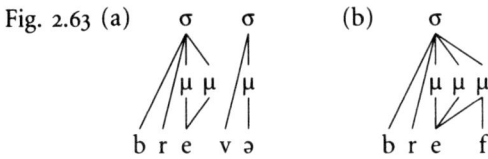

Fig. 2.63 (a)

(b)

On the other hand, generating a new mora under the first syllable node, and attaching both the vowel and the consonant to this, though technically possible, fails to relate the lengthening to the loss of the final vowel. This process is repre-sented in Fig. 2.64.

Fig 2.64 (a)   σ   σ   (b)   σ   (c)   σ   (d)   σ

b r e   v ə →   b r e   v →   b r e   v →   b r e   f

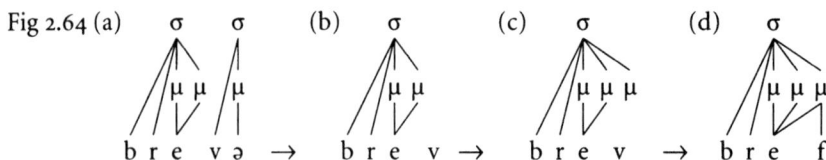

The situation is analogous to that encountered above (2.7.4.2) in the case of **finf* > *fif*, where the lengthening of the vowel appears unrelated to the loss of the consonant, since the loss is in the coda but the branching is in the nucleus. It will be recalled that Lass (1984: 260) relates the two processes by invoking branching as a 'structural primitive', applying to the syllable as a whole, so that loss of a branch in one part may cause branching in another; indeed, he uses this as an argument for the reality of the syllable. In the present case, however, the syllable is of no avail, since the loss of a branch in one syllable—here, in fact, of a syllable as a whole—results in additional branching in a different syllable. By the same reasoning, cases of this kind provide an argument for a more inclusive prosodic unit—the foot—whose overall length is preserved. The loss of one part of this unit—here the second syllable—is compensated for by further branching in another—here the first syllable.

Estonian Quantity Revisited

Length in Estonian was considered in 2.5.3.4, where we saw that attempts have been made to explain the complexities in terms of the distribution of vowel and consonant length within the syllable. A number of scholars have gone further, however, and considered the distribution of length in terms of larger units or sequences than the syllable, though there is some dispute about which units these should be. One approach (e.g. Posti, 1950; Ravila, 1962; Lehiste, 1960, 1970) is to relate the occurrence of a quantity 3 ('overlong') sound in one syllable to the presence of a quantity 1 (short) sound in the following syllable, so that there is balance between the lengths of sounds in successive syllables. In a number of publications, Lehiste (1960, 1965, 1966, 1970) claims that the true unit of length distribution in Estonian is the disyllabic sequence, where the length is determined by whether the syllable is odd-numbered or even-numbered in the sequence. All of these approaches imply a unit of quantity of which the syllable is a part, and within which there is a balance of length. An alternative solution, which may perhaps be taken to subsume this, is to relate the length distribution to accentuation, and hence to the *foot*. This is the solution put forward by Prince (1980), building on work by Lehiste and Leben.

   Prince observes that Q3 ('overlong') has a number of properties which set it off from the other quantities: it can only occur in a stressed syllable; monosyllabic lexical items must have one segment in Q3; a stressed syllable with Q3 may be immediately followed by another stressed syllable, whereas this is unusual for other stressed syllables; there are special restrictions on combinations of a vowel in Q3 with consonants in Q2, and a vowel in Q2 with a consonant in Q3; it has special intonation properties, and 'attracts the major pitch movement of the intonation pattern to its own syllable'; Q3 consonants alternate with Q2 consonants in the consonant alternation system, but never with Q1 consonants; and Q3 usually appears in the strong grade. Because of these features, Prince suggests that 'Q3 has a status in phonological representation generically different from the status of segmental length' (p. 512). His proposal is that 'a syllable phonetically associated with Q3 is in itself a minimal metrical unit [s w]—a *foot*. This prosodic status will provide the environment for the rules assigning duration to segments, and will prove to be the basis for the entire range of properties that we have just noted' (p. 513).

Following and adapting Lehiste (1965: 452), Prince represents the syllable types of Estonian as in Fig. 2.65, where C and V are Q1 segments, CC and VV, with identical C or V, are Q2, and C:C and VV: are Q3, again if the Cs or the Vs are identical. The different placement of the length-mark in C:C and VV: is explained by the fact that 'long' and 'overlong' consonants are structurally equivalent to consonant clusters which are split between two syllables, i.e. they are C·C and C: ·C respectively (· marks the syllable division), while Q3 vowels belong to a single syllable, and 'long' and 'overlong' vowels are simply VV and VV:. The syllabification of words such as *kabi* ('hoof'), *kapi* ('wardrobe'), and *kappi* ('wardrobe', partitive singular) is therefore ka·pi, kap·pi, and kap:·pi. It will be clear that this immediately disposes of Q3 in the case of consonants, since it is merely a long consonant (C:) followed by another C in the next syllable, which happens to be identical to it. Fig. 2.65 also shows the restrictions on co-occurrence which characterize Q3: a Q2 vowel cannot combine with a Q3 consonant and a Q3 vowel cannot combine with a Q2 consonant.

Fig. 2.65 I	II	III
CV-CV	CVV-CV	CVV:-CV
	CVVC-CV	CVV:C:-CV
	CVC-CV	CVC:-CV
		*CVVC:-CV
		*CVV:C-CV

From Fig. 2.65 it will be evident that Q3 syllables (column III) have exact counterparts in Q2 (column II). On the basis of this, Prince is able to see the 'overlength' of Q3 as a property of the syllable as a whole. Thus, the heavy syllables of column II can be represented as $[_\sigma CVV]$, $[_\sigma CVVC]$, and $[_\sigma CVC]$, and their equivalents in column III as $[_\tau CVV]$, $[_\tau CVVC]$, and $[_\tau CVC]$, where τ is the special kind of syllable which has Q3, as opposed to the normal syllable σ.

A further factor that needs to be introduced here is *accent*. In Estonian, the accent falls on the first syllable of native words, with subsequent secondary stresses normally occurring at intervals of two or three syllables thereafter. Prince represents the prosodic structure of Estonian words in terms of Metrical theory, with binary-branching nodes, as in the example of Fig. 2.66 (M = 'phonological word'), where the word *hilisemattele* ('later', allative plural) is given in two alternative pronunciations.

Fig. 2.66

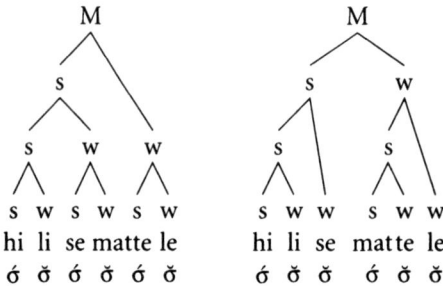

However, Q3 syllables behave somewhat differently from other syllables in respect of stress: they may be directly followed by another (secondary) stressed syllable, as in *káu:kéle* ('far away'), or *júl:késse* ('bold', illative singular). These are represented by Prince in the form given in Fig. 2.67. As can be seen, he treats Q3 syllables as comprising both the strong and the weak nodes and thus, in a model which regards such pairs of nodes at the lowest level as a *foot*, as constituting feet in their own right.

Fig. 2.67

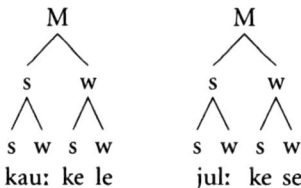

The Estonian foot, in Prince's interpretation, may be disyllabic or trisyllabic. Given an assumption that all branching is binary, these two structures can be defined by means of the two rules of Fig. 2.68, where 'F' = foot, 'u' = syllable, and 'm' = short syllable. Rule (a) caters for disyllabic feet, and rule (b) for trisyllabic feet, with an upper limit of 3 syllables overall.

Fig. 2.68 (a) F → u u
          (b) F → F m
          Condition: F contains no more than 3 syllables

In addition to the syllable, we may also introduce the mora here, so that although the foot can consist of two syllables, in certain cases it may consist of a single syllable with two moras. The rules of Fig. 2.68 can be reinterpreted in this light, so that *u* ranges over syllable and mora, while *m* is actually a mora. The rules thus define the five foot types of Fig. 2.69.

Fig. 2.69 (a) (b) (c) (d) (e)

```
                              F                 F                 F  /\
       F        F(σ)       F  \              F(σ) \            F(σ) \  \
      /\       /\        /\   \            /\    \          /\    \  \
     σ  σ     m  m      σ  σ   m          m  m    m        m  m    m  m
```

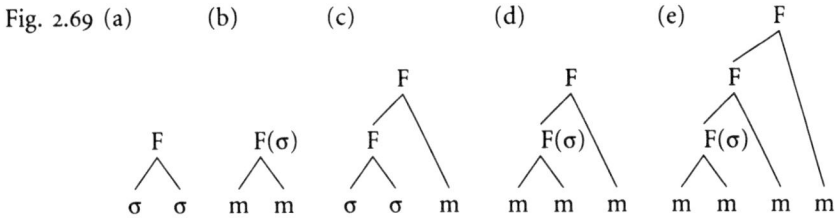

Structure (a) of Fig. 2.69 is the simple case of a disyllabic foot, such as *kappi*, while (b) represents either a monosyllabic foot consisting of two moras, as in *maa:*, or a disyllabic foot with two single-mora syllables, when it would be equivalent to (a). Structure (c) is a trisyllabic foot, such as *noorikku*, while (d) is either a trisyllabic foot with single-mora syllables or a disyllabic foot with an initial bimoraic syllable, as in *kap:pi*. Finally, structure (e) represents a trisyllabic foot with an initial bimoraic syllable (the structure [$_F$ m m] cannot be disyllabic here, because of the three-syllable rule), such as *kau:kele*. Many of the other properties of Q3 syllables can be seen as following from this analysis. For example, since each foot must contain a stressed syllable, a monosyllabic foot, with the structure [$_F$ σ], will consist of a Q3 syllable; the peculiar pitch features of Q3 syllables can be said to derive from their status as whole feet, and so on.

In more general terms, the significance of this analysis lies not particularly in the specific formalisms given here, but in the recognition that the properties of 'extra-long' syllables derive from the larger prosodic context in which they occur. Thus, according to Prince (1980: 559), 'the quantity system is essentially the product of multiplying a segmento-syllabic distinction (heavy/light) by a prosodic distinction (foot/nonfoot)'.

2.9.5 THE RELEVANCE OF PROSODIC STRUCTURE

In all the cases discussed in 2.9 it is evident that an adequate understanding of quantity requires us to go beyond the immediate context of the syllable and place the syllable itself in a larger structure. Exactly what this larger structure should be is a matter of some controversy, and the factors involved are rather poorly understood. When we go above the syllable we need to take account of the way in which syllables are organized in different languages, and this inevitably involves a consideration of rhythm. Rhythm itself is, however, a disputed territory; many scholars subscribe to the stress-timing/syllable-timing typology which, as we have seen, provides for the foot or the syllable, respectively, as the basic unit of timing in different languages, but the absence of experimental corroboration of this typology is a reminder that we are here dealing with phonological abstractions, and that a variety of factors are involved in determining the actual length of such units.

In any case, it is clear that length is not just a matter for segments; whatever higher units of prosodic structure we postulate, they have extent in time, and the temporal structure of utterances is a reflection of the timing relations present at the different levels within this structure. Furthermore, since timing relations at every level are manifested along a single dimension, *time*, the actual lengths of individual segments and syllables are the complex result of combining factors of different kinds.[88]

2.10 Conclusion

2.10.1 THE STRATIFICATION OF LENGTH

A salient feature of length that has been emphasized in the discussion so far is that it is not a unitary phenomenon but has implications at different levels of phonological structure. Some length contrasts may be appropriately handled at the segmental level, while others clearly require reference to the syllable or to larger units such as the foot. Length can thus be regarded as *stratified*, in the sense that it is distributed over several layers of structure. The difficulty is that these different layers of length are ultimately manifested in the same phonetic dimension. The phonological analysis of length must therefore involve a process of abstracting out simultaneously occurring, and phonetically indistinguishable, phenomena that belong to different layers of phonological structure. Conversely, in the formal specification of length, mechanisms are required which are able to superimpose the length relations at different levels upon one another.

In addition to the discussion earlier in this chapter, further evidence that several different layers are required for length is provided by Hayes (1995: 299–305). He draws attention to problem cases where certain syllables—for example, those containing geminates—may be regarded as light for some purposes and heavy for others. 'What is needed', he notes (1995: 299), 'is a theory that allows such dual distinctions of weight to be made, but which retains the advantages in predictive power that moraic theory holds over alternatives.' Hayes's solution is to adapt the principles of the metrical grid to moras, so that the mora-count may differ on different layers. Thus, in a language in which CV syllables are always light, and CV: syllables are always heavy, but CVC syllables may be light or heavy for different processes, he suggests representations such as those of Fig. 2.70, with two layers of moras. In such a language, according to this principle, 'processes that treat CVC as heavy may be expressed as referring to the lower layer of the syllable-internal grid, while processes that treat CVC as light would refer to the higher layer' (Hayes, 1995: 300). Hayes conjectures that 'the requirements of syllable-external prosody (e.g. footing, word minima, tonal docking) are characteristically enforced on the higher moraic layer, while

---

[88] Further discussion of the relationship between rhythm, accentuation, and length will be found in 3.5.3.

syllable-internal requirements (e.g. mora population limits) are characteristically enforced on the lower layer' (ibid.).

Fig. 2.70 (a) CV: (b) CVC (c) CV

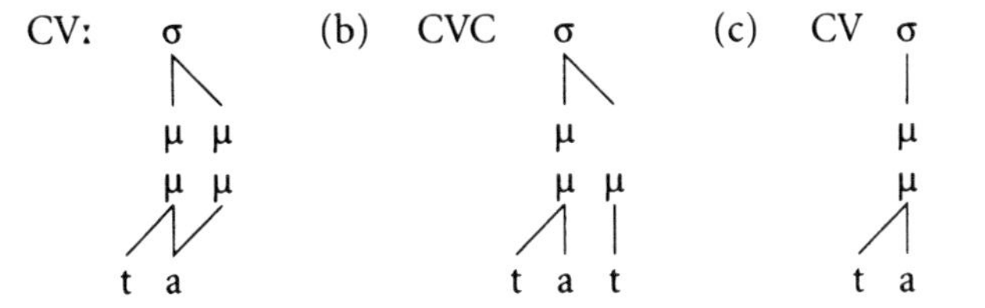

Hayes's dual representation of weight is an acknowledgement of the need for representation of quantity relations on more than one level, though it is doubtful if two layers of moras are the best way to formalize these relations, since the mora remains tied to syllable weight. As an illustration of a possible alternative, consider the allocation of length in an utterance such as 'That is very easy' (/'ðæt iz 'veri 'iːziː/), as represented in Fig. 2.71. We may display this utterance on the foot, syllable, and segment levels; by adding moras to the syllable level, we represent the weight of the syllables and the length of the vowels. But there is still something missing, since the length of the syllables depends not only on their weight but their 'quantity', in the sense of Abercrombie (1964). The first foot has an internal syntactic boundary and is of type C, with the pattern — ∪; the second has an initial light syllable which produces a type A foot with the pattern ∪ —, while the third has an initial heavy syllable, giving a type B foot with the pattern ∩ ∩. It is only in terms of these quantities that the distribution of length at the lower levels can be effected, since they determine the lengths of the individual moras.

Fig. 2.71

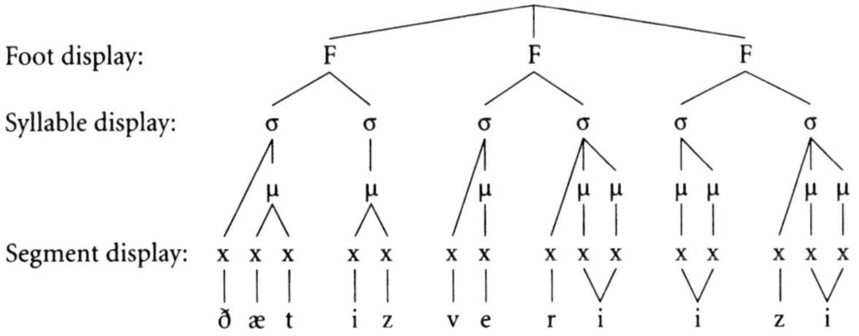

Foot display:

Syllable display:

Segment display:

How this information is to be included is, however, uncertain. It cannot be incorporated by having two layers of moras, since the issue is not the number of moras but the length of the mora itself, as determined by the quantity of the syllables, which in turn depends on the length of the foot and the number and quantity of the syllables it contains. One possibility is to include a measure of quantity at the foot level, parallel to the moraic representation at the syllable level. A word such as *never*, for example, when pronounced as a single foot, would consist of two single-mora syllables, but would be of Abercrombie's type A ($\cup$ —), while *tea for* (*two*) would be of type C. Using a unit of syllable quantity Q, and assuming, with Abercrombie, that English disyllabic feet are in triple time, we could represent these words as in Fig. 2.72.

Fig. 2.72

```
        F                      F
      / | \                  / | \
     Q  Q  Q                Q  Q  Q
     |   \/                  \/   |
     σ    σ                 σ     σ
    /µ   /µ                /µ µ  /µ
   / |  / |               / \/  / |
  n ε  v ə              t i f ə
      never              tea for (two)
```

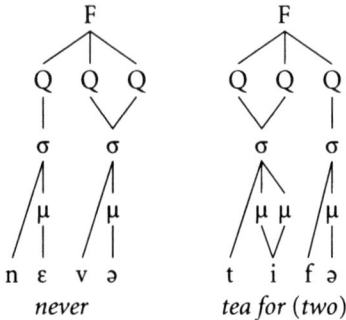

Such representations have other uses. They might be employed, for example, in cases of 'compensatory lengthening by vowel loss' where, as we saw above, the motivation for the compensatory lengthening is the preservation of the foot length rather than the syllable length. Thus, in preference to Fig. 2.59, we could have Fig. 2.73, which attributes the process to maintenance of the Q-count at the foot level rather than the mora-count at the syllable level.

Fig. 2.73

```
      F                     F                     F
    /   \                 /   \                 /   \
   Q     Q               Q     Q               Q     Q
   |     |               |                      \   /
   σ     σ     →         σ          →            σ
   ta    lə              ta    ı                 taːl
```

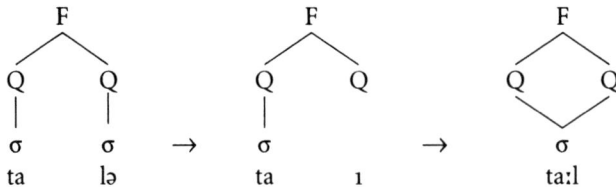

The purpose of this discussion is, however, not to propose a specific formalization for the representation of syllable quantity but rather to emphasize that length is a property of units of different levels. How this property is to be represented is a different, and secondary, question. Units such as the mora and a possible Q(uantity) unit may form part of such a formalization. The mora has been regarded by a number of scholars as a legitimate prosodic unit, alongside the syllable and the foot. McCarthy and Prince (1995), for example, set out the prosodic hierarchy as in Fig. 2.74(a). However, this hierarchy is not necessarily appropriate; as we have seen, the mora is more properly regarded as a measure of the weight of a syllable rather than as a constituent of it, and hence not a unit proper. Weight is not a unit, any more than, say tone or stress are units; it is merely a *property* of a unit, and therefore does not qualify for inclusion in a hierarchy of units. This is reflected in the fact that the mora does not conform to principles such as strict layering (Selkirk, 1984: 26; Nespor and Vogel, 1986: 12), since onset consonants are excluded. The same reservation would apply to the Q-unit, though at a higher level; syllable quantities are not constituents of the foot but properties of it. In Autosegmental terms, both the mora and the Q-unit constitute autosegments rather than units, and they are *associated* with units (Brentari and Bosch, 1990). A more appropriate representation than Fig. 2.74(a) would therefore be Fig. 2.74(b), which recognizes the foot and the syllable as 'true' units, and the Q tier and μ tier as dependent tiers, linked to these units.[89]

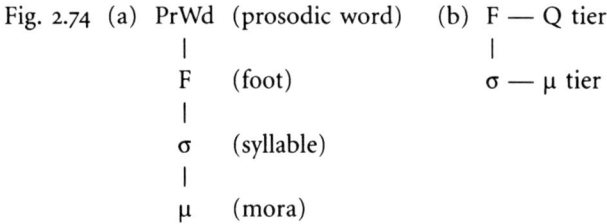

Fig. 2.74 (a) PrWd (prosodic word)   (b) F — Q tier
               | |
               F   (foot)   σ — μ tier
               |
               σ   (syllable)
               |
               μ   (mora)

2.10.2 THE TYPOLOGY OF LENGTH

In this chapter we have considered the analysis of length in a number of languages, and attempted to sketch out a general framework in terms of which it may be described. We have also identified a number of differences in the way in which length is used, for example in respect of timing and the role of the foot. As we have seen, the basic unit of timing in languages may be the foot, the syllable, or the mora; while some languages have feet and others do not. Such differences can be accommodated by the establishment of a *typology* of length, which recognizes that there are differences, but restricts them to a limited set of factors or parameters.

Prague scholars identified several typological parameters which have relevance for length. Jakobson (1931), for example, distinguishes *monotonic* and *polytonic* languages; in the former the scope of the accent is limited to the length of the syllable nucleus, while in the latter it may exceed it, having a distinction between a one-mora and a two-mora accent, or else between an accent on the first mora and the second mora of the syllable, or even both. From this follows Trubetzkoy's principle (1935) that polytonic languages must always have a length distinction in the vowels, which can be analysed in terms of an opposition between one and two moras, and Jakobson's thesis that monotonic languages—those with a free dynamic accent—cannot co-exist with such a distinction. The distinction overlaps with Trubetzkoy's division (1935) into *syllable*

---

[89] For further discussion of the principles of prosodic structure, and the relationship between units of the hierarchy and other dependent features, see 6.2.

languages and *mora languages*, later (1939: 174) *syllable-counting* and *mora-counting languages*); in the latter, but not the former, the mora plays a role.

According to Trubetzkoy (1935: 28–9), syllable languages can be classified into types according to the co-existence of length and accent. Both of these can be 'free' or 'bound' (i.e. fixed or predictable), giving four types:

(A) Both accent and length are bound: the place of the accent is fixed and the length follows the accent (e.g. Polish).

(B) The accent is free, but length is automatic (e.g. Spanish, Italian, Greek, Bulgarian, Rumanian, Ukrainian, Russian).

(C) Quantity is free, but the accent is bound, and either falls on a particular syllable in the word (e.g. Finnish, Hungarian, Czech) or depends on the quantity of the syllables (Latin).

(D) Both accent and quantity are free (English, German, Dutch).[90]

Mora languages cannot be so readily subclassified; as far as length is concerned, in these languages there is normally just a distinction between one and two moras.

There have been few other attempts to provide such a comprehensive typology in respect of length, with the exception of Pike's (1945) division of languages into 'stress-timing' vs. 'syllable-timing' (and the later addition of the category of 'mora-timing'). Though of course virtually every description of length in specific languages differs in some respect from the others, these differences relate to details of whether and how individual languages exploit the same basic categories. Some languages do not make use of a length distinction at the segmental level at all; some languages distinguish 'heavy' and 'light' syllables while some do not; and, of those that do, some treat CV̌C syllables as 'heavy' and others as 'light'. It would be possible to establish a typology on the basis of a variety of criteria of this sort. In the light of the discussion in this chapter, however, it may be suggested that the typologically most significant features for the specification of length can probably be reduced to two: (i) the presence or absence of specific units of the phonological hierarchy, and (ii) the use of specific units as the basis of timing.

For example, the model for English discussed in 2.10.1, above, includes provision for the foot as a basic unit of timing. This would be inappropriate for French or Japanese, neither of which includes such a unit in its phonological structure.[91] On the other hand, English, French and Japanese all make use of the syllable (which is in all likelihood a phonological universal), but of these only French makes use of it as the basis of timing. The mora is a measure of syllable length in many languages, but Japanese is one of the few (perhaps even the only

---

[90] It should be recalled that length, for Trubetzkoy, is a superficial manifestation of 'deeper' oppositions. For these languages, the true opposition is of 'contact' rather than length.

[91] Claims to the contrary, some of which have been included in our earlier discussion, are discounted.

one) to base its timing on it. Overlaid on these basic typological differences are other differences of length assignment in different languages, many of which have been exemplified in the present chapter.

The typology of length has been pursued further by a number of scholars, especially Hayes. Hayes (1995) deals with quantity differences in terms of an inventory of foot types, which are maximally disyllabic, and reduces this inventory to three possibilities: the Syllabic Trochee, the Moraic Trochee, and the Iamb. The difference between a trochee and an iamb—these terms are from classical metrics—is that the former is 'left-strong' and the latter 'right-strong' (i.e. accented on the first and the last syllable, respectively); the syllabic and moraic trochees differ in the unit (syllable or mora) that is involved. These categories therefore reflect a combination of accentual and durational patterns in languages. Hayes gives extensive examples of these different types from a wide range of languages, though it is not clear to what extent and in what way his typology can be related to others, such as that of Pike. His approach will be considered further in connection with accentual features in 3.5.3, below.

3

Accent

3.1 Introduction

3.1.1 THE STATUS OF ACCENT

'Accent' has proved to be one of the most controversial of the prosodic features, generating a considerable amount of theoretical debate. There has been—and continues to be—disagreement about the phonetic nature of the phenomenon, its phonological role, and the appropriate mode of its description, as well as its relationship to morphological and syntactic features in specific languages. In particular, much attention has been given to the rules required for assigning accentual features to English words and phrases. The aim of the present chapter is to examine some of these issues, and to evaluate the more important claims made and views expressed as to the nature and role of accent, and the means of representing and specifying it.

The complexity of the issues raised here is reflected in the variety of terms used to refer to accentual phenomena. We find, for example, in addition to 'accent' and 'accentuation', such terms as 'stress', 'prominence', 'emphasis', 'salience', 'intensity', and 'force', among others; we also encounter terms for different *kinds* of accent: 'syllable accent', 'word-accent', 'sentence accent', etc., and for different kinds of stress: 'word–stress', 'sentence stress', 'nuclear stress', 'contrastive stress', 'primary stress', 'secondary stress', and so on. The significance of many of these terms can only be appreciated in the context of the particular theory or descriptive framework within which they are employed, and they will therefore be discussed, where appropriate, later in this chapter. Other terms are of more central importance to the topic, and it is therefore necessary to consider them at the outset. Since there is inevitably considerable arbitrariness in how the various terms are defined and used, no claim is made that the usage adopted here is the 'correct' one, but merely that this usage, in providing designations for the central concepts, is helpful in attempting to understand the topic.

The term *accent* is used in a number of legitimate ways by different scholars, and many of these uses are mutually incompatible. As an illustration, we may note that Bolinger (1958a) and Jassem and Gibbon (1980) regard 'stress' as an abstract category, as potential accent, and 'accent' as its observable manifestation. Abercrombie (1976) and, following him, Laver (1994), on the other hand, regard 'accent' as potential for stress and 'stress' as the actual physical occurrence of it. Cutler (1984), among several others, sees 'stress' as a property of words and 'accent' as a property of sentences. Given such conflicts of usage, it is hardly possible to propose a terminological scheme which all scholars would find acceptable. In the present book, 'accent' is intended as the most neutral superordinate term, to refer to the linguistic phenomenon in which a particular element of the chain of speech is singled out in relation to surrounding elements, irrespective of the means by which this is achieved. Since accent may be realized by a variety of phonetic features, more specific terms will be used to refer to different *types* of accent, primarily *stress* (or *stress–accent*), and *pitch–accent*. The intended scope of these two terms will be considered in more detail in the course of this chapter; for the moment we may adopt the traditional view that stress is a *dynamic* and pitch–accent a *melodic* manifestation of accent. This view will need to be refined and somewhat revised as we proceed, however.[1] The term *accentuation* may also be used, in the rather broader sense of the overall organization of speech in respect of accents; we may therefore assert, perhaps tautologically, that accentuation is achieved by means of accents.

Of the other related terms mentioned above, 'emphasis' is too general to be used in this context, as it may refer to a wide range of linguistic devices, lexical and grammatical as well as phonological, which serve to draw attention to parts of an utterance or to give greater weight to the utterance as a whole. 'Prominence' is also wider than 'accent' or 'stress', as words or syllables may be made prominent by a number of different features, and it is preferable to keep these apart from accentual features proper (cf. Jones, 1967: 137 ff.). 'Intensity', 'force', and other similar terms, on the other hand, are too specific, as they refer to particular articulatory or acoustic features which are not necessarily appropriate to the phenomenon as a whole.

For the present, therefore, the terms 'accent', 'stress' and 'pitch–accent' will suffice, where the first of these includes the other two. The use and significance of these terms will be considered further below.

3.1.2 BACKGROUND TO THE STUDY OF ACCENT

Current views on accent have grown out of, and are built upon, an extensive descriptive tradition, which, since it still informs to a considerable extent the conceptual and terminological apparatus of current approaches, is not irrelevant to an understanding of the phenomenon itself. Accent is a traditional prosodic category, which was already known to ancient grammarians, even if their pronouncements on it are not always clear and unambiguous. Ancient Greek grammarians describe the accentual phenomena of their language using musical

---

[1] In particular, we shall note below that pitch is also a significant component of the dynamic manifestation of accent, and hence the stress vs. pitch–accent distinction needs to be drawn rather differently. See especially 3.2.4, below.

terminology; syllables are described as ὀξύς (*oxýs* = 'sharp') or βαρύς (*barýs* = 'heavy'), and it is concluded, therefore, that the Greek accent was essentially a matter of pitch,[2] a view that is supported by the descriptions of the related Vedic Sanskrit by the ancient Indian phoneticians. An element of uncertainty is provided, however, by the fact that the pitch–accent of classical Greek was subsequently replaced by a non-pitch (stress) accent, giving scope for different interpretations both of the phenomenon itself and of the remarks of the grammarians.

As in other matters, Latin grammarians took over the Greek terms and concepts and applied them rather uncritically to their own language. The Latin terms *acutum* ('sharp') and *grave* ('heavy') are direct translations of their Greek equivalents, and the Latin *accentus* corresponds to the Greek προσῳδία (*prosodía*, whose meaning seems to have been something like 'sung accompaniment'). Since, however, in the view of most current scholars, the accentual features of Latin are based on stress rather than pitch, the meaning of the terms has little relevance to the nature of Latin accentuation (Allen, 1965: 84). That the Latin accent was one of stress rather than pitch is clear, for example, from the evidence of vowel reduction in unaccented syllables in early Latin, and also from subsequent Romance developments, such as the loss of unaccented syllables, which are more readily explained in terms of a stress-based accent than of pitch.

Regardless of the particular facts of Greek and Latin accentuation, the legacy of this terminological misappropriation has been a degree of uncertainty and confusion in the European linguistic tradition about the nature of accent itself. Despite evidence to the contrary, scholars persisted until relatively recent times in the assumption that accentuation in languages is a matter of pitch alone, and only slowly recognized that other features might also be involved. As a result of this recognition, the term 'accent' gradually acquired a wider meaning, to include non-pitch features associated with accent, such as quantity and, eventually, 'dynamic' features such as 'strength' or 'force'. Ultimately, described as *anima vocis*, or *anima verborum*, it came to embrace not only virtually all of the prosodic and rhetorical devices of speech but the segmental features as well, a sense which is preserved in our use of the term in such expressions as 'a Northern accent', 'a French accent', and so on, which refer to a whole way of speaking.[3]

Nevertheless, language scholars periodically returned to the original Greek usage, which refers to a means of making one syllable more prominent than others, though they inevitably encountered the problem that in most of the modern European languages such prominence is signalled by other features too,

---

[2] Cf. Allen (1974: 106–7). Exactly what sort of pitch phenomena are involved is, however, not completely certain. Allen draws parallels with Scandinavian 'word-accents' (see 4.7.3, below), though these are interpreted differently here. Allen also argues that, in verse recitation at least, there must have been a 'stress-accent', too.

[3] For a survey of these developments, with reference to German usage, see especially Saran (1907).

especially quantity and stress. Grimm (1822: 20 ff.) refers to accent as 'the raising and lowering of the voice which accompanies the sound', but late nineteenth-century historical linguists such as Brugmann (1886–90: 530) accept that accent can be both 'dynamic' and 'musical', though the proportion of each element may vary in different languages. According to this view, in ancient Greek and in the ancient Indo–European languages generally, it was predominantly musical; in the modern European languages it is predominantly dynamic, though there are some languages—such as Lithuanian and Serbo–Croat—in which a musical accent is still found.[4] The shift from a musical to a dynamic accent is considered to be very general in the Indo–European languages; Verner's famous 'law' (Verner, 1875), which accounts for alternations in consonant voicing in the Germanic languages in terms of the position of the original Indo–European accent and a subsequent accent-shift, attributes the phenomenon to such a change,[5] while Lehmann (1955: 109 ff.; 1993: 58–61) continues this tradition by postulating a number of shifts between pitch–accent and stress–accent in early Indo–European in order to account for the vowel alternations known as 'Ablaut'. Since these alternations are a matter partly of vowel quality and partly of quantity, they are assumed to have arisen as a result of differences of pitch–accent and stress–accent respectively, and different historical stages can therefore be postulated in the development of early Indo–European where each of these was dominant in turn.

In the late nineteenth and early twentieth centuries, this philological tradition was challenged from several quarters. In the first place, the developing discipline of phonetics raised doubts about the physical reality of a phenomenon to which, apparently, no consistent phonetic properties could be assigned. Phoneticians such as Sweet, Jespersen, and others, champion an approach which takes actual phonetic features and describes their linguistic uses, rather than the older approach which takes a traditional philological label and attempts to interpret it.[6] Sweet (1877, 1906), for example, effectively ignores 'accent', while giving detailed descriptions of *force* on the one hand and *pitch* on the other, as separate phenomena. The 'musical accent' of some Baltic and Slavic languages is dealt with under 'intonation', and grouped together with tone in such languages as Chinese. Though recognizing that force and pitch may often go together, Sweet (1906: 72) explicitly warns against equating them: 'it is a mistake to suppose . . .

---

[4] In the present book, the pitch features of these languages are accounted for in a different manner (see 4.7.3), and the concept of 'pitch–accent' is employed more narrowly. See 3.3.4, below.

[5] Verner notes that 'for the older period of Germanic we have to start with an accent which was not purely chromatic like the accent in Sanskrit and the Classical languages, but which, like modern accentuation, had something expiratory about it, that is, was based on greater activity of the muscles of expiration and to the subsequently stronger exhalation of air'. He attributes the occurrence of voiceless consonants to this expiratory accent: 'the stronger expiration of air is an element which the expiratory accent has in common with the voiceless consonants' (translations from Lehmann (ed.), 1967).

[6] Sievers (1901), on the other hand, maintains the distinction between 'expiratory' or 'dynamic' and 'musical' or 'tonic' accent.

that high tone and strong stress can be regarded as convertible terms'. A similar separation of the two is found in the works of other phoneticians, such as Jespersen, who explicitly rejects the term 'musical accent': 'what I here call tone is often called "musical accent", which is inappropriate, since in music not only pitch but also length and intensity . . . play a significant part (just as quantity and force, as well as tone, do in speech)' (Jespersen, 1913: 225). Jespersen expresses the hope that he has contributed to 'opposing the careless use of expressions such as *Ton, betont, Hochton, Akzent, guttural,* etc.' Thus, 'accent' is considered to be in principle an inadmissible concept, since it has no consistent phonetic basis.

The traditional accentual dichotomy also came under scrutiny from within the philological tradition itself, most notably in the works of the German scholars Saran and Schmitt. Saran (1907) affirms the essential unity of accent because of its role in ranking the syllables within the word. Because of this role, 'it is understandable how quantity and strength could be substituted for pitch without destroying the content of the concept "accent" '(p.18). This naturally requires us 'to separate conceptually accent as such from the means of producing it, to distinguish accent and accentual factors'.[7]

Nevertheless, Saran does attempt to establish some sort of physical basis for accent, first by the elimination of pitch; for him 'melody' is different from 'accent'. But we cannot identify accent with 'strength of articulation', either; Saran therefore prefers to use 'heaviness' or 'weight' ('Schwere', 'Gewicht') as more general terms for the physical basis of accent.[8] Thus, ' "heaviness" (weight) is a component of accent, a significant feature of the concept, "strength" (loudness) one of the phonetic factors through which among others the mental impression of heaviness is produced' (p. 20). The reference to 'mental impression' here demonstrates the dangers of this approach, with its tendency to lapse into a vague psychologism. Saran ultimately has to invoke the somewhat mystical view of accent as *anima vocis*: 'accent is therefore the soul of speech, which is not identical with the phonetic material' (p. 19).

Schmitt (1924) explores the concept of accent from a similar perspective. He identifies three main relevant definitions of 'accent' in the usage of the day.[9] First, the term is used to refer to a *property of the syllable itself* ('syllable-accent'), for example 'rising accent', 'falling accent', 'circumflex accent', etc. Second, it can refer to the character of a syllable *in relation to others*, when one syllable is made more prominent than the other syllables in the word; and third, it can refer to *the relationship between all the parts of a word or sentence to one another*, or the way in which the utterance as a whole is structured.

---

[7] Translations here and passim by AF.

[8] This notion of 'weight' has nothing to do with the concept of 'syllable weight' discussed in Ch. 2.

[9] Schmitt actually lists five different types, but two can be eliminated without comment: a way of pronouncing ('a French accent', etc.) and a graphic mark ('acute accent', etc.).

According to Schmitt, the last of these, which has some relation to the very general view of accent as a 'way of speaking' that developed in traditional theory, can be termed 'accentuation' rather than 'accent'. The first definition applies to cases of the so-called 'musical accent' in languages such as Lithuanian or Serbo–Croat, which can again be eliminated terminologically by using the term 'intonation', traditional for this phenomenon in Baltic and Slavic linguistics.[10] We are left, therefore, with the second meaning: the character of a syllable in relation to others. Since 'accent' in this sense depends on the overall accentuation of the utterance, Schmitt defines it as an 'accentuation peak'.

But there are further difficulties here. As Schmitt notes, 'accent', even in this more restricted sense, can still be defined in different ways, either as a *psychological* or as a *physical* (physiological or acoustic) phenomenon. The first sees accent as an element of 'internal speech', the latter as an element of 'external speech', that is, as the means by which accent is realized, as stress, pitch or length. The psychological sense is regarded as derivative, however, since although there is a 'perceived accent' it is merely the sensation of a possible articulation. Furthermore, if 'accent' is an 'accentuation peak', then it cannot be a matter of either pitch or length, since neither of these can—according to Schmitt—form a peak; in his view, pitch can only form a *scale*, and there cannot, therefore, be a 'pitch–accent' which is independent of stress. This leaves us with stress[11] alone as the manifestation of accent. There is a further problem in this, however, since stress is speaker-based, and therefore irrelevant for the hearer. Schmitt achieves a compromise—somewhat in contradiction to his rejection of psychological factors—by assuming that hearing involves 'an active inner reproduction of what is spoken' (1924: 38).

Some attention has been devoted here to the work of Saran and Schmitt, not because of its intrinsic merit—though their discussion is by no means devoid of interest—but because it presents particularly clear evidence for the problem of defining accent, as it was perceived in the early decades of the twentieth century. Both philological work such as this and the phonetic work of Sweet, Jespersen, and others, point towards a dissatisfaction with the traditional approach to accent, and constitute an attempt to establish the nature of 'accentual' features on a sounder basis, though the specific solutions proposed differ considerably. In both cases, however, the scholars concerned appear to be groping for an adequate terminological and, more importantly, conceptual framework for accent; reluctant to accept the validity of the traditional view, with its dichotomy

---

[10] This term is now widely used in a different sense, of course, which will form the subject of Ch. 5. Schmitt notes this usage, but deplores it.

[11] There are some translation difficulties here, though the problems lie somewhat deeper. Schmitt's term is *Druck*, which translates literally as 'pressure', but he relates it to Jespersen's term *Exspirationsstärke* ('expiratory strength') and also claims that it is synonymous with 'intensity'; the term 'stress' is therefore a somewhat arbitrary compromise translation here. These terminological uncertainties are symptomatic of the conceptual confusion surrounding accent.

between dynamic and musical accent, they attempt to establish the phonetic correlates of accent, only to find that they are elusive and ambiguous.

Seen from the perspective provided by subsequent developments, these discussions appear to lack an important element: the phonological dimension. Without recourse to phonological concepts, there is no way of unifying the disparate phonetic features attributed to accent under a common heading, other than by an appeal to vague psychological principles. Though concerned to eliminate such 'unscientific' vagueness, these earlier scholars appear to have nothing to put in its place. We shall see in the course of this chapter how, and to what extent, the injection of phonological concepts can resolve these difficulties.

3.2 The Phonetic Basis of Accent

3.2.1 INTRODUCTION

We have seen that the traditional approach to accent failed to resolve adequately the problem of its phonetic nature. Determining the phonetic basis of accent, unlike that of other prosodic features, is evidently not merely a matter of identifying the physiological mechanisms responsible for producing the relevant acoustic feature and its auditory effect; the phonetic characterization of accent is as much a matter of theory as it is of phonetic fact.

A number of different approaches have been adopted here. As we have noted, phoneticians such as Sweet and Jespersen sought a solution to the problem by identifying phonetic parameters of speech production, specifically 'force' and 'pitch', and systematizing these in preference to pursuing phonetic correlates of an assumed 'accent'. This approach has continued to be developed, with the application of more sophisticated experimental techniques. Other scholars have looked for the nature of stress in the sound itself, a task that has also become easier with the development of the appropriate instruments. Since stress is assumed to be a reality for the hearer, experimental techniques have also been used to determine which features are perceptually relevant. Ideally, the results of these different approaches should coincide, or at least converge, but this is not always the case, and it is often evident that the findings with respect to the nature of accent tend to reflect the initial assumptions. Nevertheless, as the following discussion will show, it has been possible to clarify a number of important issues.[12]

3.2.2 ACCENT AND THE SPEAKER

From the late nineteenth century onwards, phoneticians have considered 'stress'

---

[12] For a survey of some views on the phonetic aspects of stress up to the late 1960s, see also Crystal (1969: 113–20).

to be an essentially physiological, and therefore speaker-based, phenomenon. Jones (1967: 134) states that 'stresses are essentially subjective activities of the speaker', and thus 'in actual language it is often difficult, and may be impossible, for the hearer to judge where strong stresses are' (p. 135). Allen (1973: 83) contrasts this with pitch: 'the criteria of stress are to be sought primarily in the speaker, but those of pitch primarily in the listener'.

Sweet and his contemporaries considered that stress reflects the 'force' put into the utterance by the speaker, but the nature of such force is open to a variety of interpretations, according to where it is assumed to be localized. Sweet (1906: 47) asserts that 'it is synonymous with the effort by which the breath is expelled from the lungs', and therefore a matter of respiratory activity. Jespersen (1913: 119), on the other hand, while endorsing this in principle, claims that stress cannot necessarily be localized; it is 'energy, intensive muscular activity, which is not limited to a single organ, but puts its stamp on the whole articulation'. A similar view is expressed by Jones (1967: 134), who considers it to be 'force of utterance', involving greater overall effort on the part of the speaker.

Other phoneticians have attempted to make this more precise by the application of experimental methods. Stetson (1928) proposes a theory of articulation which assumes that every syllable is accompanied by a ballistic 'chest pulse' produced by the internal intercostal muscles, and that in stressed syllables this pulse is reinforced by the activity of the abdominal muscles. Though espoused by a number of linguists, including Abercrombie (1967) and Allen (1973), this theory has not been supported by later work; Ladefoged (1967: 2–3) asserts that it is merely 'an hypothesis attempting to explain how the respiratory muscles might be involved in speech, rather than an account of the observed action of these muscles'. In his own work, Ladefoged, like Sweet, relates stress to the respiratory mechanism, and, using electro-myography, finds an increase in the activity of the intercostal muscles just before the stressed syllables, which results in an increase in subglottal pressure (Ladefoged *et al.*, 1958; Ladefoged, 1967). Because the effect of this on the acoustic features (intensity, duration, and fundamental frequency) is complex and variable, he concludes that 'stress is best described in physiological rather than acoustic terms'. A similar conclusion is reached by Fónagy (1958), who again defines stress in terms of force, and relates it to the activity of the internal intercostal muscles. Like Ladefoged, he rejects an acoustic definition of stress, and considers it misleading to distinguish 'dynamic' and 'musical' accent; for him *all* accents are dynamic.

Another attempt to determine the physiological basis of stress is made by Catford (1977: 84–5), who concludes that 'there seems to be little doubt that initiator power is the organic-aerodynamic phonetic correlate of what is often called "stress"'. 'Initiator power' is defined as 'the product of initiator-velocity and the pressure-load against which the initiator is acting' (91–2). Since one component of this is the force exerted by the respiratory muscles, this definition is evidently not unrelated to the earlier views of Sweet and Jones.

Not all investigators are convinced about the general validity of such physiological correlates, however. Lehiste (1970: 106) concludes that 'there is no single mechanism to which the production of stress can be attributed', while Ohala (1977) asserts that many of the claims about the physiological factors in stress relate only to emphatic stress, and not to normal stress: 'the data obtained so far do not support the notion that there must always be an appreciable expiratory pulse accompanying the production of ordinary (non-emphatic) stressed syllables'. He does concede, nevertheless, that in the case of emphatic stress, 'the involvement of the respiratory system is quite apparent'.

The speaker-based view of stress is also reinforced by a number of other observations. Several scholars link stress with rhythm: Sweet (1906: 50) refers to the 'rhythmic character' of stress as one of its most important properties,[13] while Catford (1977) incorporates the rhythmical foot into his principle of initiator power, the foot corresponding to a 'quantum' of such power.[14] Rhythm is here assumed to be speaker-based rather than perceptual. A further piece of evidence that stress is bound up with other aspects of speaker activity is the observation that stressed syllables are often accompanied by gestures (Jones, 1967: 135; Vanvik, 1955a). We may also note that some scholars attribute a physiological dimension even to the auditory perception of stress. We have already seen that Schmitt (1924) interpreted a perceived accent as the hearer's sensation of a possible articulation, and Ladefoged *et al.* (1958) also remark that when a listener thinks he hears stress he is probably perceiving how his muscles would have reacted in producing it.

3.2.3 ACCENT AND THE HEARER

Most discussions of the phonetic basis of accent have been concerned with its acoustic and auditory properties rather than with their physiological cause. Acoustic properties are much more accessible to observation and measurement than physiological properties, which generally require invasive techniques. Acoustically, sounds can differ from one another in *quality, duration, intensity,* and *fundamental frequency*, and attention has been paid to determining which of these is present as the acoustic manifestation of accent or stress. From an auditory perspective, duration, intensity, and frequency correspond to *length, loudness,* and *pitch,* and investigations have here been directed towards establishing which of these features contain the perceptual cues to the identification of accented syllables.

Apart from some earlier studies, such as that of Panconcelli-Calzia (1917),

---

[13] Sweet is, however, somewhat ambivalent here, sometimes insisting (1889) that 'English stress is not rhythmic, but logical'.
[14] The view of accent as rhythm has a long history; it is found in the work of Joshua Steele (1775). It has been adopted more recently by a number of phonologists, especially in the metrical framework (see below).

serious investigation of these issues begins in the 1930s. Muyskens (1931) investigates the acoustic correlates of accent in English, Parmenter and Blanc (1933) also examine them in French, while Chiba (1935) undertakes a wide ranging study covering eleven different languages of various prosodic types. Although, given the general conclusion from physiological studies that stress depends on some sort of expiratory effort, we would expect acoustic studies to identify intensity as its major correlate, in fact this is not so. Muyskens finds evidence that the realization of accent includes pitch, and the same is true, according to Parmenter and Blanc, for the accent in French and English. They assert that pitch is the most significant feature of accent in French, though intensity is more significant in English. Chiba's investigations, on the other hand, confirm the more traditional view of accent, allowing him to establish three kinds of languages, according to the predominant acoustic feature of accent: Chinese, Japanese, Korean, and Mongolian have a pitch–accent; Russian, German, English, and Hindustani have a stress–accent; French has a 'sonority accent'.

Later investigations, such as those discussed by Schramm (1937), are more revealing, however. Schramm reports on a number of experiments to determine the acoustic correlates of accent in American English; they show that 'as a general rule, the more prominent a syllable is, the greater will be its length, intensity, and range of inflection, and the higher its average pitch', but that increased duration and changes in the fundamental frequency are generally more important than intensity in differentiating accented from unaccented syllables. This view is supported by Mol and Uhlenbeck (1956), whose experiments demonstrate that 'in so called dynamic stress intensity cannot be considered as a factor, regardless whether this term is taken in an acoustic or in an articulatory sense'. Whatever the physiological basis of accent, therefore, it cannot be correlated with acoustic intensity; fundamental frequency is more important and reliable. Similar conclusions are drawn in relation to Polish stress by Jassem (1959); though traditionally considered to be of the 'dynamic' variety, it is found in Jassem's analyses to be 'melodic', with fundamental frequency playing the major role, and intensity and duration being only incidental. Similar results are reported for French by Rigault (1962).

In a number of perceptual studies, it has also been confirmed that pitch is far more important than intensity as a cue to the identification of accented syllables. An early experiment by Scott (1939) attempted to prove this, eliminating pitch cues by placing the relevant words (the pair *im'port* (verb) and *'import* (noun)) in a position where they would receive no intonational prominence. His test sentences were 'Are you sure Wood imports wood?' and 'Are you sure wood imports would?', with the intonational nucleus ('sentence stress') on *sure*. He found that errors of interpretation by listeners were frequent, and concluded that 'there seems to be a strong indication that stress, unaided, is not very efficient as a distinguishing feature in English'. In a number of classic experiments, Fry (1955, 1958) used similar pairs to demonstrate that duration is a much better

cue than intensity to the identification of the accented syllable, but that pitch is
the overriding factor. Comparable experiments were carried out by Lieberman
(1960), using similar pairs of words; his ranking of perceptual cues being pitch,
amplitude, and duration. Morton and Jassem (1965) use nonsense syllables and
come to the same conclusion.

Taking this one step further, Bolinger (1957, 1958a, 1958b, 1958c, 1965) puts
forward a theory of 'pitch–accent' in English, which not only recognizes that
'pitch is our main cue to stress', but defines different kinds of accent in terms
of pitch prominence of various kinds. Thus, the pitch pattern of an utterance
is characterized by various prominent pitch features ('corners') which can signal
stress in different ways. Bolinger (1958a) recognizes three such pitch–accents:
Accent A, in which there is a drop in pitch either within or immediately following the accented syllable; Accent B, which involves a rise in pitch, either before
or after the accented syllable; and Accent C, which is 'a kind of anti-accent A',
in which the accented syllable is 'skipped down to' (see Fig. 3.1). Accent is
here defined entirely in terms of pitch, and intensity is regarded as 'at best
unnecessary'.

Fig. 3.1. *Bolinger's 'pitch–accents'*

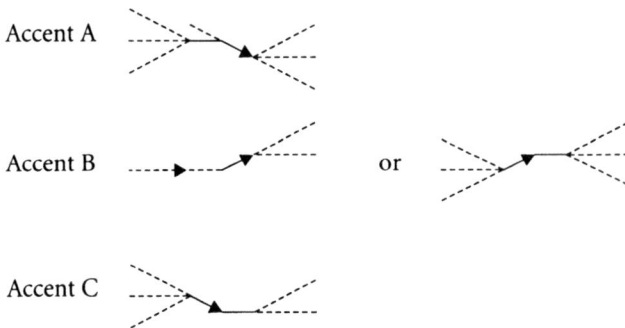

Definition of accent in terms of pitch, or as the combined effect of a range
of acoustic features, of which pitch is the most significant, naturally poses problems for the physiological view of accent or stress as extra 'force'. Lehiste (1970)
suggests that we should restrict the term 'stress' to the physiological properties,
and use 'accent' in a wider sense to include the various other features which
may contribute to the creation of 'prominence'. However, this still leaves open
the question whether this 'stress' is actually the phonetic basis of 'accent', and
whether 'accent' can be defined phonetically at all.

3.2.4 CONCLUSION: WHAT IS ACCENT?

The fact that different scholars identify different phonetic correlates of 'accent' suggests two different, and not necessarily mutually exclusive, conclusions. On the one hand, we might conclude that there are different kinds of accent, each with different phonetic manifestations, and that different investigators are therefore examining different phenomena. There is some evidence for this, since some claims relate to 'emphatic' rather than 'normal' accent, while some speak of 'word-stress' and others of 'nuclear stress'. It is by no means certain that all of these kinds of 'accent' are linguistically the same phenomenon. On the other hand, we may draw a different conclusion from the different results obtained: that accent does not have a consistent phonetic manifestation, and cannot, therefore, be defined in phonetic terms. Again, there is evidence to support such a claim.

We have seen that the traditional view assumes that accent may be manifested in two forms, dynamic and musical, where the latter includes the accentual features of languages such as Lithuanian, Latvian, Serbo–Croat, Swedish, and Norwegian. Some scholars also include Chinese and other tone languages in the same category, but these can legitimately be eliminated, as tone is in principle independent of accentuation. The accentual phenomena of Lithuanian, Swedish, and the other languages just mentioned, can also be excluded here, as they can be interpreted as a 'tonal accent', i.e. a restricted tone-system superimposed upon an accentual system, in such a way that only accented syllables are susceptible to tonal differentiation (cf. 4.7.3, below). This means, therefore, that the traditional category of 'musical accent' could be eliminated altogether from the discussion of accentual phenomena.

However, more recent work has identified a further language whose pitch features can be regarded as accentual: Japanese. Though earlier thought to be tonal, the pitch–accents of Japanese cannot be compared either to the tones of Chinese—they do not form a system of contrasting pitches in the way that Chinese tones do—or to the 'tonal accents' of Serbo–Croat or Swedish. In fact, they are in many ways comparable to the 'dynamic' accentual features of a language such as English.[15]

Beckman (1986), in a detailed study of the phonetic manifestations of accent in English and Japanese, is able to draw some significant conclusions regarding the phonetic basis of accent in general. Her investigations are based on two presuppositions: (1) 'that there is such a thing as accent that can be identified and separated from other phonological phenomena in a language', and (2) 'that phonological categories are not necessarily phonetically uniform across languages or even within a language' (p. ix). On this basis she puts forward, and substantiates, the 'stress–accent hypothesis', which claims that 'stress–accent' (i.e. the type of accent found in English or Dutch) differs phonetically from 'non-stress accent' (the type of accent found in Japanese) in that 'it uses to a greater extent

---

[15] For a more detailed discussion of Japanese accent, see 3.3.4, below.

material other than pitch'. In other words, we can identify a single phonological phenomenon, 'accent', which can be manifested either as stress–accent or as non-stress accent, the difference between these two being a matter of the use made of features other than pitch; in the latter, the accent is primarily, and perhaps exclusively, based on pitch; in the former, other phonetic features contribute. Beckman attempts to show that there is an essential unity to accent and that it is distinct from both tone and intonation. The unity is not, however, in the phonetic manifestation of accent but in its functional role as an 'organizational' feature of utterances (see below). Since pitch is a constituent element of 'accent' (whether 'stress' or 'non-stress'), the differences between accent and tone, and accent and intonation, do not lie in their phonetic basis at all, but in this difference of function.

Though Beckman appears to be returning to the traditional distinction between 'dynamic' and 'musical' accent, she in fact rejects this distinction (1986: 3–4) since it is based on phonetic features identified a priori; her distinction recognizes, like the traditional one, a unitary 'accent', but on the one hand excludes—unlike the traditional view—tonal and intonational features, and on the other hand regards the different manifestations not as the use of one phonetic feature as opposed to another but rather as the greater or lesser use of the same phonetic material.

Beckman's approach appears to solve many of the problems that we have encountered in trying to identify the phonetic basis of accent. It enables us to conclude that 'accent' is not, in fact, definable in phonetic terms but only in terms of its phonological role, which is taken to be an 'organizational' one. Attempts to base a definition on phonetic features, whether physiological, acoustic, or auditory, are therefore in principle bound to be unsatisfactory. Nevertheless, we can, with Beckman, identify two main phonetic manifestations of accent, 'stress–accent' and 'non-stress accent' (which we may call 'pitch–accent'), where the latter is almost exclusively a matter of pitch, and the former a combination of a number of features, including pitch, duration, intensity, and perhaps other properties. On this view, therefore, 'accent' is, phonetically speaking, a kind of 'place-holder' for a number of features which contribute both to its realization and to its identification. Furthermore, one such feature, 'stress', is not a phonetically consistent phenomenon, but is itself a cover-term for a set of phonetic properties, including, as its major but not exclusive component, pitch. This approach will be taken as the starting point for the discussion of the phonology of accent in the remainder of this chapter.

From the terminological point of view, this means that we can make a little more precise the use of the terms 'accent' and 'stress' in this chapter. The former will continue to be used as the general term, while 'stress' can now be used in the sense of Beckman, to mean accent manifested by a number of phonetic features, but *not* exclusively pitch. Since 'pitch–accent' (Beckman's 'non-stress' accent) is apparently rare, and the majority of languages use stress as a realization of accent, the terms 'accent' and 'stress' can often be used interchangeably.

3.3 The Phonological Basis of Accent

3.3.1 INTRODUCTION

We saw in 3.1.2 that late nineteenth and early twentieth century scholars attempted to find a suitable conceptual and terminological framework for accentual phenomena. The traditional descriptive categories—'musical' and 'dynamic' accent—appeared to be unsatisfactory, in part because their phonetic basis was unclear, and in part because the concept of 'accent' was itself vague. Both of these problems can probably be traced to the lack of a *phonological* dimension, which allows phonetically disparate phenomena to be subsumed under a single linguistic entity, yet avoids dubious psychological assumptions.

The phonological dimension was provided from the 1930s onwards with the reinterpretation of traditional categories in structuralist terms. It is possible, though at the risk of some over-simplification, to identify three main approaches to accentuation within the structuralist paradigm. First, Prague School linguists developed a framework which can legitimately be seen as the direct successor of traditional descriptive practice, though interpreted in a characteristically Praguian way. This involves the strict application of *functional* principles, and therefore approaches accent in terms of its different roles in distinguishing or characterizing words. American structuralist linguists, on the other hand, eschew functional concepts as mentalistic and procedurally inadequate, and apply *distributional* criteria to the individual phonetic features involved. A third approach, which is not so easily characterized in terms of any coherent theoretical orientation or consistent methodological precepts, is found among pedagogically oriented scholars, principally teachers of English pronunciation in the British phonetic tradition. Their concern is less with theoretically adequate formalization than with the identification of pedagogically useful categories. Other contributions to the debate on the nature of accent have, of course, been made which lie outside these general groupings. In what follows, we shall consider some of the salient characteristics of accentuation from the perspective of these different approaches.

3.3.2 THE PARADIGMATIC ANALYSIS OF ACCENT

If 'accent' is considered to be phonologically distinctive, then one approach to the phonological description of accent and stress is to establish a set of mutually contrasting 'degrees' or 'levels', thus treating accent *paradigmatically*. Most traditional treatments are concerned only with accent as a feature which gives prominence to a single syllable in the word; by implication, therefore, a two-term system is recognized with 'accented' and 'unaccented' syllables. Some scholars go further; Sweet (1906), for example, recognizes three degrees of 'force': 'level', 'increasing', and 'decreasing', as well as three main degrees of stress: 'strong', 'half strong', and 'weak'. In addition, there may be 'very strong' or 'extra strong' stress, and 'a weak stress slightly stronger than another weak one'. The three main degrees of stress are exemplified in expressions such as *contradict* or *come at once*, each of which is claimed to have one occurrence of each 'degree'. However, in the absence of a phonological framework, these degrees are clearly purely phonetic, and indeed Sweet acknowledges that the degrees of stress are 'really infinite'.

It is also not completely clear on what basis these degrees are established. Sweet states (p. 50) that the word 'impenetrability' has, 'roughly speaking', two stresses, 'a strong one on the fifth and a medium one on the first', but he notes that if we divide it into two parts we observe that the syllables of each part (*impenetra-* and *-bility*) have different degrees within them. Putting them together, we can assign the sequence 2 3 7 5 1 6 4 (where 1 is the highest) to the word as a whole. However, he does not consider whether the stress relations of the parts are actually preserved phonetically when they are put together, and indeed advocates pronouncing the syllables *mentally* in order to establish their order. The phonetic status of the stress levels is therefore somewhat doubtful. In any case, Sweet does not claim any linguistic significance for the different degrees. His lead is followed by other phoneticians, such as Jespersen (1913), who recognizes four degrees, but admits that they are arbitrary.

A more elaborate set of levels is established by Saran (1907). As we saw above, he distinguishes 'heavy' and 'light' syllables; he goes on to recognize three degrees of each, giving the six degrees of Fig. 3.2, and adds two further degrees, *überschwer 2* ('over-heavy 2') and *überschwer 1* ('over-heavy 1') to deal with cases of emphasis and contrast. Again, however, there is no concept of phonological distinctiveness here, and the levels are merely what are assumed to be phonetically recognizable gradations.

Fig. 3.2   *schwer* (heavy):
      1. *vollschwer* (full-heavy) ´
      2. *mittelschwer* (middle-heavy) ``
      3. *halbschwer* (half-heavy) `
      leicht (light):
      4. *halbleicht* (half-light)
      5. *volleicht* (full-light)
      6. *überleicht* (over-light)

The pedagogical tradition, reflected, for example, in the works of Jones and his followers, is both more sophisticated and more linguistically informed, with a conscious appeal to phonological relevance, though the focus is not primarily theoretical. This approach is more sparing in its use of different 'degrees' of stress, often recognizing, in addition to a simple 'stressed' vs. 'unstressed' distinction, an additional 'secondary stress', which appears in longer words, effectively giving three 'degrees', though the distinction between 'primary' and 'secondary' is not always consistently drawn. Thus we find transcriptions such as /ˌsentrəlaiˈzeiʃn/ (*centralisation*) and /ədˌminisˈtreiʃn/ (*administration*), with a secondary stress—indicated by the subscript ˌ —preceding the primary stress, and /ˈfutˌpæsindʒə/ (*foot-passenger*) and /ˈketlˌhouldə/ (*kettle-holder*), where the secondary stress follows (Jones, 1956: 256, 258). According to Jones, a long word such as *intellectuality* may have two secondary stresses (/ˌintiˌlektjuˈæliti/), though the alternative pronunciations /ˌintilektjuˈæliti/ (with a single secondary stress) and /ˈintiˌlektjuˈæliti/ (with two primary stresses) are also given. In addition, a distinction is sometimes made between 'word-stress' and 'sentence stress', though this is not generally regarded as involving a further 'degree'. Further differences are provided by 'emphatic' and 'contrastive' stress, but these are not usually seen as part of the stress system proper. Jones explains away further degrees of stress as cases of 'prominence' rather than stress, where prominence is an auditory effect which may result from a variety of characteristics of a syllable, including inherent qualities of the sounds themselves as well as stress and pitch (Jones, 1967: 137 ff.). He is thus left with just two degrees, with an occasional 'secondary stress', though he does not attach much importance to the latter, since the position of the secondary stress has no linguistic role.[16]

More theoretically oriented scholars have also attempted to establish systems of distinctive stresses. Bloomfield (1935: 90–2) identifies 'stress' with loudness; in English words of more than one syllable, stress 'consists in speaking one of these syllables louder than the other or others'. He goes on to establish a system of contrasting stresses: 'loudest stress' (marked "), as in *That's "mine!*, 'ordinary stress' (marked '), as in *ex'amine* or *I've 'seen it*, and 'less loud stress' (marked ˌ), as in *'milkˌman*.[17] These are considered to be 'secondary phonemes', i.e. phonemes which 'are not part of any simple meaningful speech-form taken by itself, but appear only when two or more are combined into a larger form'.

Bloomfield's successors refine and elaborate this system considerably. Trager and Bloch (1941) and Bloch and Trager (1942) establish, by means of comparisons of various word forms, a set of four stress 'phonemes' for English, again based on relative loudness: 'loud', 'reduced loud', 'medial' and 'weak', together with the corresponding diacritics, á, â, à, and a (unmarked). Examples of the application of these are given in Fig. 3.3 (cf. Bloch and Trager, 1942: 48), and their use is illustrated in the sentence *A lánguage is a sýstem of ârbitràry vôcal sýmbols.*

[16] Jones notes one exception: the word *certification*, whose meaning may differ according to the position of the secondary stress. A distinction could be made between /ˌsəːtifiˈkeiʃn/, meaning *act of certifying*, and /səːˌtifiˈkeiʃn/, meaning *granting a certificate* (Jones, 1967: 148).

[17] Bloomfield also includes the syllabicity of a syllabic consonant in the same system. It is described as 'a slight stress which makes this primary phoneme louder than what precedes and what follows'.

Fig. 3.3 cát, ánd, yés   cóntènts, rótàte   bláck-bîrd, réd-câp
          béllow, cúrrent   ùntíe, ròmánce   ôld-mán, rêd-bárn
          belów, corréct   réctifŷ, démocràt   téll(h)im-sô, stóp-thât
          énemy, pólitics   rèferée, dèmocrátic   câtan(d)-dóg, sêe(h)im-rún
          anáemic, polítely   ásk-fòrit, nòt-atáll móvie-àuditôrium, élevàtor-
                                                     ôperàtor

A virtually identical system is presented by Trager and Smith (1951), who label
the four degrees 'primary', 'secondary', 'tertiary' and 'weak'. These are exemplified in Fig. 3.4. They are again described as differences in loudness, reflecting
relative strength of articulation. The label 'weak stress' is used in preference to
'unstressed', because 'it seems better to have a positive rather than a negative
terminology' (p. 36).

Fig. 3.4 PRIMARY: /´/   yés, gó, únder, góing, abóve, allów
          SECONDARY: /ˆ/   élevàtor+ôperàtor, élevàtor+òperâtion
          TERTIARY: /ˋ/   sýntàx, cóntènts, ànimátion, hèterogéneous,
                               díctionàry
          WEAK: /˘/ or / / (the unmarked vowels in the above examples)

Newman (1946) sets up a similar set of 'stress–accents' for English, including
three 'phonemic classes' and six 'varieties' (i.e. allophones) of stress. These exclude such phenomena as 'contrastive accent' and 'rhetorical accent' which involve other prosodic features. The three phonemic classes of stress, which are
illustrated in Fig. 3.5, are 'heavy stress' (which can be 'nuclear' or 'subordinate'),
'middle stress' (which can be 'full' or 'light'), and 'weak stress' (which can be
'sonorous' or 'pepet').

Fig. 3.5   I Heavy stress (´)
              1. Nuclear heavy: ánnual, súbject
              2. Subordinate heavy: ánnual méeting, súbject of discússion
          II Middle stress (ˋ)
              1. Full middle: àntárctic, sùbdóminant
              2. Light middle: ànalógical, sùbjectívity
         III Weak stress (unmarked)
              1. Sonorous weak: ancéstral, sulfúric
              2. Pepet weak: análogy, subjéctive

It is not easy to interpret these different 'degrees', nor to relate the different
systems to one another. Bloomfield's 'loudest stress' must be eliminated from the
system as an expression of 'emphasis', so that Newman's 'heavy stress' then
corresponds to Bloomfield's 'ordinary stress' and Trager and Bloch's 'loud'/
'primary' stress. It also appears that Newman's 'middle stress' can be identified
with Bloomfield's 'less loud stress' and Trager and Bloch's 'medial'/'tertiary'
stress. Newman has no equivalent to Trager and Bloch's 'reduced loud' or

'secondary' stress, however. The 'primary stress' of the British pedagogical tradition can clearly be related—in the majority of cases, at least—to Trager and Bloch's 'loud' or 'primary' stress, but the elusive nature of the 'secondary stress' of this tradition makes it difficult to relate it consistently to Newman's 'middle stress' or Trager and Bloch's 'secondary' or 'tertiary' stress.

But there are also difficulties in interpreting these degrees within each framework. In particular, Trager and Bloch's 'secondary stress' and Newman's 'middle stress' pose problems. In the former case, the 'secondary stress' only occurs in compound words or phrases, while the 'tertiary stress' can also occur in uncompounded single words. Trager and Smith (1951) therefore make the occurrence of this stress phoneme dependent on the presence of an 'internal open juncture' ('plus juncture') /+/, which generally corresponds to a word-division or a word-internal morpheme boundary. Contrasts between secondary and tertiary stress are postulated, as in the examples of Fig. 3.6; 'tertiary' stress is recognized in cases where the two roots of the compound are closely linked, and 'secondary' stress is assumed with more loosely linked compounds or non-compounded phrases (Trager and Smith, 1951: 39).

Fig. 3.6   òld+máid ('spinster') vs. ôld+máid ('former servant')
            Lòng+Ísland vs. lông+ísland.
            bláck+bìrd vs. bláck+bôard
            Whíte+Hòuse vs. whíte+hôuse (not a brown one)

Structures such as those of Fig. 3.6 are interpreted differently by different scholars. In the case of compounds, Jones (1956: 257 ff.) treats words such as *greenhouse* (to which Trager and Smith would presumably give the primary + tertiary pattern of *White House*) as having only a single stress, while *kettle-holder* appears as either /ˈketlhouldə/ or /ˈketlˌhouldə/. Noun phrases such as *long island* have secondary + primary for Bloch, Trager, and Smith, but Jones (p. 263), and the pedagogical tradition generally, give two or more primary stresses here: /ˈtuː ˈlaːdʒ ˈbraun ˈdɔgz/ (*two large brown dogs*). Newman's distinction between heavy and middle stresses also seems to depend on morphosyntactic factors, hence the occurrence of the middle stress on the first syllable of *ànalógical*, but the non-nuclear variant of the heavy stress on the first syllable of *ánnual méeting*. For Jones, these would have a secondary and a primary stress, respectively: /ˌanəˈlodʒikl/ and /ˈanjuəl ˈmiːtiŋ/; for Trager and Bloch perhaps tertiary and secondary. But Newman's three classes of stress do not relate directly to the pedagogical tradition, since he criticizes the descriptions of such traditional scholars as Curme, who distinguishes only 'primary', 'secondary' and 'unstressed', for conflating his subordinate heavy, middle, and sonorous weak (i.e. the stresses on the first syllables of *ánnual méeting*, *àntárctic*, and *ancéstral*) and including them all in the 'secondary stress' category.

The inconsistencies here clearly demand some sort of explanation. Apart from the view, which we should probably exclude in principle, that some of the scholars involved have made erroneous observations, we could attribute the discrepancies to difference of ideolect: the different linguists have different stress systems. But although there are certainly some differences in the accentuation of individual words or even types of words, these can account for only a very small part of the problem, and do not affect the basic principles, which remain in conflict. We could also attribute the differences to the different aims of different scholars, in particular the practical orientation of the pedagogical tradition as opposed to the theoretical objectives of Bloomfieldian scholars. But the different goals should not be over-emphasized; all the scholars here aim to establish the 'truth'. It is evident, therefore, that none of these explanations will serve; we must conclude, as does Sledd (1962: 43), that 'disagreements among analyses of English stress result more from differences of theory than from differences concerning fact'. It is necessary, therefore, to examine some of the theoretical issues underlying these analyses. These issues have been discussed by Newman (1946), Arnold (1957a, 1957b), Hill (1961), and Sledd (1962), among others.

As we have already noted, the different degrees of stress observed by American phonemicists depend on the presence of certain boundaries. Specifically, the occurrence of secondary stress requires an internal open juncture (see Fig. 3.6, above), which occurs only in looser compounds or close syntactic groups, while there is only one primary stress within the 'phonemic phrase', defined as the unit bounded by external open junctures (Trager and Bloch, 1941). This means that the different degrees of stress apply to different *domains of accentuation*. However, not all scholars accept the same domains as legitimate for the analysis; Jones (1967: 149) notes that 'the semantic function of more than two degrees of stress in English appears to be confined to sentences, or to compound words of a type that cannot in my view be taken into consideration in the investigation of phonemic distinctions'. For Jones, therefore, the domain of degrees of stress is evidently the uncompounded word, with a corresponding reduction—in comparison with the American approach—in the number of degrees that can be recognized; the distinction between the American secondary and tertiary stresses requires the presence of a compound word or a syntactic phrase, while the distinction between the primary and secondary stresses needs a 'phonemic clause' which contains more than one such word or phrase, both of which are excluded by Jones.[18]

A second factor which can result in differences of analysis is the extent to which intonational features are included in the stress system. The American approach treats stress and pitch as entirely separate, though interacting, systems; the British pedagogical tradition seeks rather to combine them. Attempts to relate stress and intonation go back at least as far as Coleman (1914), who concludes that intonation is the chief factor in the expression of 'emphasis', the

---

[18] Cf. also Hewson (1980), who concludes that we can recognize three levels of stress in words, and four in sentences.

latter term including both contrastive 'prominence' and non-contrastive 'intensity'. Palmer (1922, 1924), in his description of English intonation, establishes the *tone-group* as a unit, which he defines as 'a word or a series of words in connected speech containing one and only one maximum of prominence' (1924: 13). This maximum of prominence is called the *nucleus*, which is 'the stressed syllable of the most prominent word in the tone-group'. Thus, a link is established between the stress system and intonation, with the nucleus of the tone-group, which bears the major pitch features of the intonation pattern, coinciding with the 'primary stress' of the utterance. This approach is found in all the main descriptions of intonation in the British tradition (see Ch. 5, below).

Arnold (1957a, 1957b) applies this principle to the stress system itself, by distinguishing two types of strong stress: *tonic strong* and *non-tonic strong*, but, since one of his aims is to avoid defining stress in terms of pitch, he emphasizes that this difference is not one of stress proper; it represents 'the same degree of stress associated with different pitch features'. He also points out that Jones, in his *English Pronouncing Dictionary*, marks secondary stress *before* the primary stress more consistently than *after* it, and concludes that 'any secondary stress found preceding a principal stress is in reality a principal stress which lacks the pitch prominence always associated with a principal stress'. The fact that secondary stress occurring *after* the principal stress is less frequently marked by Jones (it is generally marked on the second element of compounds but not in simple words) he attributes to the fact that this stress is always associated with a non-prominent pitch pattern. In general, then, by excluding the pitch prominence associated with the nuclear stress, we effectively eliminate the difference between primary and secondary stress. We also dispose of the distinction, sometimes drawn in the pedagogical literature, between 'word-stress' and 'sentence stress', the latter being the same as the former but associated with the intonational nucleus.

Kingdon (1939) effects the complete integration of stress and intonation, at least as far as notation is concerned. Observing that 'sentence stress and intonation in English are so interdependent that to indicate one without the other is unsatisfactory', he introduces 'tonetic stress marks' which simultaneously indicate stress and the pitch of the stressed syllables, together with that of the surrounding unstressed syllables. These marks include ' ('a level stress of the pitch appropriate to its position in the tune'), " ('a level stress raised above the pitch normal to its position in the tune'), ˇ ('a fall–rise on a single syllable'), and so on. Although this device does not add anything to the classification of stress phenomena themselves, it does indicate the extent to which stress and intonation are mutually dependent, and the difficulty of establishing a stress system which is independent of pitch.

This fact is emphasized by a number of experiments made to determine the auditory cues for the perception of stress. As we have already noted, Scott (1939) found that listeners were unable to distinguish consistently between such pairs as *'import* (noun) and *im'port* (verb) when the intonational cues were removed by putting the words in a post-nuclear position. His conclusion—that 'there seems to be a strong indication that stress, unaided, is not very efficient as a distinguishing feature in English'—appears to be supported by the experiment conducted by Lloyd James (reported in Jones, 1956: 297), which involves pronouncing the word 'mechanically' on a monotone and giving strong stress to the first and third syllables. Listeners persisted in hearing the stress on the second syllable. The general conclusion that 'stress' is not the most important feature distinguishing the 'degrees' recognized here, is endorsed by many scholars in the pedagogical tradition, including, in addition to those mentioned above, Scott (1938), Vanvik (1955b), Gimson (1956), and Hill (1960). This accords, of course, with some of the conclusions reached from experimental phonetic investigations of stress discussed above.

We have examined two different approaches to the paradigmatic analysis of stress. The one takes a single phonetic parameter—assumed to be loudness—and arranges the perceived distinctions into a 'system' of contrasting items. The other sees this system as the product of more than one set of contrasts, in particular the superimposition of intonational features, specifically the 'nucleus' of the intonation pattern, onto a simple 'stressed' vs. 'unstressed' dichotomy. Also involved here are differences of domain; different stresses characterize units of different lengths or complexity.

All of this suggests that an autonomous system of paradigmatic stress contrasts faces a number of problems. It is clear that we do not have a set of mutually contrasting items in the normal sense, since we cannot contrast all the different degrees on a single monosyllabic utterance, as we can with, say, the different vowels. We can contrast /bɪt/, /bɛt/, and /bat/, for example, as isolated utterances, but not /bát/, /bât/, and /bàt/. This fact alone indicates that the stress system of a language such as English cannot be accounted for simply in terms of a set of 'stress phonemes'.

3.3.3 THE FUNCTIONAL ANALYSIS OF ACCENT

In the paradigmatic approach to the phonology of accent that we have examined so far, attempts have been made to establish a system of mutually contrasting 'degrees'. This approach assumes that there is a specific phonetic feature—in the American structuralist tradition this feature is 'loudness', though other features can be used for the same purpose—which can be seen in scalar terms. Some of the difficulties here can doubtless be attributed to the fact that, as discussed in 3.2, above, the phonetic basis of accent evidently cannot be reduced to a single scalar feature.

The approach adopted by Prague School linguists avoids this particular problem. Its starting point is not a specific phonetic feature which is systematized phonologically in terms of its linguistic distinctiveness but rather, in accordance with Praguian precepts that we have seen in other contexts, the assumed *functions* of such features. Though in other cases this may not affect radically the resulting analysis, in the case of accent it certainly does, since it may be argued that the functional role of accent is consistent in spite of the observed variability in its phonetic realization. A functional approach is therefore able to unite these different phonetic manifestations under a single functional heading.

Prague School theory can thus maintain the traditional distinction between 'dynamic' and 'musical' accent without recourse to the dubious psychological principles to which earlier phoneticians objected. It does this phonologically, by establishing functional categories, and by not insisting that each category should have a phonetically consistent manifestation. Jakobson (1931), in an early discussion of this question, recognizes that a particular portion of the speech signal may be given prominence, but that this may be achieved in different ways. Trubetzkoy (1935, 1939) similarly notes that accent involves giving greater auditory prominence to a syllable or mora in comparison to others, but states categorically that it is phonologically irrelevant how this is achieved, whether by raising the pitch, by increasing the loudness, by lengthening, or by more energetic articulation.[19]

Nevertheless, Jakobson does not ignore the distinction between 'dynamic' and 'musical' accent, but seeks to explain it in terms of the scope of accentual contrast. For him, in languages with dynamic accent 'the scope of the accent is phonologically always the same as the length of the syllabic phoneme', whereas in languages with musical accent 'the phonological equivalence of the scope of the accent and the length of the syllabic phoneme represents only one of the possible phonological varieties or does not occur at all'. What this means in practice is that languages with musical accent are mora-languages in which the accent may fall on either mora of a long vowel, in which case its scope does not coincide with that of the vowel itself. If the accent is on the first mora, we obtain a 'falling' accent; if it is on the second mora, we have a 'rising accent'. This is not quite equivalent to the traditional 'musical' accent, however, since prominence may be given to the mora in question by stress as well as high pitch. Nevertheless this interpretation is intended to cover 'polytonic' languages such as Lithuanian, where pitch is the major component of the traditional 'accent' types. The consequences of this approach are significant, since it effectively eliminates the paradigmatic dimension of accent altogether. Even the restricted paradigmatic tonal element of a language such as Lithuanian is here interpreted in syntagmatic terms, as merely another aspect of accent *placement*, though here placement *within* the syllable, rather than placement on one syllable as opposed to another.

---

[19] *Phonologisch wesentlich ist hier nur die allgemeine Hervorhebung des Gipfelprosodems, der Umstand, daß dieses Prosodem alle übrigen überragt, während die Mittel, durch welche diese Hervorhebung erreicht wird, zum Bereich der Phonetik gehören* (Trubetzkoy, 1939: 180).

Trubetzkoy adopts a different approach to the functions of accent. Phonological functions in general are considered to be of three basic kinds (Trubetzkoy, 1939: 29): 'distinctive' (or meaning-differentiating), 'culminative' (or peak-forming), and 'delimitative' (or boundary-marking). Since the distinctive function depends on paradigmatic contrasts, accentual features are in principle not distinctive, and they can therefore exercise only culminative or delimitative functions. Which of these is involved depends, however, on whether the accent is, in traditional terms, 'fixed' or 'free'. *All* accents are culminative, in the sense that they constitute a 'peak' within the word; the role of such a peak is, in Trubetzkoy's words (1939: 29), that 'they indicate how many "units" (= words, word-combinations) are contained in the sentence in question'.[20] However, accents can only serve a delimitative function, 'indicating the boundary between two units (= close word-combinations, words, morphemes)', if they are *bound* (i.e. fixed), that is, if they occur on a specific syllable in the word (for example, the initial syllable, as in Czech or Hungarian, or the penultimate syllable, as in Polish) or if their position is predictable from other features (for example, in Latin, where the position of the accent depends on the quantity of the penultimate syllable). Only with a bound accent is the word or morpheme boundary derivable from the position of the accent; if the accent is *free*, i.e. unpredictable, this function cannot be exercised. (It should be noted, however, that 'freedom' of the accent is a relative matter, and it may be constrained within various limits.) As we saw in 2.10.2, above, since accent and quantity are closely linked, and since either of these can be 'bound' or 'free', Trubetzkoy (1935) proposes a 4-way typology of languages on the basis of these features.

By focusing on the functional aspects of accent rather than its phonetic manifestation (culminative and delimitative functions are independent of how the accent is realized, whether by greater force, higher pitch, length, or differences of articulation), Jakobson and Trubetzkoy are able to treat the traditional distinction between dynamic and musical accent as functionally irrelevant, relegating it to a matter of phonetic realization. They are therefore able to remain aloof from the controversy surrounding the phonetic nature of accent. By seeing the functional role of accent as different from that of segmental features, and by reinterpreting 'musical' accent in terms of accent placement, they are, furthermore, able to shift attention from the paradigmatic to the syntagmatic dimension. However, they do not address directly the questions raised by the different 'degrees' of stress recognized in Bloomfieldian theory. Jakobson notes that accent

[20] Not all linguists would wish to characterize prosodic features in terms of grammatical units such as words. Hjelmslev (1937), for example, while sharing many of the Prague principles, such as the unity of 'accent' and the irrelevance of its phonetic manifestations, nevertheless objects to Trubetzkoy's reference to grammatical units here, since, in his Glossematic theory, such ('plerematic') units do not correspond to phonological ('cenematic') units. Thus, accent and intonation *characterize* the speech chain without *constituting* it.

may have a double function, inasmuch as it serves both as a unifying feature for the accented unit and as a means of giving prominence to one particular unit in contrast to others. There is no implication that different 'levels' or 'degrees' are involved here. Trubetzkoy (1939: 192–3) does allude to such degrees, however, in particular in languages such as English, German, and Dutch, where words may have more than one accent. Since the culminative function of accent is assumed to be that of indicating 'how many words', there is a potential problem in having more accents than words, and Trubetzkoy concludes that 'naturally only one of these syllables can be regarded as the word-peak, while the others are only subordinate accents'.[21] He distinguishes cases where unaccented syllables have certain gradations due to automatic factors such as rhythm, with, for example, alternate syllables receiving 'a secondary ictus', from cases of phonologically relevant subordinate accents, such as those found in German compounds like *Eísenbàhn, Hóchschùle,* etc., or in pairs such as *übersètzen* vs. *übersétzen.* In the latter case there is an opposition 'main accent' vs. 'subordinate accent'. Since this phenomenon occurs in Germanic languages, with their 'predilection for compound words', and in certain polysynthetic languages of America, Trubetzkoy links the occurrence of such subordinate accents with morphological compounding, a conclusion which, as we have seen, is comparable with that reached by scholars in other traditions. He does not follow up its consequences for a culminative theory of accent, however.

Later scholars in the Prague tradition have attempted to clarify the principles set out by Jakobson and Trubetzkoy, drawing out some of the implications of the functional approach. Martinet (1954, 1968) notes that although the distinction between segmental and prosodic features is widely considered to be fundamental, it is not significant from a functional point of view, since some prosodic features, especially tone, have exactly the same functions as segments, viz. they distinguish different words. But accent has a quite different function. In spite of the existence of some minimal pairs, its function is primarily contrastive (i.e. syntagmatic) rather than distinctive (paradigmatic), marking particular units in the chain of speech. Thus, it makes no sense, functionally speaking, to group together tone and accent phonologically.

Garde (1965, 1967, 1968) endorses Martinet's points and takes them further. He notes that the distinction between bound and free accent is of considerable importance for Trubetzkoy's theory since the two accents exercise very different functions. In fact, in spite of the recognition by Trubetzkoy of three different phonological functions, in practice the distinctive function is considered the most important, and the role of the free accent, since it may serve to distinguish different words, is more distinctive than that of the bound accent. However, Garde, like Martinet, argues that the function of the free accent should not be regarded as distinctive. Treating the free accent as distinctive, on a par with

---

[21] Translation by AF.

segmental features, would entail a vast complication of the vowel system, with the recognition of separate accented and unaccented vowel phonemes. However, this would not apply in a language with a bound accent. This inconsistency is anomalous, especially since it may often be a matter of historical accident whether the accent is bound or free,[22] and it 'breaks the unity of the notion of accent' (1968: 7). For Garde, however, in spite of the acknowledged differences between free and bound accent, they have the same (non-distinctive) function. Unlike distinctive features, where the functional issue is 'is it there or not?', accent is a question of 'is it there or elsewhere?' Its function is thus syntagmatic, a matter of contrast rather than opposition.

This discussion shows something of both the strengths and the weaknesses of the functional approach to accent. On the one hand, it allows us to accommodate the different phonetic manifestations of accent in different languages, by recognizing that these manifestations have the same functional role: that of making one syllable (or other relevant unit) more prominent than its neighbours. On the other hand, the functional emphasis may result in the separate classification of identical accentual phenomena on the basis of whether they happen to be fixed or free.

3.3.4 PITCH–ACCENT

Pitch has so far been considered in relation to accent in a number of ways. First, we have considered the traditional 'musical accent' (here called 'tonal accent') of languages such as Serbo–Croat and Lithuanian; this phenomenon will be considered further in 4.7.3, below. Second, we have seen that pitch is a consistent part of the so-called 'dynamic accent' in languages such as English. Third, we have noted that pitch, as intonation, has a close relationship to accentual features, and is by some linguists included as part of the accent itself. In another case, to be discussed in 4.7.5, tone has been regarded as accentual, since a single tone pattern is differently aligned with the syllables of the word, thus fulfilling a culminative function (Goldsmith, 1976). Each of these cases requires a different treatment, but in no case is it necessary to define accent itself in terms of pitch alone; tonal accent and intonation are distinct from accent proper, while the 'accentual' use of tone claimed especially for certain Bantu languages (see 4.7.5) is here interpreted merely as a restricted tone-system. Accent itself is considered to be more general than any specific phonetic manifestation.

There is one further case, however, where pitch has a more legitimate claim to be considered accentual, and where the term 'pitch–accent' may be appropriately used. This is the infrequent case where pitch alone is employed for the

---

[22] Martinet (1968) points out that the free accent of some Romance languages, such as Spanish and Italian, arose through the loss of the length distinctions of Latin which determined the position of the accent.

purposes of accentuation, but without forming part of a tone or intonation system. This is the situation found in Japanese.

Japanese

The accentual system of Japanese has long been the subject of scholarly interest. Traditional analyses attempt to interpret the pitch features of the language in terms of the tones of Chinese, equating the high pitch of the accent with the first (high level) tone of Mandarin, but Chinese is clearly not the best of models. More satisfactory analyses only emerged in Japan under Western influence after the turn of the century (see Shiro, 1967; Nishinuma, 1979), when the matter was deemed to be of sufficient seriousness to warrant an official investigation by a Japanese government committee (Jimbo, 1925). One interpretation that emerged from this, e.g. in the work of Jimbo (1925), establishes three pitch levels, low, mid, and high; other scholars have been able to reduce the distinctive levels to two (cf. Nishinuma, 1979).

The orthodox treatment appears with Miyata (1927), who identifies an 'accent kernel' at the point immediately before the fall in pitch. From that time, the basic principles of Japanese accentuation have been fairly clear, though its theoretical interpretation still remains the subject of debate. Apart from the phonetic studies of, for example, Fujisaki (Fujisaki and Sudo, 1971; Fujisaki, Hirose, and Ohta, 1979) and Beckman (1986), phonological interpretations are given from an American structuralist perspective by Bloch (1946) and Martin (1952, 1967, 1970), from the viewpoint of classical generative phonology by McCawley (1968, 1977) and Shibatani (1972), and in non-linear terms by Haraguchi (1977), Poser (1984), Pierrehumbert and Beckman (1988), and others. More general summaries and discussions are found in Vance (1987), Shibatani (1990), and Tsujimura (1996).

The 'facts' of Japanese accent can be summarized as follows. The basic prosodic unit in Japanese is the mora rather than the syllable (cf. 2.5.4; 2.8.3); one mora in each accentual unit is 'accented', this taking the form of a high pitch, followed by a low pitch on the following mora (unless the accented mora is the final one). All moras preceding the accent are also high, with the exception of the first mora in the phrase, which is low to mid (unless the first mora itself bears the accent). The accent can fall on various moras within the word, though some words have no accent; in this case, if such words are uttered as phrases in their own right, after the initial low pitch the pitch remains high until the end.

This pattern can be represented graphically, as in Fig. 3.7(a), which shows the pitch of the word *aozóra* ('blue sky'), spoken in isolation. Here, (i) is the low or mid initial mora, (ii) the first of the pre-accentual high-pitched moras, (iii) the high accented mora, and (iv) the post-accentual low-pitched mora. This structure is found in longer phrases, such as *arewa-umái* ('that was nice'), represented in Fig. 3.7(b). Cases with an initial and a final accent, which lack parts (i) and (ii), and part (iv), respectively, are represented in Figs. 3.7(c) and 3.7(d), which show the words *kárasu* ('crow') and *kotobá* ('word'). Fig. 3.7(e) shows the pattern of an unaccented word, *kimono* ('robe'), which lacks parts (iii) and (iv) altogether. It will be noted that these last two patterns are identical; a phrase with a final accented mora is identical to one with no accent at all. However, the two become distinct if we add a particle such as *ga*; this has a low pitch in the case of *kotobá-ga* (Fig. 3.7(f)), and a high pitch in the case of *kimono-ga* (Fig. 3.7(g)).

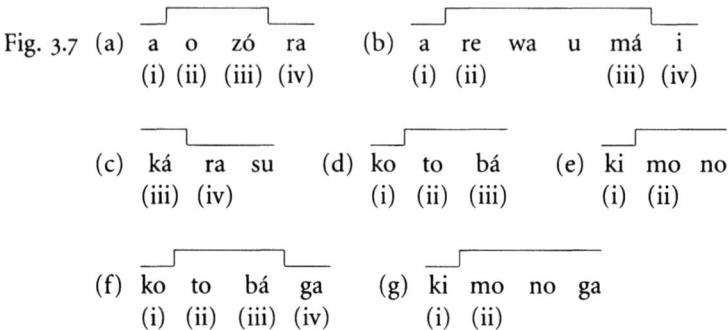

Fig. 3.7 (a) a   o   zó   ra   (b) a   re   wa   u   má   i
              (i) (ii) (iii) (iv)   (i) (ii)   (iii) (iv)

         (c) ká   ra   su   (d) ko   to   bá   (e) ki   mo   no
              (iii) (iv)   (i) (ii) (iii)   (i) (ii)

         (f) ko   to   bá   ga   (g) ki   mo   no   ga
              (i) (ii) (iii) (iv)   (i) (ii)

It must be noted that the Japanese accent is a *phrase accent*; only a single accent is possible for each phrase. When potential accentual phrases are concatenated, potential accents are 'suppressed' in favour of the first such accent, though if any such phrase does not contain an accented word it cannot bear the phrase accent. For example, the phrases *usi-ga* ('the cow') and *inú-ga* (the dog), of which the first is unaccented and the second accented, can be combined with the phrase *imásu-ga* ('. . . is here') into a single phrase. In the first case we get *usi-ga-imásu-ga*, in the second *inú-ga-imasu-ga*, with the phrase accent differently located in each. The accent falls on the first accentable part in each case.[23] Similarly, the unaccented word *kimono* ('robe') can be combined with the unaccented *kiru* ('to put on') and the accented *kíru* ('to cut') in various ways, as in Fig. 3.8. The marks ⌐ and ¬ indicate the position of the pitch rise (before part (ii) of Fig. 3.7) and the pitch drop following the accent (after part (iii) of Fig. 3.7), respectively.[24]

Fig. 3.8 ki⌐mono-o-kiru   'to put on a robe'
          ki⌐mono-o-kí¬ru   'to cut a robe'
          ki⌐ru-kimono   'a robe to be put on'
          ⌐kí¬ru-kimono   'a robe to be cut'

These phenomena have a superficial resemblance to tone; different positions of the accent produce minimal pairs distinguished by pitch. For example, *hána*

[23] Data from Martin (1952).   [24] Data from Kawakami (1961).

('beginning') and *haná* ('flower') have the pitch patterns HL and LH, respectively. However, pitch is here being used *culminatively* rather than *distinctively*, since, in accented phrases, the occurrence of the high pitch contrasts not with its absence but with its occurrence elsewhere. This is, as we saw above, characteristic of accent. Nevertheless, since high pitch is not restricted to the 'accented' mora (*aozóra* has the pattern LHHL, for example), it is not high pitch itself that has a culminative function, but rather the H + L pattern (although again it will be observed that the final L disappears if the accented mora is final).

The Japanese situation must also be distinguished from that which has led a number of scholars to propose accentual analyses for tone in some Bantu languages (see 4.7.5, below). Unlike the latter, Japanese has further characteristics typical of accent languages, such as the suppression or subordination of potential accents in compound phrases illustrated in Fig. 3.8. It therefore differs from other accent languages only in the *realization* of accent: pitch is used rather than stress.[25]

The validity of the 'pitch–accent' approach to Japanese is generally accepted, though a number of different interpretations have been put on it. One area of disagreement has been the number of pitch levels involved. The pitch–accent itself requires only two levels, but, as we have already noted, there are analyses which employ three. However, even more levels have been recognized, especially in the Bloomfieldian tradition. When Bloch first wrote on Japanese (1946),[26] he was happy simply to mark the accented syllable of a phrase as an indication of high, as opposed to low, pitch. But in his later work (Bloch, 1950), and also in the work of his students Martin (1952) and Jorden (1955), we find a more rigorously Bloomfieldian interpretation. Thus, whereas in his earlier work Bloch is prepared to distinguish phrases accented on the final syllable (Fig. 3.6(iv)) from unaccented phrases (Fig. 3.6(v)), because they are distinct when a particle follows, he later rejects this as morphophonemic rather than phonemic; phonemically, he recognizes four pitch levels. Jorden (1955) goes further, recognizing five pitch levels. The high pitch associated with the accent can have two distinct levels, according to the position of the accent within the utterance; the first phrase will have the highest level, and subsequent highs will be one step lower. We find a similar approach in Jorden and Chaplin (1963) and Chaplin and Martin (1967). The former recognize four levels, and use a special notation to indicate the rises and falls, as in Fig. 3.9(a). The expression *ookii ie desu* , 'it's a big house', can be represented as in Fig. 3.9(b), showing that there is a high pitch on -*oki*- and a medium high pitch on -*e*-.

---

[25] It will be recalled, however, that 'stress' is here considered to be a cover term for a combination of a number of different phonetic features, including pitch.

[26] Miller (ed.) (1970: xiii) reports that when Bloch began studying Japanese in the 1940s he wrote that 'the phonemics are a cinch . . . except for the tones (which I am sorry to say are no cinch at all)'.

Fig. 3.9 (a) *Symbol*   *Meaning*

⌈	Rise from neutral to high pitch
⌉	Drop from high to neutral or low pitch
⊦	Rise from neutral to medium high pitch
⊣	Drop from medium high to neutral or low pitch

(b) oʃoki⌉i i⊦e⊣ desu

It is evident that the example of Fig. 3.9(b) contains two accentual phrases, each with an accent (*-ki-* and *-e*), the difference between the two being a matter of intonation rather than accent; the first accent in the utterance has the highest pitch. The fact that both accent and intonation share the same phonetic parameter (pitch) makes the demarcation of the two difficult, and intonational features are here included in the specification of pitch–accent. Jorden and Chaplin also recognize that the rises, being automatic and predictable, are actually phonologically redundant, and only need to be marked where the boundaries between accent phrases are not clearly indicated.

The basic principles of accentuation in Japanese have been endorsed by many other scholars, in a variety of theoretical frameworks. McCawley (1968), in a classical generative framework, uses cyclical rules to determine accents and accent reduction (see 3.6.2, below). The accents are then interpreted as pitch by the rules of pitch assignment. Like Jorden and Chaplin, he is able to differentiate two degrees of height for the high pitch of accent phrases, according to the position of the phrase in the utterance as a whole. Within a non-linear framework Haraguchi (1977) and Pierrehumbert and Beckman (1988) specify the accent by associating a High-Low tone pattern on the tonal tier with the accented

Fig. 3.10 H associated with accented vowel:

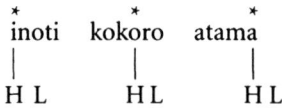

Remaining vowels associated with tones:

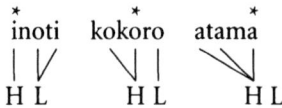

Initial H lowered to L before another H; final unattached L deleted:

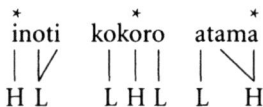

mora, though they do so in different ways. Haraguchi uses the 'star' convention of Goldsmith (1976)—see 4.7.5, below—which links the High tone to the accented mora and the Low tone to the following mora and 'spreads' the tones to the remaining syllables, and finally lowers the tone of the initial mora. This gives the derivations of Fig. 3.10 for the words *'inoti* ('life'), *ko'koro* ('heart'), and *ata'ma* ('head').

Pierrehumbert and Beckman also associate a HL pattern with the accented syllable. They use principles derived from Pierrehumbert's analysis of English intonation (Pierrehumbert, 1980) to assign the pitch pattern; the High pitch on the second mora is a 'phrasal H' and the initial Low tone is a boundary tone (L%). A similar boundary tone is inserted at the end of the phrase. The pitches of other syllables result not from 'tone-spreading', as in Haraguchi's analysis, but from phonetic transitions between the specified tones. The word *yamazakura* ('wild cherry') is therefore derived as in Fig. 3.11. Again different pitch heights for the accents are accommodated by establishing different sizes of unit. 'Accentual phrases' are grouped into 'intermediate phrases', and these into 'utterances'; there is a gradual fall during the intermediate phrase, producing lower pitch for successive accents (for further discussion of Pierrehumbert's approach see Chapter 5.)

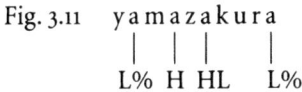

Fig. 3.11   y a m a z a k u r a
             | | | |
             L% H HL   L%

Despite the different modes of representation, however, these different analyses agree in regarding the accentual features of Japanese as a matter of pitch rather than stress.

3.4 Accentual Structure

3.4.1 INTRODUCTION

From the above discussion of accent from a phonetic and a phonological point of view (the latter in terms of structuralist phonology up to the 1960s), a rather confused picture emerges of its nature and the way in which it can be systematized phonologically. Nevertheless, it is possible to draw a number of tentative conclusions which can serve as a foundation for further discussion. In the first place, it seems evident that no adequate definition of accent as a phonological phenomenon can be based primarily on phonetic criteria. Not only are the phonetic correlates of accent elusive and inconsistent, but a restriction to a specific phonetic manifestation of accent proves to be inhibiting when we attempt to make generalizations both within and across languages. Second, it is clear that accent cannot be satisfactorily systematized on a paradigmatic basis; accentual contrasts do not involve systems of mutually substitutable items at a single point but rather differences between the occurrence of the accent at one place and at another; they therefore belong to the syntagmatic dimension. Third, accent is multi-layered, in the sense that there are—in some languages, at least—different kinds of accentual contrast, arranged hierarchically. This is not, however, to be construed as the endorsement of a paradigmatic view of accent; it is a matter of syntagmatic contrasts operating on different levels simultaneously. Thus, as we saw above, English has an intonational nucleus superimposed upon a basic accentual pattern, giving the appearance of a paradigmatic accentual system. What we have is accentual peaks at two different levels rather than an opposition at a single level.

Taken together, these conclusions point to accent not as a prosodic *feature* as such but rather as the indispensable component of a complex accentual *structure*. Since other prosodic features—pitch, length, intonation—are also involved here, this accentual structure is evidently a crucial—perhaps the major—component of prosodic structure itself. Two further points can be made which do not directly follow from the above discussion but which seem indispensable for our understanding of this accentual structure. First, the structure is a *phonological* one, based on phonological relationships; it is therefore not properly a direct reflection of morpho-syntactic structure but is *autonomous*. Second, it is not to be expected that the structures found in all languages will be the same; there is scope for typological differentiation here. In the remainder of this section we shall consider some of the implications of this view of accent in more detail.

3.4.2 ACCENTUAL UNITS

A syntagmatic view of accent requires us to consider the *domains* within which accentual contrasts operate. Each occurrence of an accented element, together with the unaccented elements with which it contrasts, constitutes an accentual unit.[27] If, as we have concluded above, there is a hierarchical aspect to accentual contrasts, then we will expect to be able to identify units differing in extent or scope.

3.4.2.1 Level 1: Accent as Rhythm

At the lowest level of accentuation, English and many other languages have a regular succession of accented syllables, usually, but not necessarily, separated by one or more unaccented syllables.[28] This provides us with a basic accentual unit, comprising the accented syllable and any following unaccented syllables,

[27] Garde (1968: 12) distinguishes between an *accentable* unit and an *accentual* unit. The former is the unit which bears the accent (usually the syllable) and the latter the unit within which accentual contrasts are created (e.g. the foot).

[28] Some scholars, e.g. Selkirk (1984), define rhythm as an *alternation* of strong and weak syllables, but this is unsatisfactory, since it excludes the occurrence of a sequence of stressed monosyllables, as in English *four large black dogs*, which is perfectly rhythmical.

and this unit is usually termed the *foot*. This basic accentual level will here be called *Level 1 accentuation*. Accent at this level is sometimes referred to as 'word-stress', but this is misleading, since although words are often characterized by a single accented syllable this is by no means always the case. Words may have more than one accent or none at all. Lexical words are more likely to have such an accent than grammatical words, but a significant factor in determining whether a word is accented or not is also its length: long words are likely to have more accented syllables than short ones. This is because Level 1 accentuation in English is primarily a matter of *rhythm*.

Though phoneticians from Sweet onwards have remarked on the rhythmical basis of English accent, this factor has often been ignored in discussions of the phenomenon. It is only relatively recently (and especially in Metrical Phonology—see below) that the rhythmical principle has received due recognition in discussions of stress and accent. We have already considered English rhythm in discussing syllable quantity (2.9.3), and noted that it is based on the principle of *isochrony*: accented syllables have a strong tendency to occur at approximately equal intervals of time, so that the feet are of more or less the same length.

One factor that must be taken into account here is the difference between *actual* and *potential* accents. Though in principle accents are likely to occur on lexical items and not on grammatical items, the rhythmical basis of accentuation in English means that potential accents may not be realized, and the accents may occur on syllables which might be expected not to have them. The actual occurrence of accents will therefore depend on the particular juxtaposition of words, as well as on the speed of utterance. This difference between the potential for accent and the actual occurrence of accent may well be the major factor in creating the impression of different degrees of accent or stress, since such 'degrees' reflect a hierarchy not of accents themselves but of potentiality for accent.[29]

Consider, for example, the expression *elevator-operator*, which for Trager and Bloch (1941) exemplifies their four degrees of stress (/élevâtor òperâtor/). Analysing this in terms of a rhythmical view of accent, we can recognize two accents here: 'elevator-'operator. At a slower speed, more accents will appear: 'ele'vator-'ope'rator, while at a rapid rate of utterance, especially if this expression is included in a larger one, we may have only a single accent: *the 'elevator-operator's 'car*. It can be seen that a hierarchy of accentability emerges, displayed in Fig. 3.12, which corresponds point by point with the degrees of stress recognized in the American tradition, but which in fact requires no more than an accented/unaccented distinction based on rhythm, and a variable which reflects

---

[29] How the notion of 'potential accent' can be satisfactorily incorporated into a linguistic description is a difficult question. It has some relationship to the competence/performance distinction of Chomsky (e.g. Chomsky, 1965), though Chomsky makes it clear that competence is not simply potential performance. The underlying/surface distinction may also be relevant here, though we cannot simply take every potential accent to be underlyingly present, since in some styles of speech *every* syllable is accented.

speed or style of utterance. If only one syllable is accented, it is *e-*; if two are accented, then we will add *o-*; if four are accented then we add *-va-* and *-ra-*.

Fig. 3.12   the | elevator operator's | car
                | elevator | operator
                | ele | vator | ope | rator

A number of other facts can be explained in these terms. If accent is primarily rhythmical, then the actual phonetic features associated with it can be rather variable; indeed, since rhythm involves, as Gimson (1956) suggests, a 'mental beat', there is no requirement that it should have *any* phonetic manifestation. This is true of musical rhythm as well as speech; the regular beat of a piece of music is not necessarily marked by any specific dynamic feature, but is nevertheless perceived by both performer and listener. This also explains the occurrence of so-called 'silent stress' (Abercrombie, 1971), where the accented syllable is not audible at all. This is found not only in verse reading (silent beats are found at the end of most lines with an odd number of feet),[30] but also in speech, as in the expression ['k̩kju] ('(than)k you') (Jones, 1956: 245; Abercrombie, 1967: 36).

Thus, a major aspect of accentuation is explicable in terms of a rhythmic beat, and this is able to account for most of the accentual phenomena in a language such as English. Some other apparent accentual distinctions, such as those of Trager and Bloch, are arguably spurious, and arise from the inclusion either of potential accents or of non-accentual features such as quantity or vowel reduction.

3.4.2.2 Level 2: Accent as Intonation

The rhythmic 'beat' provides us with Level 1 accentuation in a language such as English, but the structure is further elaborated by intonational features. As we have already noted, intonation patterns have a structure, which includes a peak or *nucleus*, and this is superimposed on the basic accentual framework just outlined. Since this peak has to coincide with an accented syllable, this syllable is often considered to be more strongly accented than the others, as we have seen in our earlier discussion. This form of 'higher' accent will here be called *Level 2 accentuation*. This is the basis of the distinction made by Arnold (1957a, 1957b) between *tonic strong* and *non-tonic strong* syllables, and of the traditional distinction between 'sentence stress' and 'word-stress'. However, there is no evidence that the intonational nucleus (Level 2 accent) is actually dynamically 'stronger' than the Level 1 accent; its prominence is attributable to its role in the intonation pattern. The difference between the two accents is simply that the Level 2 accent has a larger domain than the Level 1 accent.

Whether or not the Level 2 accent is properly considered to be an 'accent' is

---

[30] The reader may test this with, for example, a children's rhyme such as 'Three blind mice', which has three syllables in several lines, including the first, but four beats in each line.

a terminological issue rather than a matter of phonological fact. There is no doubt that the intonational nucleus is prominent, and it could therefore be said to have a culminative function in the same way that Level 1 accent does. Some scholars in fact reserve the term 'accent' for precisely this phenomenon, and use the term 'stress' for the basic rhythmical accent of Level 1. In this terminological framework, Arnold's 'non-tonic strong' syllables have stress but no accent, while 'tonic strong' syllables have both stress and accent. However, this usage adds yet another source of potential confusion, and will be avoided here.

This structure, with a Level 1 accentual pattern consisting of rhythmical beats and a superimposed Level 2 pattern with an intonational peak, is found in many languages which have a 'stress-timed' rhythm. Given the interpretation of 'degrees of stress' just outlined, there is no need for any further structure in such languages to describe accentual phenomena. However, in languages without a stress-timed rhythm the accentual structure may be different. In French (see 2.9.3.4) there is no rhythmical accent or 'word-stress', and the intonational peak occurs on the final syllable[31] of each intonational phrase. If we follow the principle that the intonational peak is not in itself an accent, then French has no accent. However, we could describe this peak as a 'phrase accent', or—coinciding with French usage (cf. Garde, 1968: 3)—a 'tonic accent'; in this case French has a Level 2 accent but no Level 1 accent.

The situation in other languages, especially those with a different kind of rhythmical structure, is less clear, in spite of detailed studies, since terminological and conceptual differences make the interpretation of the findings difficult. We shall here examine Spanish and Italian.

Spanish and Italian

In Spanish, as we saw in 3.9.3.4, there is a syllable-timed rhythm, but there are also accented syllables, and the place of the accent in Spanish words is variable, giving contrasts such as *'termino* ('term'), *ter'mino* ('I terminate') and *termi'no* ('he terminated'). Taken in isolation, it is, of course, impossible to say whether such accents are at Level 1 or Level 2, since the word is here equivalent to a phrase. However, several studies (Navarro Tomás, 1936; Trager, 1939; Delattre, 1965; Macpherson, 1975; Pointon, 1980) not only demonstrate a non-rhythmical word-accent within Spanish utterances, but suggest that, unlike the situation in French, there may be more than one such accent for each phrase. Indeed, Alarcos Llorach (1968: 202–3), from the Praguian perspective, notes that each part of complex words may have its own stress, e.g. *fuérte-ménte, así-mísmo, déja-se-ló, explíca-me-ló.* Other scholars, however, starting with Stockwell, Bowen, and Silva-Fuenzalida (1956) and extending to generative accounts such as those

---

[31] As pointed out by S. Jones (1932), among others, the accent in French is not necessarily strictly on the final syllable; where the final syllable has an articulated [ə], the accent is on the penultimate syllable.

by Harris (1969, 1983) and Brame (1974), treat the first of these stresses as subordinate, giving patterns such as *fuèrteménte, fòrmalísmo, Àcapúlco*. Stockwell, Bowen, and Silva-Fuenzalida in fact explicitly recognize three 'stress phonemes' for Spanish, albeit reluctantly, since they 'still "feel" that two stresses ought to be enough for this language'. All of this is reminiscent of the debates about degrees of stress in English, and it suggests that there are similarities between the accentual structures of English and Spanish, to the extent that there is a basic Level 1 'non-tonic' accent and a superimposed Level 2 'tonic accent'. However, it is difficult to reconcile this with the syllable-timed rhythm of Spanish, which precludes a rhythmically-based accent, and we would have to conclude that the Level 1 accentual unit (the foot) in Spanish is not, as in English, a rhythmical unit. There is admittedly some uncertainty here, however, since it is also claimed that some accentual phenomena in Spanish do have a rhythmical basis. Navarro Tomás (1936) suggests that stressed and unstressed syllables alternate, while Harris (1983: 86) notes that non-primary stresses can occur 'on even-numbered syllables counting leftward from the primary stress, subject to the condition that nonprimaries cannot occur adjacent to each other or to the primary'. If this interpretation is valid, it suggests that a rhythmical principle of some sort is involved.

A similar conclusion may be appropriate for Italian. Agard and di Pietro (1965), in a strictly Bloomfieldian interpretation, establish four degrees of stress (though only three in individual words); Vogel and Scalise (1982) identify the regular occurrence of a 'secondary stress', which is predictable partly on phonological and partly on morphological grounds once the position of the primary stress is known. We thus have such forms as *impossíbile, lìberaménte, pròbabìlitá*, etc. Since these stresses are evenly spaced, largely occurring on alternate syllables, a rhythmical principle would appear to be operative here, in spite of the fact that Italian is generally said to have a syllable-timed rhythm. Vogel and Scalise do not consider the accentuation of word groups or phrases, so it is not clear what structures they would recognize at higher levels, or whether their primary stress is, in fact, a Level 2 phrase accent.

For Spanish and Italian, then, the nature of the accentual system is somewhat unclear. On the one hand, much evidence points to a situation similar to that of French, with a syllable-timed rhythm and a single (Level 2) non-rhythmic accent for each phrase; on the other hand, the interpretations just given suggest a rhythm-based (Level 1) accent. The co-existence of a syllable-timed rhythm and a rhythm-based stress does not seem plausible. A possible solution is suggested by Bolinger (1962), and much later by Roca (1986) in a metrical framework (see below). Bolinger claims that '(1) the secondary [stress] is too fickle to be located positively between primary (stress) and weak (non-stress), and (2) so far as I know, it differentiates nothing'. He argues that 'it would therefore be better not to suggest phonemic status by referring to "secondary stress"'. In a similar vein, Roca demonstrates that 'secondary stress, in languages like Spanish and Italian at least, is but a manifestation of phrasal rhythm', and therefore a predictable phenomenon. This view results in 'freeing lexical stress from the pressures of prosodic rhythm, and postlexical rhythmic stress from the idiosyncrasies of lexical determination'. The rhythmical 'secondary stress' discussed here can therefore be seen as a rather superficial phenomenon overlaid on the syllable-timing of the language, and therefore quite different from the rhythmical stressing of English, which is fundamental to prosodic organization.[32] 'Primary stress' in Spanish and Italian, on the other hand, remains a manifestation of non-rhythmical Level 2 accentuation at the phrasal level.

Other languages display other accentual phenomena. Mandarin Chinese has both a tonal and an accentual system; the accentual system is similar to that of English, with a rhythmical Level 1 accent. The question here is whether Mandarin also has a Level 2 'tonic accent' comparable to that of English. Such an accent is difficult to detect, since intonation has different characteristics in a tone language and a non-tone language (Fox, 1995). Cantonese differs from Mandarin in having no stress-based accentual system; in this case, the lack of a tonic accent—if true—would mean that the language arguably has neither a Level 1 nor a Level 2 accent, and therefore no accentual structure at all. Finally, we may consider the accentual units of Japanese. As we have noted, Japanese has a pitch–accent consisting of a fixed falling pitch pattern, preceded by a high pitch. This accent is not based on rhythm, and the pattern cannot be interrupted by subordinate accents. Hence, Japanese has, like French, only a Level 2 phrase accent.

In English, however, we may claim that accentuation at Level 1 is a matter of rhythm and at Level 2 a matter of intonation. It is possible, moreover, for there to be more than one 'level' of intonational prominence, so that we might consider there to be a 'Level 3' accentuation. This is because intonational units may be subordinated to one another, creating a hierarchy of prominence of the 'tonic accents' (see 5.7, below). However, it may be terminologically undesirable to extend the concept of 'accent' further into intonational phenomena in this way.

3.4.3 THE ACCENTUAL HIERARCHY: ACCENT AS PROSODIC ORGANIZATION

We have seen that accent can be described in terms of a recurrent prominence. However, the fact that this is a syntagmatic, culminative phenomenon means that it is not to be equated with paradigmatic, distinctive, segmental features, such as voicing, lip-rounding, nasalization, etc. Accent has the effect of dividing

---

[32] Endorsing Roca's interpretation, Halle and Vergnaud (1987a: 99–100, 1987b) recognize the special status of these 'secondary stresses' in Spanish, and generate them by means of a special 'Alternator Rule'. However, they also use this rule for English where, evidently, its status is very different.

the utterance into units within which the accentual contrasts operate. As a result, it has, as Beckmann (1986) suggests, an 'organizational' role, whose implications go beyond the occurrence of the accent itself.

This organizational role has been observed at several different points in the present book; indeed, it is difficult to talk about *any* prosodic feature without some reference to accent or stress. As we saw in Chapter 2, length interacts in numerous ways with accentual phenomena. Length and syllable weight distinctions are often restricted to accented syllables, while syllable quantity is determined, in languages such as English, on the basis of stress-timed feet. Although tone is in principle independent of accent, the two interact in many ways, as discussed in detail in 4.7, below. There may be different tonal systems in accented and unaccented syllables, or tonal contrasts may be restricted to accented syllables, as in tonal accent languages. Here, the accentually defined foot may become a unit of tone as well as accent. In virtually all cases it seems to be the case that tone is subordinated to accent, rather than the reverse; accent is the controlling feature.

We have already seen, and this will be developed in Chapter 5, that there is also a close link between accentuation and the structure of intonation patterns, with accent again being the dominant partner in the interaction. The location of the intonational nucleus can be regarded as a form of accentuation, and in some languages this is the *only* form of accent that occurs. Where this tonic accent occurs in addition to the non-tonic accent, an *accentual hierarchy* is created, with Level 1 and Level 2 accents. But this hierarchy is not to be identified with the stress systems devised by Trager, Bloch, Smith, and others; it is essentially a matter of structure rather than of paradigmatic contrasts.

There is thus considerable justification for seeing accent as a fundamental determinant of prosodic structure as a whole in many languages. Since accent is not a universal feature of languages, it clearly cannot be an indispensable part of this structure, and we shall therefore need to consider alternative principles, too. These matters will be considered further in the final chapter of this book.

3.5 The Representation of Accent

3.5.1 INTRODUCTION

The view of accent and accentual structure sketched out so far has been an informal one, in the sense that it has not taken account of how this structure is to be described in more explicit and formal terms. There are two different but related questions here. First, we must determine how accentual features are to be *represented*, that is, what particular units, features, structures, etc. are appropriate for the description of accent. Second, we must consider how accents are to be *specified*, that is, what mechanisms are to be employed for determining the accentual features and accentual structure of utterances. Though ideas on these topics have evolved in tandem, they are nevertheless different questions, and it is appropriate to consider them separately.

3.5.2 DISTINCTIVE FEATURES OF ACCENT

The representation of accent depends on what we take accentual features to be. The pedagogical tradition takes accent to be a property of the syllable, and simply marks the accented syllable with a raised ´. Where 'secondary stress' is required, a subscript ˌ is used. In the American structuralist approach, stress is considered to be a 'suprasegmental phoneme' which occurs simultaneously with segmental phonemes. As noted above, the four 'stress phonemes' of this tradition are represented with the three symbols /´/, /ˆ/, and /`/, the fourth degree being unmarked. Distinctive feature theory, on the other hand, regards prosodic features as part of the segments with which they occur (Jakobson, Fant, and Halle, 1952: 13). In this framework, a binary feature [±stress] is employed. Neither of these approaches is particularly successful in representing accentuation, since both imply that 'stress' or 'accent' is comparable to segmental features such as 'voiced' or 'nasal', and they fail to accommodate the 'organizational' role of accent that has been discussed above.

In classical generative phonology, epitomized by Chomsky and Halle (1968), a feature framework is also used. The rules for stress assignment (see 3.6, below) assign the feature [1 stress], but because of the cyclical operation of the rules, this in fact produces a multivalued feature, with [2 stress], [3 stress], etc. These correspond to the Trager–Bloch–Smith levels, and therefore do not conform to the view advanced in 3.4. But there is a further problem, since Chomsky and Halle's degrees of stress differ from those of Trager and Bloch in one crucial respect: there is no theoretical limit to the number of degrees. This framework therefore appears to be in principle incompatible on two counts with the approach presented in 3.4: not only does it recognize a paradigmatic set of stress levels (or its equivalent); this set is *unlimited*. Some of the implications of this will be discussed below (3.6.4).

Vanderslice and Ladefoged (1972) propose a different analysis which, though it shares the drawbacks of other feature-based approaches, nevertheless comes somewhat closer to accommodating the hierarchical approach adopted here than do analyses which recognize a set of degrees. They break down these 'degrees of stress' into a number of binary distinctions, which apply to syllables and are related in a hierarchical fashion: [±heavy], [±accent], [±intonation], [±cadence], [±endglide], and [±emphasis]. These features fall into two groups; the first two and the last are regarded as accentual, while the third, fourth and fifth are intonational. Thus, accent and intonation are distinguished, though integrated into a common set of suprasegmental features. The distinction between [+heavy] and [−heavy] ('light') reflects whether the syllable is 'full' or 'reduced'; it is, therefore, not one of accent in the sense in which this term has been used above, though, as Vanderslice and Ladefoged note, 'a light syllable corresponds to an unstressed or weakly-stressed syllable in several important traditions of stress analysis'. In fact, it corresponds to the 'pepet' of Newman (1946). The distinction between [+accent] and [−accent] is the basic accentual one, so that [+accent] 'corresponds roughly to IPA primary stress'.[33] Syllables which are [+accent] are always [+heavy], so that the [±heavy] distinction applies only to [−accent] syllables.

Of the intonational features, [±intonation] is of interest to us here, since it corresponds to the 'nuclear' or 'tonic' accent. Thus, according to Vanderslice and Ladefoged, 'only one syllable in a sense group can be marked [+intonation], and it is always the last accented one'.[34] However, this feature simply marks the location of the tonic accent, and does not in itself have phonetic correlates; these are supplied by the features [±cadence] and [±endglide], which replace [+intonation]. The final feature, [±emphasis], is also intonational, in that it involves an 'extra-large pitch obtrusion on an accented heavy syllable'; it is also considered to be accentual, but it applies not at the 'word-accent level' but at the 'sentence accent level', where it may signal contrast.

Thus, apart from this last, there are three different features in Vanderslice and Ladefoged's system which account for what has often been regarded as accent, and these features are hierarchically ordered, in the sense that only a [+heavy] syllable can be [+accent] and only a [+accent] syllable can be [+intonation]. However, Vanderslice and Ladefoged do not regard these as three 'degrees of stress', but as binary contrasts involving different dimensions. Thus, they 'factor out' the feature [±intonation], and regard complex words such as *hand-made, archbishop, anticlimax*, etc. as having two accents ('hand-'made, etc.), where the second accent is also [+intonation]. They see no reason to distinguish these cases from words such as 'photo'graphic, 'relax'ation, etc. which are traditionally given a secondary and a primary stress. On the other hand, words such as *foot-passenger, kettle-holder*, etc., which are often transcribed with a secondary stress *following* the primary stress (see above), are regarded as having only a single accent, the second 'accent' being interpreted as an unaccented heavy syllable. If both [±intonation] and [±heavy] are excluded, then accentuation in English is reduced to a single feature: [±accent].

3.5.3 THE METRICAL REPRESENTATION OF ACCENT

The reduction of accentuation to the occurrence of a single feature is compatible with the approach advocated above, in which—for English, at least—accent is

---

[33] This statement is not, in fact, true, since the IPA does not endorse any particular phonological analysis but merely provides symbols for representing categories.

[34] The last part seems to be an unnecessary and illegitimate requirement. Accented syllables can occur after the tonic accent, though, as Arnold (1957a) notes, they will lack the pitch prominence of those occurring before it and may often fail to be marked as 'secondary stresses'. Cf. also Scott's experiments (1939) which show that listeners have difficulty perceiving the position of post-nuclear accents.

regarded as a rhythmical phenomenon, characterized by the regular occurrence of a 'beat'. However, it remains a paradigmatic representation, and therefore unsatisfactory as a means of specifying the culminative role of accent in utterances.

A different approach is presented by Liberman (1975), and especially Liberman and Prince (1977), introducing a *Metrical* representation of accentual phenomena.[35] This approach has proved to be extremely influential, and its use can be seen in other areas of prosodic representation, such as length (2.7 ff.) and tone (4.5). A fundamental innovation here—at least in the generative tradition—is to regard English stress as a purely *relational* property, reflecting *relative prominence* among sentence constituents. This can be represented graphically as in Fig. 3.13, which shows these relations not as an opposition between different 'degrees' (e.g. *rèd cóws*, or *stréss-shìft*), but as a local relationship between sister nodes, where one is 'strong' (*s*) and the other is 'weak' (*w*). Liberman and Prince emphasize that this 'strength' is relational, so that *s* or *w* are meaningless in isolation, independent of the relationship.

Fig. 3.13

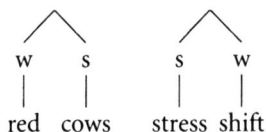

```
   w    s      s    w
   |    |      |    |
  red  cows  stress shift
```

This approach can be extended to cover more complex structures, such as those of Fig. 3.14. Here, there is embedding of syntactic constituents, and hence a more complex metrical tree. It can be seen that each branching node dominates a pair of nodes, one of which is strong and the other weak, producing a hierarchical structure.[36]

Fig. 3.14

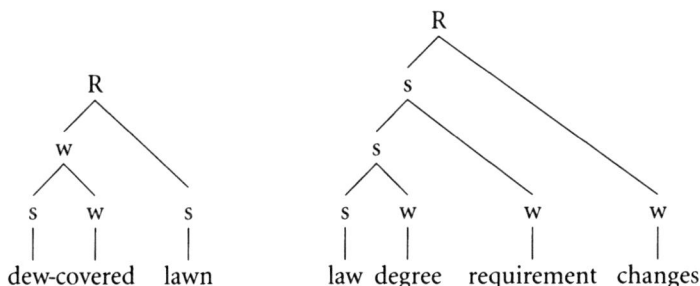

```
              R                              R
             / \                            / \
            w   \                          s   \
           /\    \                        /\    \
          s  w    s                      s  w    w    w
          |  |    |                      |  |    |    |
    dew-covered  lawn            law degree requirement changes
```

[35] For useful discussion of metrical theory see Hogg and McCully (1987), Goldsmith (1990: ch. 4), Kenstowicz (1994: ch. 10), Kager (1995).

[36] It is interesting to note that a remarkably similar representation of stress relations was given much earlier by Rischel (1964), who describes the stress pattern of *livelihood* in terms of + and - on two levels, one superimposed upon the other. Liberman and Prince refer to Rischel's article, but they had no access to it.

Although this hierarchical arrangement of strong and weak nodes—which reflects the hierarchical syntactic structure of the phrase—appears to produce a ranking of syllables with regard to strength, and therefore a paradigmatic analysis of stress, this is not the intention, and Liberman and Prince make it clear that the relationships here are syntagmatic. The 'root node' R of the tree, therefore, 'will of course be neither *s* nor *w*, since it is not in a syntagmatic relation with any other node'. It is nevertheless possible to derive the 'degrees of stress' of theories such as that of Chomsky and Halle (1968) from the metrical tree by application of an algorithm, as follows:

If a terminal node *t* is labelled *w*, its stress number is equal to the number of nodes that dominate it, plus one. If a terminal node is labelled *s*, its stress number is equal to the number of nodes that dominate the lowest dominating *t*, plus one.

In the case of an expression such as *labour union finance committee president*, for example, which is represented in Fig. 3.15, the application of this algorithm would give the 'degrees of stress' indicated for the strong syllable of each word. However, this is dismissed as mere 'numerology', and is not regarded as significant; 'there is nothing inherent in the relational method of representation that would lead one to the particular rank-ordering of terminals implied by Fig. 3.15, expressing the notion "degree of stress"'.

Fig. 3.15

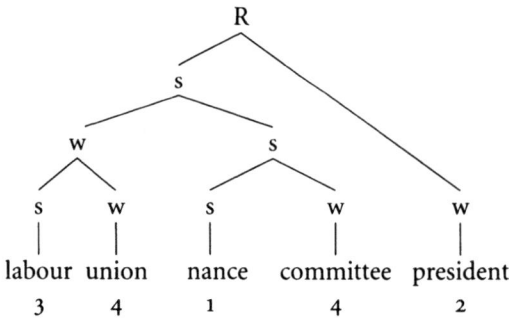

We have so far seen how Liberman and Prince represent the accentual structure of phrases and compounds. In order to determine the position of the accented syllable in *words*, they use an additional device: a binary feature [±stress], assigned to vowels. If a syllable is metrically strong, its vowel will be [+stress], but the converse is not necessarily true; not all [+stress] vowels will be in metrically strong syllables, so that, for example *gymnast* and *modest* have the same metrical structure but different values of [±stress], and similarly with *raccoon* and *balloon*, as shown in Fig. 3.16. Thus, apart from its role in determining the metrical structure, the feature [±stress] appears to relate to vowel reduction, and therefore to the feature [±heavy] of Vanderslice and Ladefoged, discussed above; it does *not* represent a phonetic property of accent as such.

Fig. 3.16

s w	s w	w s	w s
gym nast	mo dest	rac coon	bal loon
+ +	+ −	+ +	− +

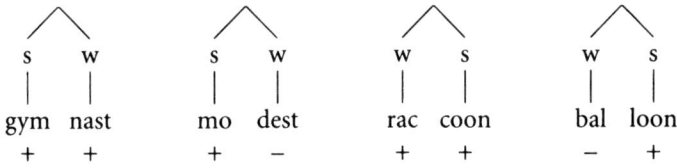

One further means of representing stress is provided by Liberman and Prince: the *metrical grid*. Although in principle the tree representation used so far incorporates a rhythmical principle, with an alternation of strong and weak nodes, there are a number of cases where rhythm needs to be invoked more directly in order to determine the distribution of accented syllables. One such case is the so-called 'stress-clash' which can occur in expressions such as *thirteen men*. Although, when spoken in isolation, *thirteen* is accented on the second syllable, in *thirteen men* the accent occurs on the first syllable. A standard explanation for this is that retention of the final accent in *thirteen* would result in two adjacent stresses, on *-teen* and *men*—a 'stress-clash'—and the stress pattern is adjusted accordingly. To effect this adjustment, we need to be able to recognize such stress-clashes, and Liberman and Prince achieve this by displaying the various 'levels' of stress occurring on particular syllables in a series of columns, as in Fig. 3.17. The consecutive numbers are here used as 'placeholders', indicating the occurrence of stress on that syllable at the level in question. In Fig. 3.17(a), stress is placed on the second syllable of *thirteen* at level 2, giving two adjacent stresses at that level with no unstressed syllable intervening. The 'clash' is resolved in Fig. 3.17(b) by shifting the stress to the first syllable by means of the *Rhythm Rule*.

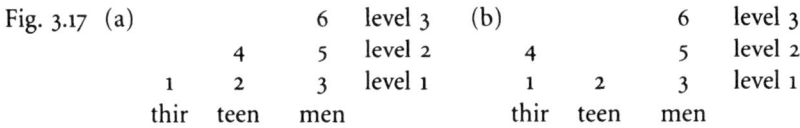

Fig. 3.17 (a)

		6	level 3
	4	5	level 2
1	2	3	level 1
thir	teen	men	

(b)

		6	level 3
	4	5	level 2
1	2	3	level 1
thir	teen	men	

Liberman and Prince therefore provide three different ways of representing accent: in terms of *features, trees,* and *grids*. The feature [±stress] is described as 'a relational feature of constituent structure rather than an intrinsic feature of phonological segments'; in fact, as just noted, it appears to be more of a technical device to facilitate the drawing of the trees than a phonetic property. The tree 'encodes relative prominence', while the grid represents 'hierarchies of intersecting periodicities'. Given three different modes of representation, it is natural to ask whether all of these are actually necessary, and whether any of them could be considered derivative or redundant.

The first of these representations that has been regarded as unnecessary is the feature [±stress]. Liberman and Prince (1977) use it to determine the 'strong' syllables in order to draw the trees and also to distinguish between unreduced and reduced syllables, as with the words of Fig. 3.16, above. Nespor and Vogel

(1979) are able to dispense with this feature in Italian, since there is no vowel reduction in this language, but even for English it is possible to do without it, as demonstrated by Selkirk (1980), Hayes (1981), Giegerich (1983), and others. Selkirk (1980) is able to achieve this by introducing an important new concept into the theory, or rather by formalizing an existing concept in a new framework: *prosodic categories*. These are simply phonological units larger than the individual segment: *syllable* (represented by σ), *stress foot* (represented by Σ),[37] and *prosodic word* (represented by ω). These units are not new, as all had been employed before in various phonological frameworks, and indeed all are used by Liberman and Prince, but Selkirk incorporates them more formally as major determinants of prosodic organization. She is able to deal with the distinction found in such pairs as *gymnast* and *modest*, which for Liberman and Prince require the feature [±stress], by considering the former, but not the latter, to have two feet, as in Fig. 3.18.

Fig. 3.18

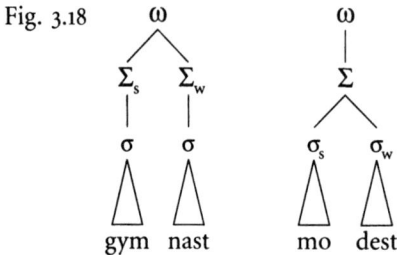

Hayes (1981) adopts the same principle, separating *metrical feet* from the remaining structure with a horizontal line, as in Fig. 3.19, representing *rabbi* and *happy*.

Fig. 3.19

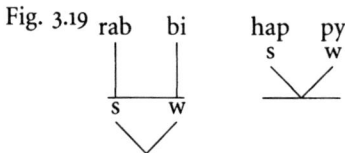

Another category is the *prosodic word*. This appears in Liberman and Prince's approach under the title *mot* (M), where it is used to ensure that words are treated as single units in the assignment of stresses in compounds or phrases. Liberman and Prince's 'Compound Rule' assigns stress to the first element of a compound unless the second element branches, so that, for example, *labour union member* has the main stress on the first element (*labour*) but *labour union*

---

[37] Selkirk deliberately uses this term in preference to the simpler 'foot' in order to distinguish her unit from that of Abercrombie (1964), though it is by no means clear that the two are actually as different as she implies. Selkirk's later development of these ideas (Selkirk, 1984: 42–3) suggests that she has misinterpreted Abercrombie's intentions here (see below). Some clarification is provided by Cutler and Ladd (ed.) (1983: 143–4), who suggest that Selkirk's 'foot' is smaller than Abercrombie's, and that the latter corresponds more closely to Selkirk's 'prosodic word'. For further discussion, see Ch. 6.

finance committee has the main stress on *finance* because its second part branches (see Fig. 3.20).

Fig. 3.20

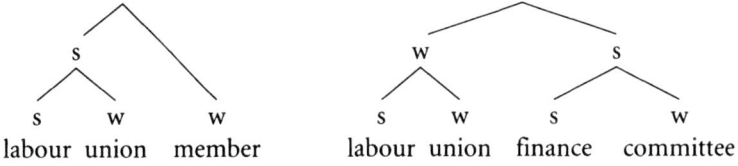

However, each component of these compounds consists of more than one syllable, and could therefore be said to branch. The rule only works if we treat each word as a single unit when applying it. In order to ensure that this is so, Liberman and Prince label each node at the word level 'M', as in Fig. 3.21. The Compound Rule can now be revised to assign stress to the first element of a compound unless the second element branches *at the same level*; it ignores branching structure *below* this level.

Fig. 3.21

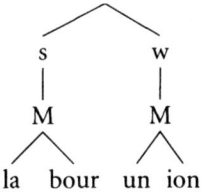

Selkirk (1980), Hayes (1981), and others, also incorporate the word ('prosodic word') into their models in a similar way. Hayes, for example, gives the tree for *reconciliation* shown in Fig. 3.22 (Ft = 'Foot', Wd = 'Phonological Word').

Fig. 3.22

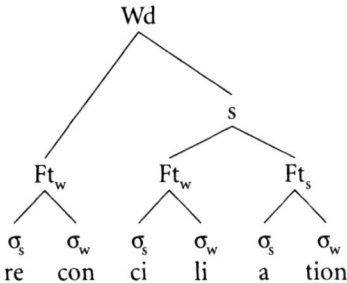

Selkirk insists on binary-branching in the trees, and thus cannot cater directly for feet which have more than two syllables. Such feet will need two levels of structure with a higher and a lower node, as in the word *America*, given in Fig. 3.23. The upper, and more inclusive, node is designated 'stress superfoot' (Σ'). This unit consists of a disyllabic foot followed by another weak syllable.

Fig. 3.23

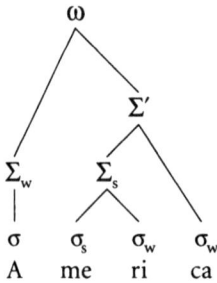

As we noted above, Liberman and Prince have two means—apart from [±stress]—of representing the accentual pattern of utterances: the tree and the grid. Since metrical strength relations are represented by the tree, some scholars have questioned whether the grid is required. The motivation for the grid is, as we have seen, to enable 'stress-clashes' to be identified and rectified by means of the 'Rhythm Rule', but Kiparsky (1979) claims that this rule is 'an operation on metrical trees', and does not need the grid for its operation. Thus, instead of the grid representation of Fig. 3.17, Kiparsky formalizes the process in terms of trees, as in Fig. 3.24. Similarly, Giegerich (1980, 1984) considers the grid to be superfluous, since it can in any case be derived from the tree. For him, it is reduced to the status of an 'illustrative device' with no independent contribution.

Fig. 3.24

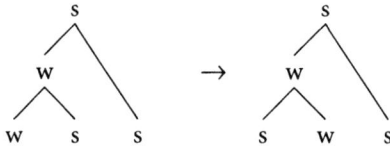

Many other scholars working in the metrical framework, including Prince, Selkirk, Halle, and Vergnaud, have taken the opposite course, however, and regard the *tree* as superfluous, resulting in *grid-only phonology*. The original idea of the grid, as set out by Liberman and Prince (1977), was to provide a means of formally identifying stress clashes. The grid is constructed as follows (note that we shall now adopt a more usual and more convenient formalism, and use stars instead of Liberman and Prince's consecutive numbers). If we take an expression which is subject to stress-clash and the Rhythm Rule— for example, *achromatic lens*—consisting of a number of syllables, we may represent each syllable at the bottom level of the grid (level 1)[38] by a star (see

---

[38] These 'levels' are, of course, not identical with the Level 1 and Level 2 accentuation discussed earlier.

Fig. 3.25). To represent this expression on higher levels, we apply a fundamental principle, the *Relative Prominence Projection Rule*, which runs as follows:

Relative Prominence Projection Rule
In any constituent on which the strong–weak relation is defined, the designated terminal element of its strong subconstituent is metrically stronger than the designated terminal element of its weak subconstituent.

This rule states that terminal syllables which are 'strong' in the metrical tree will also be 'strong' in the grid. We therefore move up the tree (given upside-down in Fig. 3.25), putting a star on each strong syllable at the next-higher level—on level 2 the strong syllables are *a-*, *-ma-*, and *lens*, on level 3 *-ma-* and *lens*, and finally *lens* on level 4.[39] The result is given in Fig. 3.25(a).

Fig. 3.25

(a)

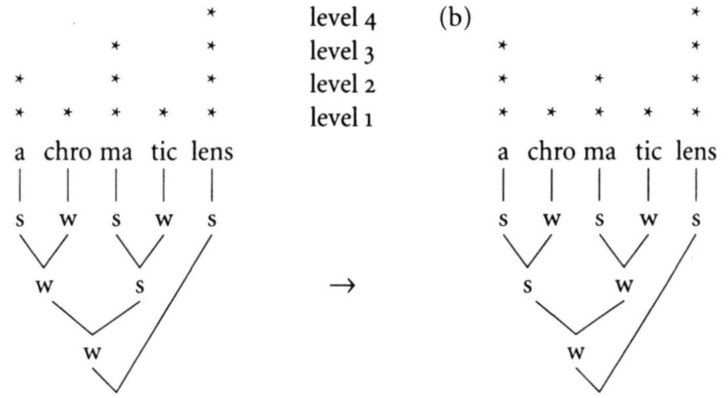

```
                        *      level 4   (b)                          *
                 *      *      level 3          *                      *
          *      *      *      level 2          *         *            *
          *   *  *   *  *      level 1          *   *     *   *        *
          a chro ma tic lens                    a  chro  ma  tic    lens
          |   |  |   |  |                        |   |    |    |     |
          S   W  S   W  S                        S   W    S    W     S
           \ /    \ /   /                          \ /      \ /      /
            W      S   /          →                 S        W      /
             \      \ /                               \        \  /
              \      S                                 \       W
               \    /                                   \     /
                 W                                        W
                  \ /                                      \ /
```

Given a grid such as this, we can define grid marks which are next to each other *on the same level* as *adjacent*. 'Stress-clash' can then be defined as a case where adjacent grid marks have no intervening grid mark on the level below—in the case of Fig. 3.25(a) this applies to *-ma-* and *lens*, which have stars on level 3 with no intervening star on level 2. In Liberman and Prince's theory such a clash will trigger the reversal of the stresses, to give the representation of Fig. 3.25(b).

It is clear that the grid and the tree represent different things. Liberman and Prince (1977) argue that the tree representation is superior to the previous numerical characterization of 'degrees of stress' because it is *relational*: 'strong' is only strong in relation to 'weak', and does not reflect an absolute measure of anything. Selkirk (1984: 16ff.) suggests, however, that stress is not entirely relational, since it is possible to have a string of adjacent stressed syllables which have no unstressed syllables to be stronger than, and 'main word stress' is always stronger than ordinary stress. She therefore argues that the metrical grid theory of stress caters for both the relational and the non-relational aspects of stress,

---

[39] Lens gets an extra star at Level 4 because it is stronger than the weak node with which it is paired. Note that these levels are not equivalent to those used earlier in 3.4.

while the tree representation deals only with the relational aspects, unless it is supplemented by a set of 'prosodic categories' which—in her later work—she rejects.

Prince (1983) also rejects the tree theory. He notes that the standard metrical model devised by Liberman and Prince (1977) involves a 'two-stage mapping between syntactic structures and the grid: first, a translation into (binary-branching) *s/w* trees; second, an interpretation of the *s/w* relations thus derived in terms of alignment with the grid'. However, Prince attempts to show that the middle stage is unnecessary, and that the grid can be derived directly from the syntactic structure, 'without the intervention of a level where calculations with *s* and *w* take place on trees'. For example, given a right-branching structure in which the right-hand constituent is always strong (as, for example, in the 'Nuclear Stress Rule' of Chomsky and Halle (1968)), we could draw a tree in which there are pairs of *w* and *s* sister nodes. These could then be converted into a grid in which the rightmost element is the strongest. But, Prince argues, the information provided by the tree is actually irrelevant here, as we can proceed directly to the construction of the grid on the basis of the terminal nodes. The same will be true if the pattern of prominence is *s* + *w*.

This general approach, which dispenses with trees and represents accentual patterns in terms of grids, has been widely adopted; it is found, for example, in the theoretical framework of Halle and Vergnaud (1987a, 1987b), and the later work (1995) of Hayes (though Hayes, 1984, argues that both the tree and the grid are necessary, as they have different roles: the tree indicates stress and the grid indicates rhythm). In their influential work, Halle and Vergnaud (1987a) take up the metrical model of Liberman and Prince (1977), but without the tree representation, and add to it a number of typological ideas from Hayes (1981), applying the grid theory to a range of languages with different principles of stress-assignment. However, they do not entirely abandon the information contained in a tree representation, since they incorporate the notion of *metrical constituent structure*, recognizing metrical constituents (in effect, feet), and identifying the *heads* of these constituents. The head is the element which bears the stress. This gives a *bracketed grid* rather than a tree. In Maranungku and Weri, for example (Hayes, 1981; Halle and Vergnaud, 1987a: 17ff.), stress falls on alternate syllables, commencing with the initial syllable in the phrase in the case of Maranungku and with the final syllable in the case of Weri. The metrical constituents are therefore 'left-headed' and 'right-headed', respectively, and can be represented as in Fig. 3.26. Here, each syllable is represented by a number on the bottom level of the grid (line 0 in Halle and Vergnaud's representation), with the head given the number 1 and the sequence reflecting whether the constituents are left- or right-headed, and the stresses are indicated by an asterisk on line 1, coinciding with the head of each constituent. Since in Maranungku the main stress is on the initial syllable, and in Weri on the final syllable, an additional asterisk is provided on line 2 on these syllables. Such representations therefore reflect not only a basic stress pattern (Levels 1 and 2 accentuation of the scheme presented in 3.4.2, above), but also differences of accentual organization in different languages.

Fig. 3.26 (a) *Maranungku*

```
      *                    *              line 2
   *    *    *       *    *    *          line 1
  (1   2) (3 4) (5)  (1 2) (3 4) (5   6)  line 0
  lángka ráte  tí    wéle péne mánta
  ('prawn')           ('kind of duck')
```

(b) *Weri*

```
            *                   *         line 2
     *    *        *    *    *             line 1
   (4 3) (2 1)   (5) (4 3) (2 1)          line 0
   ulú  amít      á  kuné tepál
   ('mist')       ('times')
```

An important factor in these representations is the *typological* dimension, which allows the 'parametrization' of stress rules—i.e. an approach in which languages differ according to the particular 'settings' of basic parameters that their grammars embody.[40] This approach has been developed especially by Hayes, who is concerned with the establishment of different foot types in languages, which in turn reflect different accentual structures. Hayes (1981) establishes two parameters for feet: Quantity-Sensitivity and Dominance. The former is concerned with the relationship between stress and syllable-weight; in some languages stress assignment depends on whether the syllable is heavy or not. The latter is concerned with the location of the stressed syllable within the foot; the foot may be 'left-dominant' or 'right-dominant'.

Halle and Vergnaud (1987a) use a different set of parameters, which is determined by their use of metrical constituents. First, they distinguish cases where the head of the constituent (and therefore the stressed syllable) is at the edge of the constituent from cases where it is not. This provides a typological feature 'Head Terminal' ([±HT]). Second, they distinguish *bounded* from *unbounded* constituents, with the feature [±BND], according to whether there is a limit on the number of syllables the constituent may contain. However, they suggest that no language can have [−HT] constituents which are also [−BND] (i.e. constituents where the head is neither initial nor final and where the number of syllables is unlimited), since this would violate their 'Recoverability Condition', which stipulates that heads and constituent boundaries must be mutually predictable. Bounded constituents can be either *binary* or *ternary* (two and three syllables, respectively).

---

[40] On the role of parameters see Chomsky (1981: 3–4).

In more recent work, Hayes (1995) greatly simplifies the set of possible foot-types permitted by the theory, effectively reducing them to three: the Syllabic Trochee, the Moraic Trochee, and the Iamb. The terms trochee and iamb, derived from traditional verse metrics, refer to feet which are left-strong and right-strong, respectively, while the syllabic and moraic trochees differ in the unit involved. Hayes (1995: 71) represents these feet as in Fig. 3.27. It can be seen that both moraic trochees and iambs can also appear as single syllables. This is a consequence of Hayes's insistence on feet being maximally disyllabic; a phrase with an odd number of syllables will thus have a 'stray' syllable which constitutes a foot.

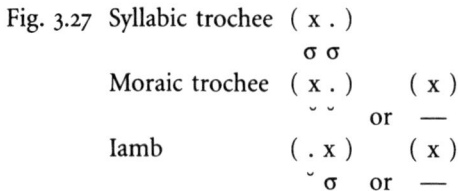

Fig. 3.27 Syllabic trochee (x .)

                        σ σ

        Moraic trochee (x .)   (x)

                      ˘ ˘   or —

        Iamb   (. x)   (x)

                      ˘ σ or —

Hayes gives extensive documentation and analysis of the stress systems of languages where these different foot types occur. According to Hayes (1985: 182), 'stress systems based on the syllabic trochee tend to be fairly simple'; the foot consists of two syllables, of which the first is strong. The examples from Maranungku given as Fig. 3.22(a), above, are of this type; other languages which Hayes places in this category include Icelandic, German, Hungarian, Czech, Modern Greek and Polish, as well as various languages of Australia and America. Moraic trochees can be illustrated from various forms of Arabic, as well as some American, Indo–Aryan, and Australian languages. Here, the foot consists of two moras, and stress assignment is therefore a matter of mora-counting (Hayes, 1995: 125ff.). Iambs are found primarily, though not exclusively, in America, including the Algonquian and Eskimo families; other languages included here are dialects of Bedouin Arabic, Ossetic, Cambodian, and other Mon–Khmer languages. The 'canonical form' of such feet, according to Hayes (1995: 205), is /˘⁻/, with a light syllable followed by a heavy one. Other languages, such as Weri (illustrated in 3.22b, above), Turkish, Malay, and Tiberian Hebrew, may possibly belong here, though Hayes concedes that such 'right-to-left iambic systems' may be analysable as trochees.[41]

Hayes is also able to postulate a general principle which goes beyond these categories, and relates the accentual system to the quantity system of the language. Drawing on 'a tradition of psychological experiments on rhythmic grouping' (1995: 79), Hayes provides evidence that, when presented with an alternating series of sounds, listeners group them into pairs differently according to whether

---

[41] The brevity of the discussion here is not a fair reflection of the extensive documentation of these various categories given in ch. 6 of Hayes (1995).

the alternation is of intensity or duration. Thus, given the patterns presented in Fig. 3.28, listeners group the sounds of Fig. 3.28(a) into pairs commencing with the louder sound, and those of Fig. 3.28(b) into pairs with the longer sound last.

Fig. 3.28 (a) . . . x́ x x́ x x́ x x́ x x́ x x́ x x́ x x́ x x́ x . . .

(b) . . . - — · — · — · — · — · — · — · — · — . . .

This principle obviously has some relevance to the theory of foot types, and Hayes formulates it as the 'Iambic/Trochaic Law', which runs as follows (Hayes, 1995: 80):

The Iambic/Trochaic Law
(a) Elements contrasting in intensity naturally form groupings with initial prominence.
(b) Elements contrasting in duration naturally form groupings with final prominence.

Part (a) of this law covers the trochaic foot types; the iambic type is catered for by part (b). Since the latter depends on duration, this predicts that iambic feet are likely to be based on moras rather than syllables, with a short (light) syllable followed by a long (heavy) one; hence the canonical iambic foot given above. Trochaic feet should, according to this principle, have equal length syllables, or have syllables which are independent of quantity or weight. This is, according to Hayes (1995: 81ff.), typically the case with moraic trochees and syllabic trochees, respectively.

3.5.4 EVALUATION

In spite of the influential nature of the metrical theory of stress, in its various versions, there are a number of characteristics of the theory which give rise to doubts. At several points, the theory entails claims about the nature of stress and accentual structure which do not correspond with the conclusions reached earlier in this chapter. Though not all of these problem areas can be examined here, some of the major difficulties can be mentioned.

A major advance of metrical theories on previous generative approaches is the recognition that stress is primarily a matter of *rhythm*. Rhythm is included in the model of Liberman and Prince (1977), and is the main motivation for the grid, which allows for stress shifts by the 'Rhythm Rule'. The grid is thus 'fundamentally a formalization of the traditional idea of "stress-timing"'. For them, however, rhythm is only one factor in the specification of stress, hence their use not only of the grid but also of the tree, and of the feature [±stress], each of which caters for different factors. These different ways of representing stress appear to be the source of one of the most unsatisfactory aspects of metrical approaches: the retention of unnecessary and spurious 'degrees of stress'. As we shall see, these are generally susceptible to a non-accentual analysis.

The feature [±stress] is used by Liberman and Prince largely as a means of accommodating the distinction between reduced and non-reduced vowels and syllables (see Fig. 3.12), and therefore does not belong in the accentual system at all. We saw that it can be eliminated in a number of ways; Selkirk (1980) and Hayes (1981) do so by treating syllables to which it would apply as separate feet, as in Fig. 3.16 and Fig. 3.17, above. According to Selkirk (1980), this solution ensures that the second syllable of words such as *gymnast* or *rabbi*, unlike that of *modest* or *happy*, will retain some prominence, and thus be assigned secondary stress. But it may be seriously questioned whether this is an appropriate solution, since the second syllable of *gymnast* or *rabbi* does not, except in very exceptional circumstances, bear Level 1 accentuation at all, including 'secondary stress'. Rhythmically, both these syllables form a single foot with the first syllable of the word, as in *The / gymnast / drove the / rabbi's / car*, where feet are separated by /, and are thus unaccented, though they are *unreduced*. The foot solution may eliminate the need for the feature [±stress] but at the expense of the inclusion of a spurious accent in these words.[42]

More serious, however, are the cases where, effectively, a paradigmatic system of stresses is recognized, in spite of the insistence that stress is here interpreted syntagmatically. The main source of this problem is the view, unambiguously expressed by Liberman and Prince (1977), that 'relative prominence tends to be preserved under embedding'. Thus, to give their example, the relative stresses of a simple compound such as *whále-òil*, with a stronger stress on *whale* than *oil*, is preserved when this compound forms part of a larger expression, such as *whàle-oil lámp*.[43] Since the syntactic structure of phrases and sentences allows for (theoretically) unlimited amounts of recursive embedding, this provides for a correspondingly unlimited amount of stress subordination. An inevitable consequence of this view of stress is that the model still retains—in somewhat weakened form—the concept of a paradigmatic system of 'degrees of stress'.

This is particularly evident in Halle and Vergnaud (1987a), who simply repeat the claims of Chomsky and Halle (1968) that 'degrees of stress' are a reflection of syntactic embedding, and, since this is unrestricted, so are the number of degrees. They give the examples of Fig. 3.29, including the sentence *formaldehyde is a powerful poison*, in which, they assert, there are six degrees of stress (note that 0 = weakest and 5 = strongest). In isolation, *formaldehyde* is given the contour 1 3 0 2, and it retains this in Fig. 3.29(a); the 'Nuclear Stress Rule' increases the stress level on the rightmost element, so that this word has the contour 1 4 0 2 in Fig. 3.29(b); in Fig. 3.29(c), Halle and Vergnaud argue that 'the main stress of *formaldehyde* is less than that of *poison*, yet greater than that of *powerful*'; hence the six degrees of stress represented here.

---

[42] That some means of specifying the reduced/unreduced dichotomy is necessary is, of course, not in dispute here. The point being made is that this dichotomy is not a matter of 'accent' and should therefore not be specified by features of accent or stress.

[43] Actually, this example appears to be flawed, since—according to the rules of Liberman and Prince themselves—the main stress is normally on the first element, since the second element does not branch: *whále-oil làmp*.

Fig. 3.29   1   3   0 2   0 0   4   0
          (a) formaldehyde is a poison

                 0   3   0   0   1   4   0 2
          (b) the poison was formaldehyde

                 1   4   0 2   0 0   3   0 0   5   0
          (c) formaldehyde is a powerful poison

In terms of the approach adopted here, however, a representation with six degrees of stress is an impossibility, indeed an absurdity. Though this sentence could be pronounced in a number of different ways, none of them require more than the two levels of accentuation discussed above (possibly three, if we include intonational subordination as a matter of accentuation). Assuming, with Halle and Vergnaud, a single accentual phrase, and adopting a grid notation, the sentence of Fig. 3.29(c) can be represented as in Fig. 3.30. There is no evidence that the stress on *-hyde* is less than that on *pow-*, or that that on *mal-* is greater than these. The extra accent on *poi-* is the phrase (Level 2) accent, and is thus a matter of intonation.

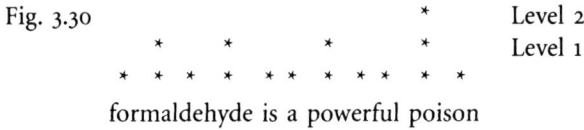

Fig. 3.30   *   Level 2
                 *   *   *   *   Level 1
          *   *   *   *   * *   *   * *   *   *

          formaldehyde is a powerful poison

Given an alternative phrasing, with a separate phrase for *formaldehyde*, we would, of course get the rendering of Fig. 3.31, with an additional phrase accent on *-ma-* (the phrase boundary is indicated by ||). The first phrase would be subordinated intonationally to the second, which could lead us to 'rank' the second phrase accent higher than the first, but this is no longer a matter of accent, but of intonation structure.

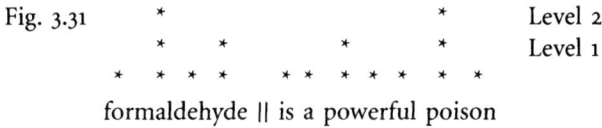

Fig. 3.31   *   *   Level 2
                 *   *   *   *   Level 1
          *   *   *   *   * *   *   *   *   *   *

          formaldehyde || is a powerful poison

Hayes also rejects multiple paradigmatic stress levels, and interprets the different 'degrees' rhythmically. He gives, for example (1995: 28), the representation of Fig. 3.32 for the phrase *twenty-seven Mississippi legislators*, which appears to incorporate three levels of stress.[44] Hayes expressly rejects the view that there is a multi-valued stress feature here, since the grid represents a rhythmic structure. However, this representation is still based on a false assumption, which leads to the incorporation of spurious degrees.

---

[44] Hayes's use of 'x' rather than '*' is retained here.

Fig. 3.32   x
            x   x   x
            x   x   x   x   x   x
            x x x x   x x x x   x x x x
            twenty-seven Mississippi legislators

In terms of the approach taken here, this phrase could again have several different pronunciations, of which the most straightforward is one with six accented syllables at Level 1, and a single Level 2 accent, as in Fig. 3.33.

Fig 3.33   x   Level 2
            x   x   x   x   x   x   Level 1
            x x x x   x x x x   x x x x
            twenty-seven Mississippi legislators

Hayes's distinction of stress levels *within* each of the words *twenty-seven* and *Mississippi* is, in the model advocated here, not possible if the whole phrase constitutes a single accentual phrase. This distinction has two possible sources; first, it may result from regarding *potential* accents as subordinate degrees, as discussed earlier. Thus, a rendering with fewer accents, as in Fig. 3.34, would eliminate the accents on *-se-*, *-si-*, and *-la-*, which are then merely potential accents. Under this interpretation, the version given in Fig. 3.32 is a non-existent conflation of Figs. 3.33 and 3.34.

Fig. 3.34   x   Level 2
            x   x   x   Level 1
            x x x x   x x x x   x x x x
            twenty-seven Mississippi legislators

An alternative source of the version given in Fig. 3.32 is a rendering with three shorter accentual phrases, increasing the number of Level 2 accents, as in Fig. 3.35(a) (phrase boundaries are indicated by ||). In this case, 'Iambic Reversal' is less likely, and the version of Fig. 3.35(b) is perhaps more usual, in spite of the 'stress-clash', though both are possible.

Fig. 3.35 (a)   x   x   x   Level 2
                 x   x   x   x   x   x Level 1
                 x x x x   x x x x   x x x x
                 twenty-seven || Mississippi || legislators

                 x   x   x   Level 2
          (b)   x   x   x   x   x   x Level 1
                 x x x x   x x x x   x x x x
                 twenty-seven || Mississippi || legislators

The claim made here, therefore, is that all cases where a hierarchy of stress 'levels' is postulated can be reduced to the two levels of accentuation recognized here. The lower level (Level 1) is the level of accentuation proper; in a language such as English it is based on a rhythmical principle. The upper level (Level 2) (as well as a possible third level, Level 3), is dependent on intonation structure, and is *not* rhythmical.

The rhythmical basis of speech has, as we have noted, been accepted by many scholars, though the way that this is interpreted may differ. Selkirk (1984) argues at length (pp. 38–52) for a similar approach to the one presented here, but she draws different conclusions at several points. She rightly attributes to Abercrombie (1964) the credit for having developed the foot as the basis of rhythm in English. She cites (p. 42) the example given by Catford (1966) of an utterance with several different renderings, with different groupings of syllables into feet (see Fig. 3.36). This is entirely comparable to the examples given above. Oddly, however, she remarks that 'the notion "foot" employed here cannot be the same one defined by Abercrombie, for each of the monosyllabic words in these examples is stressed, and so constitutes a foot on its own. The vertical marks must in fact be taken as indicating strong–weak relations on a level above that of the foot.' Selkirk assumes that the foot in Abercrombie's sense cannot be monosyllabic, because it is based on an alternation of stressed and unstressed syllables. However, she is mistaken here; Abercrombie's foot is based *not* on an alternation of strong and weak beats but on the regular occurrence of stressed syllables. He gives (1964) the example |*four* | *large* | *black* | *dogs* to illustrate precisely the occurrence of monosyllabic feet.[45] There is therefore no need to invoke a higher level in order to account for the rhythmical structure of the examples in Fig. 3.36.

Fig. 3.36 | John | bought | two | books | last | week
          | John | bought two | books last | week
          | John bought | two books | last week
          | John bought two | books last week

Selkirk (1984: 43) gives examples similar to those of Hayes (1995) where *two* levels of rhythm appear to be involved. These are reproduced as Fig. 3.37, where the vertical bars are intended to mimic the placements of Catford (1966). She claims, however, that in addition to the stresses on the initial beats of each foot, there are further rhythmic beats; all beats are italicized in Fig. 3.37. On the basis of this, she is able to claim (p. 43) that 'the intuition, then, is that rhythmic groupings are made at more than one level'. If this is so, then it represents important evidence that a simple indication of stress (Level 1 accentuation) is insufficient; a grid with multiple levels is necessary.

---

[45] Selkirk (1984: 39) in fact quotes another example with a monosyllabic foot from the same page of Abercrombie's article: | *This is the* | *house that* | *Jack* | *built*.

Fig. 3.37   (i) | Mary | purchased | twenty | pamphlets | yesterday | morning
            (ii) | Mary | purchased twenty | pamphlets yesterday | morning
           (iii) | Mary purchased | twenty pamphlets | yesterday morning
           (iv) | Mary purchased twenty | pamphlets yesterday morning

The counter-arguments applied above to Hayes's examples are equally applicable here, however. Assuming a single accentual phrase, then in so far as renderings (ii) to (iv) have rhythmical prominence on all the italicized syllables they are equivalent to rendering (i); otherwise we may claim that the assumed prominences are spurious, and are based on *potential* prominence. Again different phrasal groupings are possible, providing different Level 2 accents, as in Fig. 3.35, above. Thus, version (ii) might reflect a division into three accentual phrases, as in Fig. 3.38, accounting for the lower prominence on *twenty* and *yesterday*, as non-tonic accents, than on the tonic accents of *purchased, pamphlets*, and *morning*. But what must be emphasized here is that we do not in any case have more than one level of *rhythmical* prominence.

Fig. 3.38   *   *   *
          *   *   *   *   *   *
        *   *   *   *   *   *   *   *   *   *   *   *

Mary | purchased || twenty | pamphlets || yesterday | morning

As far as Hayes's different foot types are concerned, their status remains unclear. That, according to part (a) of the Iambic/Trochaic Law, 'elements contrasting in intensity naturally form groupings with initial prominence' confirms the view that a stress-based rhythm provides units commencing with the accented syllable. Hence, a sequence of syllables x x́ x x́ x x x́ x́ is probably always perceived as x | x́ x | x́ x | x́ x | x́ rather than as | x x́ | x x́ | x x́ | x x́ |. The difficulty comes with 'iambic' feet, formed according to part (b) of the Law, which states that 'elements contrasting in duration naturally form groupings with final prominence'. If for 'intensity' in part (a) we read 'stress', then what is the 'prominence' associated with the final long element of an iambic foot, if this type of foot has no stress? Though length has frequently been identified as one of the features which characterize 'stress', it is not otherwise accorded independent status as a realization of accent. Hayes's foot typology may therefore not be a matter of different accentuation types at all. It must also be borne in mind that the original experiments reported on by Hayes (1995: 79) are not concerned with speech as such but with rhythmical perception in general, and Hayes's further justification (pp. 80–1) is based on the rhythm of verse and music; speech rhythm does not necessarily follow the same principles. As Hayes (1995: 26–8) points out, musical rhythm, in some cultural traditions at least, can be quite complex, with multi-layered hierarchical structures and simultaneous cross-rhythms. The temptation to see the rhythm of speech in equally complex terms is seductive, especially when we see that linguistic models can often be insightfully applied to music—see especially Lerdahl and Jackendoff (1983), who analyse musical structure in terms of generative grammar. However, speech rhythm seems to be much simpler than that of music, not least because, as Hayes (1995: 27) points out, only one voice is involved.

As we saw above, both Halle and Vergnaud (1987a) and Hayes (1995) give extensive illustrations of the application of their theories to a wide variety of languages. This raises further questions about the possibility of establishing general principles of accentuation. The discussion throughout this chapter has made it clear that the interpretation of accentual phenomena is more a matter of theory than of fact; the data assume remarkably different forms according to the theoretical model that is used to account for them. This view is reinforced by the observation—documented in this chapter—that linguists who are native speakers of English can come to such widely divergent conclusions about the nature of accentuation in their mother-tongue. When we turn to reports of other languages in the available literature on stress and accent the evidence is still more unreliable, not only because the quantity of the evidence is very much smaller, but also because much of it is, as Hayes (1995: 4) acknowledges, second-hand.[46] For this reason, therefore, generalizations require considerable caution, and no claims can be made about the general validity of the approach to accentuation described here.

3.6 The Specification of Accent

3.6.1 ASSIGNING ACCENT

Thus far, we have been concerned with the *representation* of stress and accent, with the assumed nature of these features and the structures into which they fit, and to which they contribute. A further question to be addressed is how these features and structures should be *specified*, that is, how the accentual patterns of words and sentences[47] are to be derived.

An initial issue here is the degree to which the accentual structure of sentences is *autonomous*, i.e. independent of the morpho-syntactic structure or lexical content. The fact that accentuation is a rhythmical phenomenon is strong evidence for the autonomy of prosodic structure, as is the possibility of assigning an accentual structure to meaningless utterances. The point here is not that the

---

[46] An illustration of the difficulty here is found in the work of Halle and Vergnaud (1987). The authors refer (p. 12) to accentuation in French, in which, they assert, 'stress is word-final', although received opinion among scholars is that French has no word–stress at all.

[47] It is a moot point whether we should here refer to *sentences* or *utterances*. The role of grammars is usually construed as the specification of sentences as abstract objects rather than of utterances as physical events. However, it could be argued that prosodic features are too context-dependent to be assigned to sentences in the abstract; they can only be assigned to actual utterances. This issue will be addressed further below.

morphological or syntactic structure is irrelevant, but rather that this structure must be mapped onto an independent well-formed prosodic structure; there must clearly be rules and principles for achieving this. The processes here can be construed in a number of ways, according to the model adopted. For example, we can devise rules for assigning stress to words and sentences, taking account of the relevant morphological and syntactic factors as well as the phonological constraints; or, using a different model, we can see these rules as principles for aligning parts of sentences with the metrical grid, perhaps taking account of the strong–weak relations of the metrical tree, and so on.

Much of the extensive discussion of these matters centres on the specific rules of individual languages, especially English. Works such as Kingdon (1958a) and Fudge (1984) give detailed information not only about the general principles involved but also about the idiosyncratic accentual features of specific morphemes. It is inappropriate to consider these language-specific principles here; what concerns us are the general principles, including the kinds of factors that influence the placement of accent, and the general characteristics of a formal model of accent assignment.

It is evident that no one single factor determines accent placement; phonological, morphological, syntactic, and pragmatic factors may all be involved, and differently in different languages. As far as phonological factors are concerned, these include such criteria as the position in the word and the weight of the syllables (which can be interpreted as 'mora-counting'—see 2.5.4). Of particular interest here is the typological dimension; different languages may employ different principles, but the possibilities are not limitless, and there are definable types. Hyman (1977) provides a useful survey of the position of the stress in 444 languages, of which 300 have a 'dominant stress placement', as summarized in Fig. 3.39.[48] It can be seen that the the majority of languages with a dominant position have the stress on the initial or final syllable, though penultimate position is also well-attested. The relatively small number with second-syllable stress is striking.

Fig. 3.39 (a) languages with dominant initial stress   114
          (b) languages with dominant second-syllable stress 12
          (c) languages with dominant penultimate stress   77
          (d) languages with dominant final stress   97

Hyman attempts to provide explanations for these figures. Initial and final stress can be explained in terms of the demarcative function (cf. 3.3.3), i.e. where stress indicates a word-boundary. According to Hyman, 'the closer stress falls to that boundary, the better it will fulfil its linguistic function'. Penultimate

---

[48] As Hyman admits, the figures are rather crude and unreliable, since they do not distinguish between position in the word, position in the phrase, and position in the stem, nor between 'syllable-counting' and 'mora-counting'.

stress demands a different explanation, however, and Hyman suggests that its source is intonation. If the basic intonation pattern is a fall, and this is analysed as High + Low, then this will ideally require two syllables for its execution, hence the High pitch (which constitutes the accent) will occur on the penultimate syllable. No such principle can be invoked in the case of second-syllable stress.

Morphological factors include accentual characteristics of individual affixes, some of which may 'attract' the accent and others 'repel' it, or which may require the accent to be placed on a specific preceding syllable. Fudge (1984), for example, refers to *autostressed* suffixes which attract stress to themselves (e.g. *-ade* in *lemo'nade*, *-aire* in *millio'naire*), and *pre-stressed* suffixes, which assign the stress to a preceding syllable (e.g. *–ic*, which places the stress on the preceding syllable, as in *pho'nemic*; or *-fy*, which places the stress two syllables before, as in *so'lidify*).

3.6.2 STRESS AND SYNTAX

Of particular significance is the role of syntactic structure in the specification of accents, as we have seen above. This has been one of the major themes in generative phonology, occupying a substantial part of Chomsky and Halle (1968). The first explicit account of stress within a generative framework is found in Chomsky, Halle, and Lukoff (1956). They start from the (then) generally accepted Bloomfieldian analysis of English stress with four contrasting degrees and concede that they 'have, on the whole, not attempted to discover new facts or to challenge the accuracy of available data'. However, their account is radically different from their sources,[49] and proposes to specify stress using only a single opposition—'accented–unaccented'—but using an elaborate set of rules and taking account of the syntactic structure of the utterance, the latter being achieved by incorporating 'junctures'. The rules given include the following:

Rule 2: The effect of internal (external) juncture is to:
(i) weaken the main stress in its right (left) domain by one
(ii) weaken the other stresses of the right (left) domain by one if main stress has been reduced by (i) to the level of other stresses
(iii) weaken the non-main stresses of the left (right) domain by one if these are equal to the main stress of the right (left) domain.

Rule 4: Given a phonemic clause,
(i) assign the value 1 to all accented vowels;
(ii) then apply each rule pertaining to accented vowels no more than once to each constituent, applying a rule to a constituent of order *n* only after having applied it to all constituents of order *n* + 1; i.e. beginning with the smallest constituents and proceeding to larger and larger constituents;

---

[49] In the discussion in Sledd (1962), conducted in terms of Bloomfieldian assumptions, this paper is dismissed as 'naive'.

(iii) next assign to each unaccented vowel the weakest stress which is
    (a) at least 3
    (b) at least 4 if the given vowel is /i/ or if it occurs before main stress with no
        intervening juncture
    (c) greater than the value of any accented vowel;
(iv) finally apply all rules which pertain to unaccented vowels.

This allows Bloch and Trager's *elevator-operator* to be derived as in Fig. 3.40.[50]

Fig. 3.40   ɛ l i v e t i r - a p i r e t i r   RULE APPLIED

1.	1				1								4i
2.	1				2								4ii, 2i
3.	1	4	3	4	2	4	3	4					4iii

A number of significant principles are incorporated into these rules. First, the stresses are allocated on the basis of syntactic structure, reflected in the appeal to external and internal junctures in Rule 2 and elsewhere. Second, the rules apply over and over again until the largest syntactic constituent is reached (Rule 4ii). Third, the stress level is a reflection of the number of times the rules have applied (Rule 2). Because the last of these principles could result in a theoretically unlimited number of stress levels (since there is no theoretical limit to the depth of syntactic embedding), Chomsky, Halle, and Lukoff introduce a final rule which sets an (unspecified) limit, depending on the style of speech and the speaker.

These principles are characteristic of the classical generative approach to the specification of stress; they are found virtually unchanged in Chomsky and Halle (1968) and other works in the same tradition. The 'stress contours' of complex words and phrases are derived by the cyclical application of rules to ever larger domains, determined by the constituent structure of the phrase. Stress is assigned by placing [1stress] on the appropriate element at each cycle, and the different degrees are obtained by a convention reducing all the other stress levels by one. Fig. 3.41 gives a three-fold example (Chomsky and Halle, 1968: 20–1): *black board-eraser* ('board-eraser that is black') *blackboard eraser* ('eraser for a blackboard'), and *black board eraser* (eraser of a black board) showing how the assumed 'stress contours' of the different phrases are derived by means of cyclical rules. The brackets indicate the constituent structure and the horizontal lines indicate the scope of application of the rule at each cycle. At Cycle I primary stress is assigned to the individual words. The innermost brackets are deleted and primary stress is assigned again at Cycle II, placing primary stress on the first element in each domain (where these are compounds) or on the final element (where they are phrases). The same rules apply again on Cycle III.

---

[50] The final stress of line 3 is given as 3 in the original; this is assumed to be an error and has been amended to 4. Note that Bloch and Trager's transcription reflects an American pronunciation.

The final stress contour thus reflects the constituent structure of each phrase.

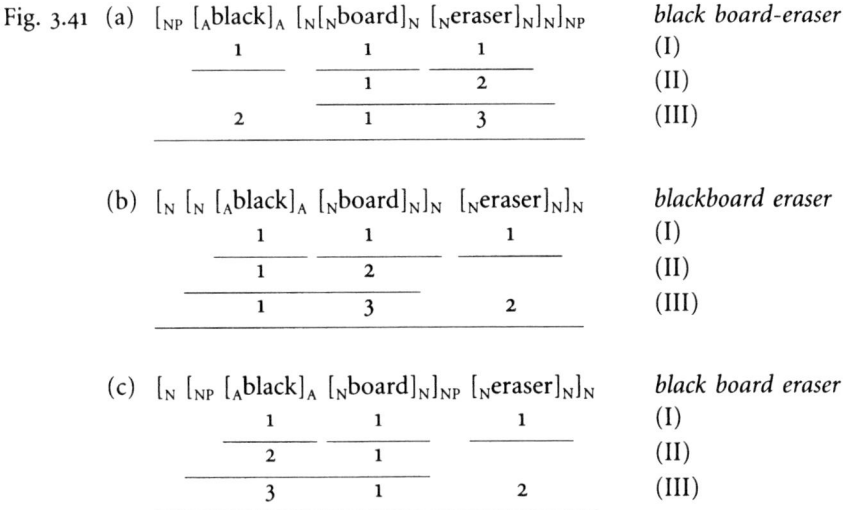

Fig. 3.41 (a) $[_{NP} [_A black]_A [_N[_N board]_N [_N eraser]_N]_N]_{NP}$ *black board-eraser*

1	1	1	(I)
	1	2	(II)
2	1	3	(III)

(b) $[_N [_N [_A black]_A [_N board]_N]_N [_N eraser]_N]_N$ *blackboard eraser*

1	1	1	(I)
1	2		(II)
1	3	2	(III)

(c) $[_N [_{NP} [_A black]_A [_N board]_N]_{NP} [_N eraser]_N]_N$ *black board eraser*

1	1	1	(I)
2	1		(II)
3	1	2	(III)

The details of the model presented here are developed by a number of other scholars, such as Halle and Keyser (1971), Ross (1972), Halle (1973), Brame (1973, 1974), and others. These revisions have generally been in order to make the rules more precise, or to simplify and generalize them. For example, Schane (1975)[51] proposes that the convention whereby non-primary stress levels are reduced by one when primary stress is assigned should be restricted to cases where primary stress is assigned to an existing primary stress rather than to a non-primary one; this amendment is incorporated in Halle's revision (1973), resulting in a greatly simplified set of rules. However, the principles mentioned above—cyclical application of stress rules to a syntactic constituent structure, producing a number of degrees of stress—remain intact.

Since the starting point for the rules of stress assignment is the syntactic structure of the sentence, there has been discussion of the relationship between stress and syntax, particularly in the case of 'sentence stress' (what has here been called Level 2 accentuation). A notable controversy in this area was initiated by Bresnan (1971), arguing that the rule assigning this stress should be included in the syntactic transformational cycle, thus blurring the distinction between syntax and phonology. The matter was not entirely clarifed in the ensuing debate (Berman and Szamosi, 1972; Bolinger, 1972; Lakoff, 1972; Bresnan 1972), which also queried the extent to which stress can be determined on syntactic grounds.

As we have noted, the basic assumptions of the model are unaffected by these revisions and controversies. In fact, as noted above, the principles appear again in metrical theory (Liberman and Prince, 1977; Halle and Vergnaud, 1987a), if

---

[51] Written in 1972, but unpublished at the time.

in somewhat diluted form. As we have seen above, Halle and Vergnaud apply their rules cyclically to a syntactically specified structure, producing an unlimited number of degrees of stress: 'the difficulty of placing an upper bound on the number of degrees of stress that need to be distinguished derives from the fact that there is no upper bound on the depth of syntactic embedding' (Halle and Vergnaud, 1987a: 37).

3.6.3 NON-CYCLICAL APPROACHES

Although the approach just outlined has become standard in generative accounts of stress, there are alternatives, which propose non-cyclical procedures for stress assignment. Schane (1975) argues that a cyclical approach is unnecessary, and stress is assigned to the whole word in one operation. Morphological boundaries are invoked in this process, but there is no need for hierarchical constituent structures. As an example of how this is assumed to work, consider the words *attestation* and *devastation*. This pair is often cited (e.g. by Halle and Keyser, 1971: 53) in support of the cyclical application of stress rules, since the second syllable is unreduced in *attestation* but is reduced in *devastation*. This is considered to reflect the presence of stress on this syllable in an earlier cycle in the case of *attestation* but not in the cases of *devastation*, since the former contains the verb *attest*, while there is no **devast*. Schane gives an alternative analysis which does not require the cycle, as in Fig. 3.42. Rule 1 is a standard rule which places the stress on the penultimate vowel unless it is a lax vowel followed by no more than a single consonant; it assigns stress to *-at-* in both words. Rule 2 places the stress by the same principle before an initially-stressed suffix; here it assigns stress to the heavy syllable before the suffix *-at-* in *attestation*, but does not apply to *devastation*, because here *-at-* is not a suffix. The alternating stress rule places [+stress] two syllables before a previously assigned [+stress] syllable, and applies to both words. The detail rule converts [+stress] into a numerical stress value according to the following principle: 'The rightmost [+stress] not on the final syllable becomes a [1 stress]; then all remaining [+stress] become [3 stress]'. Finally, in *attestation*, the rhythm rule applies, reducing one of the [3 stress] syllables to [4 stress]; it takes the form $3 \ldots 3 \ldots 1 \rightarrow 3 \ldots 4 \ldots 1$. In Schane's model, the difference between the two words is in the presence or absence of a morpheme boundary before *-at-*; no cyclical rule-application is needed.

Fig. 3.42 attest + āt + ion

		+		rule 1
	+			rule 2
+				alternating stress rule
3	3		1	detail rule
3	4		1	rhythm rule

```
devast    āt + ion
            +          rule 1
   +                   alternating stress rule
   3        1          detail rule
```

Shibatani (1972) also abandons the cycle in the specification of Japanese accent. He rejects McCawley's orthodox generative approach, which produces different levels of accent, and assigns different pitch features to them. Shibatani argues that 'there are no grades of abstract accent – it is only a question of whether or not there is an accent there'. Thus, the specification of pitch levels does not depend on an elaborate ranking of accents; it is a matter of 'surface pitch adjustment'. For English, Sloat (1974) similarly dispenses with different degrees, recognizing only primary and secondary stress. As a result, there is again no need for cyclical rules.

Schane's subsequent work (1979a, 1979b) focuses on rhythm as the prime ingredient of accentuation rules. For him, rhythm is based on an alternation of strong and weak syllables, and rules are required to determine which strong syllables have primary stress. There are also rhythmical constraints, forbidding, for example, two contiguous strong syllables. These constraints 'define the surface accentual patterns of English', rendering the cyclical rules of Chomsky and Halle unnecessary.

Though these alternative views of the specification of accent have not had the influence and acceptance of cyclical theories, it is clear that they are closer in spirit to the model of prosodic structure advocated in 3.4. The main purpose of cyclical rules is to capture the assumed principle that prominence relations within words are maintained when these words are embedded in larger structures. If this principle is abandoned—and this is the position adopted here—then the motivation for the cycle disappears. If, furthermore, accentuation in languages such as English is assumed to have a rhythmical basis, then the multiple degrees of stress generated by the cyclical model are in any case inappropriate, and some sort of recursive linear model would appear to be preferable.

This is not to say, however, that the rules for determining which syllables in an utterance are to receive accent are necessarily simple; indeed, there are many complex factors involved here, with the interplay of phonological, morphological and syntactic criteria. Rules are evidently needed to map hierarchical, multiply-embedded, syntactic structures onto rather simpler prosodic structures. Whether or not cyclical rules are required here is an open question; it is possible to take account of syntactic factors in assigning accentual structure without requiring such rules. The indications are that existing models which use cyclical rules produce an over-differentiated and unrealistic accentual structure.

3.6.4 THE STATUS OF 'STRESS CONTOURS'

A further issue is raised primarily by generative models, where accentual patterns are generated by the application of rules to syntactic structures: the status of the 'stress contours' generated. Two questions will be considered here: the 'degrees of stress' which result from such rules, and alternative accentual renderings of utterances. Both questions raise difficult and controversial issues about the nature and status of accent and, beyond this, about the status of phonological representation and derivations themselves.

We have seen that Chomsky and Halle (1968), and the tradition which follows them, devise a grammar which derives the accentual patterns of sentences from their syntactic structure, and in particular the depth of embedding of syntactic constituents is claimed to be reflected in the number of 'degrees of stress' that are generated. Since an indefinite number of degrees runs counter to all phonetic evidence (whatever we consider the phonetic nature of accent to be), the status of such 'degrees' is unclear. Chomsky and Halle (1968: 25) state that 'we do not doubt that the stress contours and other phonetic facts that are recorded by careful phoneticians and that we will study here constitute some sort of perceptual reality for those who know the language in question'; however, they also assert that 'there is nothing to suggest that these phonetic representations also describe a physical or acoustic reality'. They claim that 'a person who knows the language should "hear" the predicted phonetic shapes', while 'there seems to be no reason to suppose that a well-trained phonetician could detect such contours with any reliability or precision in a language that he does not know'. On the strength of this claim, Chomsky and Halle have no problem with an indefinite number of degrees, since they are not required to have any basis in phonetic fact. Nevertheless, they do suggest that 'it is necessary to formulate a principle for interpretation of phonetic representations that nullifies distinctions that go beyond a certain degree of refinement' (p. 23). This in itself seems contradictory; if the degrees have no physical reality, it is not clear why a limit must be set.

This approach carries many dangers, not least methodologically, since there is effectively no objective control on the analysis; the claims made about stress are shielded from any kind of empirical scrutiny or verification. It is also difficult to see what is being described if it has no objective reality.[52] Hoard (1971) complains that 'Chomsky and Halle are rather vague about just what it is exactly that a *stress* contour is as a surface phonetic phenomenon. . . . If a well-trained phonetician cannot transcribe a stress contour in a language he does not know, as Chomsky and Halle claim, then it is, by definition, not a surface phonetic phenomenon.' Chomsky and Halle's disclaimer can therefore be construed as a sign of the weakness of their analysis.

The second question to be addressed is the existence of alternative accentual

---

[52] That there is a subjective element to accentuation is not denied; accent is described in 3.4 in terms of a 'mental beat'. However, it is possible to recognize this subjective element without abandoning the phonetic reality of the phenomenon, since the phonetic basis is manifested in the rhythmical spacing of accents. Establishing a whole set of contrasting degrees with no requirement of phonetic reality is another matter entirely.

patterns for utterances. Such alternatives have been presented on several occasions in this chapter, together with the claim that the 'potential' accents have illegitimately been included as lower degrees of stress. The question at issue is whether such different versions—which do not necessarily differ substantially in meaning—should be considered a matter of *competence* or of *performance* , that is, whether they are part of the 'ideal' grammar of the speaker or merely aspects of its realization. This point is addressed by Cutler and Ladd (ed.) (1983: 143), who provide 'comparative notes' on a number of prosodic terms, including the concept of 'domains', which they describe as 'chunks of structure over which prosodic phenomena may be defined'. Commenting on the system of domains ('foot' and 'tone-group') used by Halliday (1967), they remark that 'an important characteristic of Halliday's system is that it is intended to describe utterances, and hence assigns prosodic structure not as an abstract property of words and sentences, but as a dimension of their spoken realization. Within this system it is therefore possible for a particular word or sentence to be assigned different structures in different utterances.'

If we incorporate the variant renderings into the grammar of competence, then it is clearly not possible to determine the accentual pattern on the basis of constituent structure, or, indeed, of any rule which is sensitive only to grammatical features of the sentence, since these features are constant. Models which attempt to do this must therefore relegate accentual variation to performance. If differences in accentual structure are a matter of performance only, however, then this entails establishing an ideal ('abstract') rendering; but it is very doubtful whether such a rendering exists, and it is not clear on what basis it could be established, other than arbitrarily.

3.7 Conclusion: Accent and Prosodic Structure

By way of conclusion to this chapter, we may restate some of the main conclusions that have been drawn regarding the nature of accent from the survey of views presented here. As we have seen there is still no real consensus about some of the most fundamental aspects of accent—its phonetic nature, the existence of 'degrees of stress', and the appropriate means of representing and specifying it. In this chapter, a particular view of these phenomena has been articulated, which owes debts to several of the many traditions of analysis and description. It recognizes, first of all, the unity of accentual phenomena, whether these be 'stress–accent' or 'pitch–accent'; this unity allows us to relegate the specific phonetic content of accent to a matter of secondary importance. Second, this approach separates out accentual features as such from other apparently related phenomena, such as vowel reduction and intonation. As a result, it is possible to reduce accentuation to a relatively simple structure containing two 'levels'; at the lower level (Level 1) we have features traditionally called 'word-stress' (though this term is inappropriate given the autonomy of accental structure), which can be accounted for—in English and many other languages—in rhythmical terms. At the higher level (Level 2), we are concerned with the traditional 'sentence stress'; this is a property of larger units, and is primarily a matter of intonational prominence.

As with other areas of prosodic structure, accentuation depends crucially on a hierarchical principle; the two levels recognized have different domains of relevance and they are ordered hierarchically. However, there is no place here for the elaborate paradigmatic stress systems established by a number of scholars in the American structuralist tradition, and continued through classical generative and some more recent metrical models. In particular, too, the principle of an unlimited set of 'degrees' dependent on syntactic constituency is rejected; the status of such degrees has not been satisfactorily established.

However we interpret the phonetic and phonological basis of accent, however, there is no doubt that it is—in Beckman's terms (1986)—an 'organizational' feature, whose role is essentially syntagmatic. In languages which possess it, accentual structure is the fundamental framework which supports the whole phonology. We shall return to this framework in a wider setting in the final chapter.

4

Tone

4.1 Introduction

4.1.1 THE NATURE OF TONE

Pitch is not in itself a phonological feature; it is a *phonetic* feature with a variety of prosodic functions, and it can only be interpreted phonologically in the light of these different functions. These functions are usually assigned to one of three broad types: *tone, accent*, and *intonation*. The precise definitions of these, and the criteria for delimiting them, are, however, a matter of some controversy. *Intonation* can be distinguished from the other two first because its domain of application is the phrase or the sentence, rather than the word, and second because its function is discourse-oriented rather than lexical or grammatical. *Pitch–accent* involves the use of pitch in an accentual function, i.e. to give prominence to one particular element, as discussed in Chapter 3. *Tone*, finally, has lexical or grammatical significance, as an intrinsic property of a morpheme, word, or grammatical construction.

However, these brief characterizations are neither unambiguous nor necessarily mutually exclusive. Pitch–accent, for example, may serve to distinguish different lexical items; is it then tone because it is lexical? Intonation is often assumed to have grammatical functions; for example, it is said to distinguish different sentence types. In what way does this differ from the use of tone for grammatical purposes? Syllables may be given prominence by tones or tone patterns as well as by pitch–accents. These ambiguities suggest first that pitch phenomena in languages will not necessarily be classifiable in terms of a single criterion, and second that there are likely to be marginal cases which cannot be definitively assigned to one particular category or another. We would also anticipate encountering some difficulties in defining the term 'tone-language' itself. This chapter is concerned specifically with *tone*; we shall be concerned to understand the nature and structure of tone, and particularly, in view of the overall focus and purpose of this book, how it relates to other prosodic features, and to the prosodic structure of which it is a part.

4.1.2 BACKGROUND TO THE STUDY OF TONE

Tone was not part of the European philological tradition which provided the framework for the description of languages before the twentieth century. While concepts such as 'quantity' and 'accent' were familiar to classical scholars before the rise of linguistics in the modern sense, this is not true of 'tone'. The reasons for this are clear: none of the major European languages are 'tone-languages' in the full sense,[1] and acquaintance with non-European languages was quite limited before the modern era. Nor did the historical and comparative philological study of the nineteenth century necessitate the development of a theoretical or descriptive terminology for tonal features, in spite of the fact that the early Indo–European languages, including Classical Greek, in all probability had tonal characteristics.[2] The fact that some languages, and in particular Chinese, have tones, had long been known in Europe; references to the tonal nature of Chinese go back several hundred years.[3] But no wider conclusions appear to have been drawn from this. The indigenous and extensive linguistic tradition of China[4] also had no impact on European linguists.

The role of tone in some of the world's languages had nevertheless begun to be appreciated in the course of the nineteenth century, primarily as a result of the linguistic activities of European missionaries in Africa and Asia, working in their several colonial empires. Since the majority of these missionaries had little or no linguistic training, and—it must be said—in some cases evidently even less linguistic ability, the quality of their descriptions is very variable, and tone is not infrequently ignored completely (as, for example, in Koelle's *Africa Polyglotta* of 1854). But some of these missionaries were remarkably observant and competent in describing the indigenous languages which they encountered, and the best of them produced extremely valuable descriptions and analyses which include accurate details of the tonal features of the languages concerned.[5] By the early years of the twentieth century, a number of traditions of description had developed. One evolved among German scholars working in Africa,[6] whose work includes descriptions of Ewe, Shambala, Yaunde, Duala, Sotho, Venda, and other, mainly Bantu, languages. Another tradition developed among British scholars; deriving

---

[1] As we shall see in 4.7.3, below, there are modern European languages, such as Norwegian, Swedish, Serbo–Croat, Lithuanian, and several others, which can be said to have tonal features, but these features are of a rather restricted kind, and have generally been subsumed under 'accent'.

[2] It is generally agreed that Greek had a 'tonal accent' in the classical period, as evidenced by the pronouncements of Greek grammarians, as well as descriptions of the related Vedic Sanskrit by ancient Indian phoneticians. These features are represented orthographically in Greek by the different accents—*acute, grave*, and *circumflex*—used from about 200 BC. But although the rules for the use of these accents were well known, their phonetic and phonological implications were—and are—a matter of some debate. Cf. Allen (1968: ch. 6).

[3] The tones of Chinese are clearly described in, for example, Trigaut's work of 1625 (Wängler, 1963: 7; Robins, 1997: 121–2). Abercrombie (1967: 173) also notes the use of the term 'Chinese language tones' by Robert Hooke in 1679.

[4] The nature of the Chinese tones appears to have been first explained by Shen Yue in the 5th century AD (Malmqvist, 1994).

[5] Among the notable churchmen who studied African tone-languages from the 1850s onwards are Christaller, who reported on Twi, and Crowther, who wrote on Yoruba (Wängler, 1963).

[6] These included Westermann, Roehl, Nekes, Meinhof, Endemann, and others. For a discussion of their contributions, see Meinhof (1915), and Wängler (1963).

much from the 'English School' of practical phonetics, and building on the institution of the School of Oriental (later Oriental and African) Studies in London, it produced detailed analyses of a number of tone-languages of Africa and Asia, with particular strengths in the phonetic description of tones and (in the case of African languages) their use in grammatical paradigms.[7]

Much of the work discussed so far pre-dates the development of explicit phonological principles; the gradual introduction of phonological concepts and categories provided a more sophisticated approach to tonal phenomena, as well as revealing the many differences in the use of tone in different languages. The understanding of tone still lagged some way behind that of other prosodic features, however. The contribution to this phenomenon of the major European approach, the Prague School, is disappointing, since it operates within the rather rigid typological scheme established by Jakobson and Trubetzkoy, which appears to be too narrow to accommodate the wide variety of tonal phenomena encountered, with the exception of those found in tonal accent languages of the European type. For example, it appears to be taken as axiomatic that all tone-languages are mora-counting, and that no language can have more than three distinctive levels (Trubetzkoy, 1939: 181–2).[8] Even the tonal features of a language such as Chinese are interpreted in essentially 'accentual' terms (ibid.: 179ff.). There are in any case relatively few references to non-European languages in Trubetzkoy's work, and—in stark contrast to the detailed treatment of Eastern European languages—little evidence of first-hand acquaintance with the languages concerned.

This cannot be said of the American linguistic tradition, one of whose major concerns was the description of the indigenous languages of the Americas, many of which are tonal. Early American studies of tone include those of De Angulo (1926) on Zapoteco, Hoijer (1938, 1943) on Apache and (1945) on Navaho, and Bender and Harris (1946) on Cherokee. As an American contribution to the study of African languages we may also note Sapir's description (1931) of Gweabo (Jabo), spoken in Liberia. A significant boost to the study of tonal phenomena was given by Pike's important book *Tone Languages* (1948), which not only sets out a typology of tone-languages but also provides procedures for establishing tonal distinctions, and identifies many of the problems involved. Pike uses two Mexican languages, Mixteco and Mazateco, as the main sources of his examples.

The studies of Pike and others attempt to apply the established principles of phonemic analysis, set out in, for example, Pike (1947), to the analysis of tone.

---

[7] To be noted especially here is the work of Jones, Ward, Armstrong, Beach, Doke, and Tucker. Jones published descriptions of Cantonese (Jones and Woo, 1912), Nanking Chinese (Jones, 1913), and Sechuana (Jones and Plaatje, 1916); Ward of Efik (1933), Igbo (1936), and Yoruba (1952); Armstrong of Kikuyu (1940); Beach (1938) of Hottentot; Doke of Zulu (1923, 1926) and Shona (1931); and Tucker of the Sudanic languages (1935, 1940).

[8] In Trubetzkoy's defence, it may be noted that some modern scholars have also made similar assumptions, as will be evident later in this chapter.

The resulting framework forms the foundation for much of the subsequent descriptive work in this field. However, theoretical models appropriate to segmental phonology are not always applicable to tone, and it has therefore been necessary not only to reappraise the analysis of tone in the light of further developments in phonological theory itself, but also to devise appropriate phonological concepts to accommodate tonal phenomena. A range of different theoretical approaches to tone have been forthcoming, shadowing, and more recently initiating, developments in phonological theory. The establishment of classical generative phonology led to an expansion of tonal studies in the late 1960s and the 1970s which sought to apply its principles to tonal processes,[9] but a direct result of this work was also the rise of autosegmental phonology, which challenged the basis of the conventional treatment of tone, and has gained a position of ascendancy in tonal studies—and indeed in phonological theory in general—in recent years.

4.1.3 THE PHONETIC BASIS OF TONE

The basis of tone is the pitch of the voice, and pitch itself is the auditory impression produced by the rate of vibration of the vocal cords, the *fundamental frequency*, measured by the number of cycles per second, or Hertz (abbreviated Hz). The physiological mechanisms responsible for the production of voice and for the control of the rate of vibration are complex but reasonably well understood (see, for example, Lehiste, 1970; Ohala, 1973, 1978; Laver, 1994). The significant point for the study of tone is that speakers are able to produce, and perceive, a continuously variable vocal feature which can be exploited linguistically.

Although our main focus here is the phonological framework for tone, the nature of the physiological mechanisms involved in its production is by no means irrelevant for these concerns. The significance of the phonetic basis of tone reveals itself in several ways, for example in determining the appropriate distinctive features of tone and in explaining the origin and evolution of tone-systems. The establishment of a typology of languages based on their use of tone and related features can also not be achieved on functional grounds alone, but must take account of the phonetic nature of the parameters involved. Phonetic considerations will therefore impose themselves on the discussion at several points in the remainder of this chapter.

Introductions to the study of tone generally make the point that pitch contrasts, unlike measurements of fundamental frequency, are *relative*, in the sense that we cannot assign a specific *frequency* to a tone; we cannot, for example, state that a particular tone is always pronounced at, say, 200 Hz. The identification of specific tones is relative first to the speaker's vocal range; a 'high' tone for a female speaker will be considerably higher in absolute terms than the same

---

[9] Some results of this work are conveniently presented in Fromkin (ed.) (1978).

tone for a male speaker.[10] But the relativity of tone goes further than this, since the pitch of the 'same' tone spoken by the same speaker varies from utterance to utterance, and, indeed, from one part of an utterance to another. Because of so-called 'downdrift' (see 4.2.2.3, below), the pitch of an utterance often falls gradually throughout its length, so that a 'high' tone at the end of the utterance may be lower than a 'low' tone at the beginning.

Pitch is also, for the most part, a *linear* feature, in the sense that there is a single dimension of variation—the 'height' of the voice—which can be plotted against time. Though this would appear to make pitch a relatively simple phenomenon, this apparent phonetic simplicity is, paradoxically, a source of difficulty in the phonological analysis of tone, as it provides no internal differentiation to serve as the basis for a phonological interpretation. Pitch features with a variety of different functions and domains of relevance may be combined in a single phonetic parameter, and must be abstracted out for phonological purposes. The analysis of tone therefore presents difficulties in proportion to the simplicity of its phonetic nature.

4.1.4 THE NOTATION OF TONE

There is no standard way to represent tonal features, and several different systems are in use. Informal descriptive labels, such as 'mid', 'low fall', etc., though often adequate for a general characterization of tones, need to be supplemented by more systematic notation systems, especially for the purposes of transcription. One approach is to represent the pitch graphically, using a simplified musical notation. Given the five lines of a standard musical stave, and using the lines and the intervening spaces to represent pitch levels, a total of nine steps is available, which is more than adequate for most purposes. Such an analysis is given by Jones (1913) for Nanking Chinese, Lloyd James (1925) for Yoruba, and Beach (1938) for Hottentot. A simplified, three-line stave is used by Taylor (1920) for languages of Burma, and by Chiu (1930) in describing Amoy Chinese. However, the use of musical notation can be seriously misleading, as the basis of tone is not the same as that of music. Though terms such as 'musical accent' and 'tone melody' are widely used, tone patterns are not comparable to musical melodies; they are not, for example, in a particular 'key', nor do they conform to standard musical scales or intervals. We cannot speak 'out of tune'.[11]

A different, and particularly clear, iconic device for the phonetic representation of tones is introduced by Chao (1930). This consists of a vertical line, whose height represents the pitch range, with a horizontal or sloping line adjoining it

---

[10] According to Laver (1994: 451), the maximum range of fundamental frequency in ordinary conversation is approximately 50–250 Hz for men, and 120–480 Hz for women.

[11] Tone-languages can, of course, be sung, creating particular problems where tone patterns conflict with musical pitches. For a discussion of singing in Chinese, see Chao (1924, 1956); Coleman (1924). List (1961) discusses tones and singing in Thai.

to the left, which indicates in stylized form the level, shape, and length of the tone. Examples are given in Fig. 4.1.

Fig. 4.1 *Straight*   *Circumflex*   *Short*
        tones   *tones*   *tones*

    ⌐| ∧| |

    ⌐| ∨| ┤

    ＼   ∧| ┐

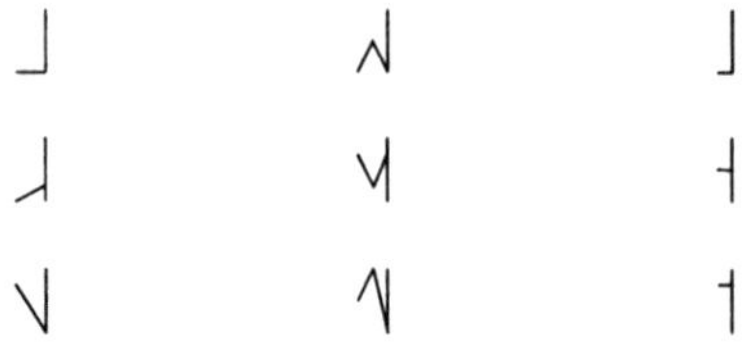

Such devices are rather cumbersome, however, and cannot be used in transcriptions. An alternative is to use integers to designate pitch levels, so that contours are described as 22, 55, 34, 41, 312, and so on.[12] The 'circumflex' tones of Fig. 4.1, for example, could be described, from the top down, as 131, 424, and 351. This has the drawback of pre-empting to some extent the phonological interpretation, since it assumes a limited number of distinctive pitch levels, and also analyses pitch contours in terms of a series of points, which may or may not be phonologically appropriate (see below, 4.3.2). Furthermore, the interpretation of the numbers depends on establishing in advance the permissible range, and scholars vary in this regard. Doke (1923, 1926) employs nine levels for Zulu; Pike (1948), restricting himself to contrasting pitch levels only, generally admits only four. More recently, five levels have been regarded as the norm.

The numerical notation can be used in transcriptions, e.g. *nta⁴hai³⁻⁴*, but a more practical solution is to use diacritic marks, and a standard set has been used, with ´ for high tone, ` for low tone, ^ for falling tone, and ˇ for rising tone; mid tone can be left unmarked, or else marked with ‾. These conventions are convenient for the standard keyboard used for Western European languages (though neither ‾ nor ˇ is commonly found),[13] but they have the disadvantage that they are not iconic; level tones are represented by sloping lines and simple rises and falls by complex shapes. Such marks may also conflict with the conventions of established romanization systems, such as the Pinyin system for Mandarin Chinese, which uses ‾ for the high level tone, ´ for the high rising tone, ˇ for the low fall–rise, and ` for the falling tone, e.g. *mā, má, mǎ, mà*. There is also no provision here for representing the tones of languages with more than three levels or, say, both high and low falling tones.

In much recent work, tones have been represented with the descriptive labels

---

[12] Most scholars number the phonetic levels from the bottom up, so that 1 = low and 5 = high; Pike (1948), and others, use the opposite convention, so that 5 = low and 1 = high. The former convention will be used here unless otherwise indicated.

[13] The widespread availability of computer fonts containing these symbols has rendered this factor increasingly irrelevant, though it was a significant one when the notations were being devised, and typewriters were used for transcriptions.

H, L, M, F, R, standing for High, Low, Mid, Fall, and Rise, respectively, though the status of these terms, as phonetic or phonological categories, is not always clear. They cannot, furthermore, be easily used in transcriptions, and they are therefore often supplemented by the conventional diacritics in the transcription of 'surface' forms. Completely phonological is the identification of the specific tones of a language by integers, giving, for example, ma^3, $shuo^1$, and so on, where the figures relate not to pitch levels but to an arbitrary system of classification of the tones of a particular language. A similarly arbitrary system is often used in historical tonology where the phonetic value of reconstructed tones is not known. In comparative East Asian linguistics such proto-tones are generally designated 'A', 'B', 'C', etc., where the labels have no phonetic values whatever, but represent assumed phonologically distinct items in the reconstructed proto-language.

Although questions of notation are in some respects trivial, and clearly subordinate to the categories that are represented, they are not entirely without significance, since an adequate notation system is both a practical necessity for the representation of forms and a tool in the formalization of the linguistically significant categories and structures. It is important, therefore, that we use a form of representation which is compatible with the analysis adopted.

4.2 Preliminaries to the Phonology of Tone

4.2.1 PHONETIC VS. PHONOLOGICAL ANALYSIS OF TONE

Early writers on the subject of tone do not make an explicit distinction between phonetic and phonological aspects of the phenomenon, though there is often an intuitive appreciation of the difference, with the recognition of a limited number of 'tones', which may have 'variants' in particular contexts. From the 1920s, however, we find the conscious introduction of explicit phonological categories, in direct imitation of contemporary developments in segmental phonology. Scholars invoke the distinction between 'phoneme' and 'allophone', though not always consistently, and the terminology occasionally provides difficulties. The term 'toneme' is used by a number of scholars, but the attempt made by Beach (1924, 1938) to relegate 'tone' to the same status as 'phone'—i.e. as a term for a purely phonetic form, rather than a phonological one—did not meet with success. Pike (1948: 4) notes that 'it has not had popular acceptance, since "tone" has strong nontechnical usage in the meaning "significant pitch unit", i.e. toneme'. Doke (1923, 1931) uses the term 'tone' in an idiosyncratic way, asserting that Zulu has nine 'tones' (the nine pitch levels that he claims are required to characterize the tones phonetically). For him, a 'toneme' is then a combination of such 'tones', such as '3–4', or '8–3–8', a use of the term to which Beach (1938), for one, takes exception.

In his study of Shona, Doke (1931) recognizes two categories of tone: 'characteristic' and 'significant', where the former refers to the pitch features peculiar to a specific language. He assumes that such features are 'not essential to the grammatical significance of the language', unlike significant tone, which 'plays an active part in the grammatical significance of the language'. Though this appears to correspond to the distinction between phonetic and phonological aspects of tone, it is not clear that pitch features which are characteristic of a particular language are necessarily non-phonological. Furthermore, he divides 'significant tone' into three categories, based on function (Doke, 1926, 1931): 'semantic tone', 'grammatical tone', and 'emotional tone'. The first of these refers to the lexical function of tones, i.e. their ability to distinguish different words; the second refers to the morphological function, i.e. in distinguishing different forms within the same paradigm; the last is concerned with special pitch features for sarcasm, surprise, etc. Though the first two of these might be seen as phonological, the last we might prefer to include under intonation rather than tone.

These terminological difficulties notwithstanding, the explicitly 'phonemic' approach to tone was firmly established by the 1930s, and received its definitive statement in the work of Pike (1948). There are, however, some difficulties in applying the principles and procedures of segmental phonology to tones, since not all tonal phenomena fit neatly into a phoneme-based theory. In order to clarify this, we shall examine some of these difficulties in more detail here. There are, of course, other phonological approaches which have their own perspective on the problems discussed here, claiming to have solved them in various ways, and to have offered new insights into tonal phenomena; we shall consider some of these later in this chapter. However, many of these difficulties persist in other theoretical frameworks, if perhaps in another form, and it is therefore also worth considering them as representative of the kinds of phenomena which any theory of tone has to accommodate.

4.2.2 'PERTURBATIONS'

The fundamental problems in the phonemic approach—and, indeed, any other phonological approach—to tone have already been mentioned above: the *relativity* and *linearity* of pitch as a phonetic feature. There is in principle no phonetic difference between a 'high' and a 'low' tone, except, of course, for the pitch level, and since the pitch level is relative and variable, and cannot be determined out of context, the identification of tones as 'same' or 'different' becomes problematic. As Schachter (1961) points out, all tones must be regarded as phonetically similar to all other tones—a circumstance that, if translated into the domain of segmental phonology, would probably render orthodox phonemic analysis all but impossible. For this reason, tonal contrasts require the application of a variety of principles which would not be usual in segmental phonology.

Pike (1948) identifies a number of the practical difficulties encountered in the course of tonemic analysis which arise from this basic characteristic of tones. Although some of these difficulties are inherent in all phonological analysis, for example, problems of defective distribution, several are peculiar to the analysis of tones. He also gives examples of what he calls 'tonal perturbations' in Mixteco and Mazateco, which include a variety of tonal processes and relationships which pose problems for the analyst. In what follows, we shall consider some of the major problems encountered here, especially those which have continued to cause difficulties in other phonological approaches, too.

4.2.2.1 'Tonemic Substitution' and 'Change Within a Toneme'

As just observed, a major difficulty in the analysis of tones is the identification of tones as 'same' or 'different', especially since tones appear to take different forms in different contexts. These 'tone-changes'[14] fall into two types: those involving the substitution of one tone for another, and those involving non-phonemic variation in the phonetic realization of the tones. These problems are, of course, familiar ones in segmental phonemic analysis, where they are regarded as morphophonemic and allophonic alternations respectively, but they take on an added difficulty in the case of tones, for the reasons given above.

In the former case, called by Pike 'tonemic substitution', a variety of factors may lead to the replacement of one tone by another. In some cases the substitution is 'mechanical', in the sense that it is determined by the juxtaposition of tones. Pike (p. 77) gives an example from Mixteco (Fig. 4.2), where the first tone of the word *bīnā* ('today') is changed from mid to high when it follows another word with mid tones (mid tones are represented by ‾).

Fig. 4.2 kīʔìn-ná žūkū   'I'm going to the mountain'
kīʔìn-ná bīnā   'I'm going today'
kī?ìn-ná žūkū bínā 'I'm going to the mountain today'

Such phenomena are widespread in tone-languages. Cheng (1973: 42ff.) describes the well-known 'tone sandhi' rule of Mandarin Chinese, where a third tone, which in isolation is pronounced as a low fall–rise, is replaced by a second (high–rising) tone before another third tone. Thus *hǎo* ('good') combines with *jiǔ* ('wine') to produce *háo jiǔ* ('good wine').[15] This process is a recursive one, so that the sentence *Lǎo Lǐ mǎi hǎo jiǔ* ('Old Li buys good wine'), in which

---

[14] On the whole, linguists in the American structuralist framework avoid terms such as 'change' for synchronic relationships, with their implications of processes rather than distribution, and prefer to speak of 'alternations'. In practice, lapses are frequent, and terms such as 'replace morph' are found (e.g. Gleason, 1961: 74). Welmers (1959) maintains a strictly distributional stance in describing tonal alternations, but even he notes that in Senari 'the last low of the stem *becomes* mid before some suffixes which have low tone' (emphasis added).

[15] It will be recalled that the standard tone marks used for Mandarin Chinese are as follows: ‾ = High level, ´ = High–Rising, ˇ = Low Falling–rising, ` = Falling. It is perhaps worth noting that Hockett (1947) treats the tone resulting from this tone sandhi rule as a phonologically distinct fifth tone.

every syllable, individually, would have the third tone, may in fact be pronounced—depending on the rate of speaking and the phrasing—with second tones on every syllable but the last.

In these cases it is possible to keep track of the tonal changes provided that the tonal context is identifiable. However, similar changes may occur where there is no phonological conditioning, so that tone differences assume an independent grammatical function. In Mixteco, for example, tone is used morphologically, to distinguish different grammatical forms, giving pairs such as those of Fig. 4.3 (Pike, 1948: 23).

Fig. 4.3 kìkū-ná 'I am going to sew'   kíkū-ná 'I am sewing'
ʃìkó-ná 'I am going to sell'   ʃíkó-ná 'I am selling'
kàkā-ná 'I am going to walk'   kákā-ná 'I am walking'

Tones may also be changed in particular syntactic contexts. For example, in the so-called 'associative' construction in Igbo (Emenanjo, 1987: 36), low tones may be changed to mid, as in Fig. 4.4 (mid tones are represented by ⁻).

Fig. 4.4 ụ́lọ̀ = 'house' + ọ̀sá = 'squirrel' → ụ́lọ̄ ọ̄sá = 'house of squirrel'

Pike (1948: 86) gives a further example from Mixteco, where the word žūù ('food'), with a mid tone followed by a low tone, has the form žúù, with a high tone and a low tone, in the expression ⁿdēžū žúù ('food made out of rocks'), but ⁿdēžū žúú, with two high tones, when it means 'rock-like food'.

The significance of these phenomena for the analysis of tone is that tone changes render the identification of individual tones difficult, since a word or syllable which has one tone in one phonological, morphological, or syntactic context may appear with another tone in another context. This may make it difficult to identify an inherent tone or tone pattern for a specific word or morpheme. We cannot necessarily assume that the basic or inherent tone is that which is found when the word or morpheme is spoken in isolation.

Other changes do not involve the substitution of one toneme for another, but rather 'change within a toneme' (Pike, 1948: 27). This may consist of the widening or narrowing of the pitch range of the utterance, a higher or lower pitch given to a particular tone under the influence of a neighbouring tone or a particular type of consonant, or at the end of an utterance, and so on. In Tiv, for example, a low tone is realized as a low fall at the end of an utterance (Arnott, 1969); in Mandarin Chinese, a third tone (low fall–rise) becomes a so-called 'half-third' tone, consisting only of a fall, before a first, second or fourth tone (Chao, 1968: 27). The problem in all these cases is that such non-phonological changes may be indistinguishable from cases of tonemic substitution. As Pike (1948: 31) puts it, 'one of the most difficult problems confronting the toneme analyst is to determine whether a pitch change is of the phonemic substituting-toneme type or, rather, of the non-phonemic conditioned-pitch type. The different types of changes combine to give so many variables that it is difficult for the

investigator to handle them discriminatingly, or even to find a solid, stable starting point from which to begin their classification.'

4.2.2.2 Distributional Problems

Another difficulty arises in languages, mostly East Asian, where some tones have
a limited distribution. In particular, the set of tones encountered in so-called
'checked' syllables, which are closed by plosives, is often more restricted than the
set found in 'unchecked' syllables, which are open or are closed by sonorant
consonants. The problem here is whether to identify the restricted tones of
checked syllables with the unrestricted tones of unchecked syllables, especially
when they are phonetically different.

   Chiu (1930) describes Amoy Chinese in terms of eight tones, two of which
(tones 4 and 8) are, however, short and are restricted to syllables which end in
/p/, /t/, /k/ and /ʔ/. It is possible to regard these tones as variants of tones 3 and
1, respectively. In Thai (Abramson, 1962), not all of the five tones found in unchecked ('live') syllables occur in checked ('dead') syllables. In checked syllables
with short vowels, only high and low tones occur; in checked syllables with long
vowels, only falling and low tones occur. A similar phenomenon is found in the
Gauri dialect of Jinghpaw (Jingpho), where Maran (1973) notes that there are
'checked' and 'unchecked' tones; the former occur in closed syllables and the
latter in open syllables. Furthermore, the occurrence of high or low tones depends on the final consonant: if this is voiceless the tone will be high; if it is
voiced the tone will be low. Whether we identify the tones occurring in
'checked' syllables with those occurring in 'unchecked' ones in such cases is a
matter on which analysts differ.

4.2.2.3 Downdrift, Downstep, and Upstep

One of the most intractable problems which confronts every theory of tone is
the appropriate treatment of *downstep*, and the related, though much less frequent, phenomenon of *upstep*. Different aspects of this problem will be encountered at various points in this chapter, and it will therefore be useful to address
it here in a general and preliminary way.

   The starting point is the phenomenon of *downdrift*. This is a reflection of a
general and almost universal phenomenon in languages which involves the gradual lowering of pitch throughout the utterance or the phrase. It is also found in
non-tone languages such as English, where it affects the intonation pattern, and
where it often goes under the name of *declination* (see Chapter 5). This gradual
pitch lowering takes a variety of different forms, depending on the nature of the
prosodic structure of the language in question (cf. Hombert, 1974; Fox, 1995). In
English, the overall pitch of successive accentual units (feet) tends to fall; in
French, where there are no such units, the pitch may fall from syllable to syllable. In tone-languages there is an additional constraint: the lowering of the pitch
should as far as possible not interfere with tonal contrasts. In practice this means

that the pitch will only fall at specific points where these contrasts are not endangered; in the majority of languages where it occurs it takes the form of a reduced pitch interval when a high tone follows a lower one. Thus, in Fig. 4.5, from Igbo (Emenanjo, 1987) we have the sequence of tones LHLHHHHLH; the interval of the pitch drop from the H tones to the following L is greater than that of the jump up from the L tones to the following H, resulting in a gradual, but step-wise, fall overall:

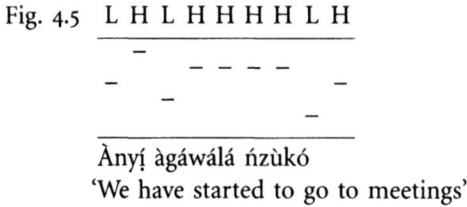

Fig. 4.5   L H L H H H H L H

Ànyị àgáwálá ńzùkó
'We have started to go to meetings'

In spite of the fact that the pitch of the last H tone of this sequence is no higher than that of the first L, the distinctiveness of the H and L tones is not endangered, since their identity is determined in relation to the previous tone: a H or a L tone is high or low in relation to the preceding L or H tone. Provided that we adopt this local view of tonal contrast, the different phonetic pitches of phonologically identical tones do not present insuperable difficulties for a phoneme-based theory of tone.

Consider now the case of tonal *downstep*. This resembles downdrift, but differs in one crucial respect: here a lowered high tone *directly* follows a higher one, without the occurrence of an intervening low tone. The data of Fig. 4.6 from Tiv (Arnott, 1964) illustrate the phenomenon; the third high tone steps down to a lower level, but this cannot be attributed to a jump up from a low tone.

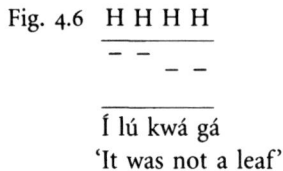

Fig. 4.6   H H H H

Í lú kwá gá
'It was not a leaf'

This phenomenon was observed early on in the study of tone-languages, for example by Christaller in the mid-nineteenth century, and again in the early twentieth century by phoneticians such as Jones and Tucker. The behaviour of this lowered high tone was noted, but the factors involved could not be identified. Jones refers to a 'curious system of tone lowering' in Sechuana (Jones and Plaatje, 1916), while Tucker (1929: 101) notes that in the Suto–Chuana languages 'there are certain places in every sentence of any length, where all succeeding high and mid tones are a semi-tone lower'. However, he cannot determine why the pitch drops, nor under what circumstances, since 'this phenomenon seems to be governed by some as yet obscure grammatical and syntactical laws'. Jones (1967: 158) discusses the same phenomenon in Chuana (Tswana), and, though he is able to specify the syntactic conditions under which it occurs, he uses it to make the point that 'it may be inconvenient and perhaps not always possible to group all the essential tonal phenomena of a tone-language into tonemes'.

We owe to Welmers (1959) a clear statement of downstep and an assessment of its significance. He notes that while in many African tone-languages each tone occurs at a specific and distinct level, without downstep, in others, such as Kikongo, Efik, and Tiv, which have downstep, the situation is more complex. Here, there appear to be three level tonemes, but there is a peculiar relationship between the two non-low ones, which are distinguished as 'same' (= 'same as the preceding non-low') vs. 'drop' (= 'lower than the preceding non-low'). Thus, after a High tone there are three possibilities: a 'same' tone, spoken on the same level as the High, a 'drop' tone, spoken at a lower level than the High, and a 'low' tone, all of which are phonologically distinct. After a Low tone there are only two possibilities: 'high' and 'low'. After a 'drop' tone, it is not possible to return to a higher level; the pitch of the 'drop' tone defines a new high level for following tones, and it may in turn be followed by one of the same three tones. This means that, confusingly, a 'drop' tone followed by a 'same' tone produces different tones spoken on the same pitch level, while a 'drop' tone followed by another 'drop' tone produces identical tones spoken on a different pitch level.

In a language with such 'downstepped' high tones, the result is a series of tonal steps, or 'terraces', with each 'drop' tone setting a new, and lower, pitch level. Fig. 4.7, from Efik (Winston, 1960), shows a series of five such terraces. Welmers uses the presence of such 'terracing' as a typological criterion: languages without downstep are 'discrete level languages' while those with downstep are 'terraced level languages'.

Fig. 4.7   L H H H H H H H H H L

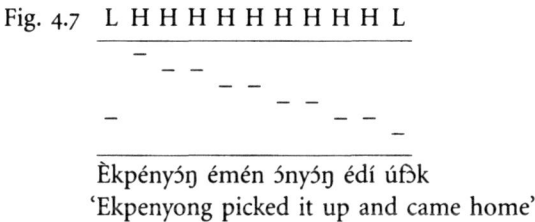

Èkpényɔ́ŋ émén ɔ́nyɔ́ŋ édí úfɔ̀k
'Ekpenyong picked it up and came home'

Downstep creates a variety of problems for the analysis of tone, as it is phonologically ambiguous. On the one hand, the occurrence of a downstepped tone is phonologically significant—there are both grammatical and lexical contrasts in some languages between a downstep and its absence—and such a tone could therefore be regarded as phonologically distinct from a *preceding* high tone. But on the other hand the downstepped tone remains a high tone for whatever comes after it, and it is therefore not phonologically distinct from a *following* high tone. The solution to this tonological conundrum is not immediately evident. We shall encounter downstep again as we examine different theoretical proposals to account for it.

4.3 The Paradigmatic Analysis of Tone

4.3.1 TONES AND TONE-SYSTEMS

As we have seen, for a tone-language we can identify two or more distinctive pitch patterns—'tones'.[16] Though each such tone may be variable, we may nevertheless usually describe it in terms of certain broad phonetic characteristics—'high', 'mid', 'low', and 'level', 'falling', 'rising', etc. Assigning *phonological* properties is a more complex task, as it depends not just on the individual tone itself but on the tone-system as a whole.

A number of other factors need to be taken into account here. First, we must determine the *domain* of tone, i.e. the unit of speech to which we may consider that tones are assigned. Pike (1948: 3) assumes that the domain is the *syllable*, and he incorporates this assumption into his widely (but not universally) accepted definition of a tone-language, as 'a language having lexically significant, contrastive, but relative pitch *on each syllable*' (emphasis added). We shall have cause to examine this assumption more critically below, but will maintain it for the time being as a working hypothesis. Our initial task will therefore be to examine the pitch patterns occurring on individual syllables.

Second, we must consider what the parameters of the description of tones should be; we can analyse tones along the dimension of sequence—i.e. in terms of a concatenation of features—and the dimension of simultaneity—in terms of co-occurring or mutually substitutable features.[17] This raises two significant and much debated questions: whether tones are divisible in temporal terms, or whether they are unitary; and how the dimension of pitch height is to be analysed. We shall consider each of these questions in turn below.

As far as the analysis of systems is concerned, it is possible first to categorize systems in terms of the *number* of tones. Many African languages, including the majority of Bantu languages, have only two tones, High and Low, but some East Asian languages are claimed to have up to a dozen, with a variety of levels, rises, and falls. However, the number of tones is not as significant as the *kind* of tones that languages have. Pike (1948: 5) makes an initial distinction between *register* and *contour* systems; the former are characterized by having *level* tones, the latter by having *gliding* tones, where a level tone is 'one in which, within the limits of

---

[16] A system with only one pitch pattern would have no contrasts, and would not, therefore, be a tone-language.

[17] These two dimensions are, of course, equivalent to the Saussurean 'syntagmatic' and 'paradigmatic' dimensions, respectively (Saussure (1967 [1916]: 170–5).

perception, the pitch of a syllable does not rise or fall during its production', while a gliding tone is 'one in which during the pronunciation of the syllable on which it occurs there is a perceptible rise or fall, or some combination of rise and fall, such as rising–falling or falling–rising'.

However, this is not an absolute distinction, and Pike has to allow for 'register–tone languages with contour overlap' and 'contour–tone languages with register overlap'. Welmers (1959; 1973), in revising Pike's typology, suggests that such mixed types may well be more common than the pure ones, while Voorhoeve (1968) concludes that by recognizing these overlaps Pike 'destroys the basis of his typological classification because on phonetic grounds alone it is difficult to distinguish between a contour–tone language with level tones and a register–tone language with gliding tones'. He thus rejects a phonetically based typology altogether.

It can be argued that the distinction between contour and register systems has wider importance. In the first place, it largely correlates with areal (geographical) factors, since the tone-languages of South East Asia are predominantly of the 'contour' type, and many languages of Africa are of the 'register' type. Second, and more significantly, the different kinds of tone-systems have been found to have rather different characteristics. Register systems, for example, tend to be rather small—typically with no more than three, and predominantly with only two, levels—while contour systems are often much larger. There are also other significant differences between the two types of languages, which will be considered in due course.

Other questions also have a bearing on the appropriate analysis of tones. Tone is generally considered to be a matter of *pitch*, but in some systems there are other features involved, too. In some languages, such as Burmese, Vietnamese, and some forms of Chinese, there are differences of *voice quality* in syllables with different tones (cf. below, 4.3.4.6). One example of this is Shanghai Chinese (Zee and Maddieson, 1980; Yip, 1992), which has five tones, two of which are accompanied by 'murmur' (breathy voice). A similar phenomenon is found in Tibetan (Yip, 1992), where a phonation contrast occurs between a 'high register', characterized in some instances by pharyngalization, and a 'low register', characterized by breathy voice.

The question raised here is whether such features constitute independent phonological parameters of tonal distinctions, or whether they can be regarded as mere phonetic concomitants of pitch features. The phonetic mechanisms for the production of different voice qualities are known to be related to those involved in the production of pitch variations themselves, as well as other laryngeal features. Whether these relationships can be properly reflected in a phonological analysis of such systems is a more difficult issue, however.

A further possible factor in the analysis of tones is the segmental context. As we saw in 4.2.2.2, some tones may be limited in their distribution to syllables with certain structures, and in particular there may be a restricted set of tones in syllables closed by a voiceless plosive or glottal stop. In these cases, it may be possible to regard this structure as part of the tones themselves, so that we may recognize not merely closed and open syllables, but 'checked' and 'unchecked' tones. A related factor here is the length of tones. Some tones may occur only in short or light syllables and others in long or heavy ones. Again it is possible, rather than ascribing the different length or weight to the syllable itself—perhaps regarding the mora, rather than the syllable, as the bearer of the tone—to locate the difference in the tones themselves, by distinguishing 'short' and 'long' tones.

In spite of all these additional factors, however, pitch remains the most important feature of tones, and pitch features must inevitably serve as the main parameters of tonal distinctions. Taking this as our starting point, therefore, we need to explore the analysis of the pitch features of tones, in terms of their syntagmatic composition on the one hand, and the available paradigmatic contrasts on the other.

4.3.2 LEVELS VS. CONTOURS

As we have noted, the distinction between level and gliding tones has been regarded as a fundamental dichotomy between tones, and hence between tone-systems. This implies that contour tones are a legitimate type of tone, different from, but of equal status with, level tones, and many scholars have made this assumption. Trager (1941) states that *all* prosodic features can be analysed in terms of 'intensity' and 'contour', the former representing a 'static' feature and the latter a 'dynamic' one. Static features are described as 'maximal', 'medial', and 'minimal'; dynamic ones as 'crescent', 'minuent', and 'constant'. For tone, the former are register features represented by 'high', 'mid', and 'low', and the latter are contour features represented by 'rising', 'falling', and 'level'. Pike similarly insists that 'the glides of a contour system must be treated as unitary tonemes and cannot be broken down into end points which constitute lexically significant contrastive pitches' (1948: 10).

With the development of distinctive feature theory, and its incorporation into generative phonology in the 1960s, more specific demands were made on the representation of tones, and the role of contours was examined more critically. Gruber (1964) and Wang (1967) devise frameworks for Asian languages in which contour tones are distinguished from others by specific features, [±rising] and [±falling] in the case of Gruber, and [±contour], [±rising], [±falling], and [±convex] in the case of Wang. However, it is always possible to regard gliding tones as combinations of levels, and we must consider the possible justification for this approach. Pike (1948: 21) warns against carrying over to contour–tone languages the analytic principles applicable to register–tone languages, citing De Angulo's description of Cantonese as a register system with three levels (1937) as a cautionary example. He argues that in many contour–tone languages the contours are 'basic tonemic units', since they are uninterruptable. Their endpoints cannot necessarily be equated phonetically with level tones, and, unlike the tones of register–tone languages, they are restricted to one per syllable.

For Pike, the register interpretation of glides is in principle not excluded, but it is admissible only where this interpretation can be shown to be justified. One such justification would be where a glide arises from the juxtaposition of two independent level tones. An example is the analysis of falling tones in Efik given by Westermann and Ward (1933). The expression *ké ùbóm* (in the canoe), with the tone pattern High-Low-High,[18] is actually pronounced *kûbóm*, with a fall on the first syllable. Here the vowel of the first syllable has been elided, but its tone has been retained, and combined with that of the following syllable. The fall here is therefore equivalent to a High–Low sequence, and it is possible to eliminate it from the phonological system of tones.

Similarly Newman (1995) argues that the falling tone of Hausa can be legitimately analysed as a High + Low sequence, first because it always occurs in heavy (2-mora) syllables, which suggests that it has two parts, and second because in many cases it corresponds to a High + Low pattern in longer words, for example, in words such as *zân* 'I will', and *mîn*, 'to me', which derive from *záanì* and *mínì*, respectively. In these cases, therefore, we can justify the elimination of contour tones from the system, even if elsewhere they are assumed to be necessary phonological elements. Such phenomena are very widespread in African languages.

Woo (1969), on the other hand, presents arguments in support of the thesis that *all* contour tones should be analysed into levels. She argues that contour tones are consistently long, and that the syllables which bear them must therefore be bimoraic or trimoraic. Contours can therefore *always* be regarded as a sequence of levels, each mora having a single level. In Mandarin Chinese, for example, the third tone, which is falling–rising, is clearly both the longest and the most complex of the four tones of the language; under Woo's proposal, this tone would consist of three levels, and syllables with this tone would be trimoraic, with one level for each mora. However, Woo's claim can easily be falsified, as there are attested cases of contour tones on short syllables, precluding a bi- or tri-moraic interpretation (Leben, 1973b). Furthermore, since quantity otherwise plays no part in Mandarin phonology, her proposal would entail considerable redundancy.

While rejecting the specific arguments presented by Woo, other scholars have nevertheless supported the view that contour tones should always be decomposed into levels. In a detailed critical review of the arguments presented on both sides, Anderson (1978) concludes that, with minor exceptions, contours should have no place in the phonology of languages but should always be represented by levels. He dismisses all of Pike's arguments for regarding contour

---

[18] Westermann and Ward actually give the pattern High-Low-Mid, but the Mid tone in this case is merely the result of the lowering of the High tone after a Low tone (downdrift).

tones as 'basic tonemic units', though largely on the grounds that they do not prove that contours should *not* be decomposed into levels. For example, in response to Pike's argument that contours in Asian languages are not interrupted by boundaries, Anderson observes that, given the fact that these languages are 'of a type in which the word, the syllable, and the morpheme are virtually co-extensive units, it seems exceedingly unlikely that we could find evidence of this kind [i.e. for the contour belonging to two adjacent morphemes], but this fact alone does not serve as a positive argument *against* decomposing their contour tones'. Anderson thus starts from the point of view that contours should be represented as levels *unless* evidence is adduced to the contrary.

There are also more positive phonological arguments in favour of the decomposition of contours, however. One of these comes from the parallel behaviour of contours and level tones in certain contexts. For example, in Mende (Leben, 1978), the tone of a nominal root is 'copied' onto following toneless syllables, such as the postpositions -*hu* ('in') and -*ma* ('on'), as in the examples of Fig. 4.8.

Fig. 4.8   *Citation form*   + -*hu*   + -*ma*
          kɔ́   'war'   kɔ́hú   kɔ́má
          pélé 'house'   péléhú   pélémá
          bèlè 'trousers'   bèlèhù   bèlèmà

Syllables with rising and falling tones have identical effects to those with High and Low tones respectively, as in Fig. 4.9.

Fig. 4.9   *Citation form*   + -*hu*   + -*ma*
          mbǎ   'rice'   mbǎhú   mbǎmá
          mbû   'owl'   mbûhù   mbûmà

Thus, only the final part of the contour tone is copied, suggesting that this final element is an independent entity, and that these tones should therefore be regarded as Low + High and High + Low, respectively. It can be argued that to regard them as unitary Rise and Fall would not permit them to have parallel effects to the level High and Low tones; in fact, we would expect that the copying would result in the following syllables having a rising or falling tone.[19]

Mende is, of course, an African tone-language, and it is mainly in Asian languages that contours have been considered unitary. Even here, however, we can point to phenomena which suggest that a contour should be regarded as a sequence of levels. In fast speech in Mandarin Chinese, a high–rising tone may become high level after a high level or high–rising tone when followed by

---

[19] Maddieson (1978) claims as a universal the non-occurrence of processes in which whole contours are copied: 'in no case has a rule been found in which a contour tone is copied through an assimilatory process'. He does admit, however, that whole contours can be copied by other means, such as reduplication.

another tone (Cheng, 1973). Graphically, this can be represented as in Fig. 4.10.

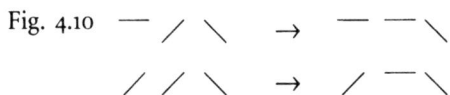

Fig. 4.10   ‾ ╱ ╲   →   ‾ ‾ ╲

╱ ╱ ╲   →   ╱ ‾ ╲

This is evidently an assimilatory process, where the pitch differences are smoothed out in rapid speech. It can be argued that the process can only be understood as such, however, if we assume that a high–rising tone is Mid + High; this allows us to say first that the Mid of the high–rise is raised to High, and second that the change takes place after a High tone (whether high level or high–rising). We can now express the assimilatory rule in a natural way:

... High Mid High ... → ... High High High ...

Similar examples can be found in other forms of Chinese; Chen (1996) gives examples of 'sandhi' phenomena in Wenzhou which involve the 'spreading' of the final pitch of the tone to an adjacent tone. He concludes that 'the fact that a syllable can give away part but not all of its tonal material argues for the compositional nature of contour tones'.

Though apparently persuasive, these arguments are not necessarily overwhelming. The fact that such assimilatory processes take place is certainly evidence for specific pitch levels as *phonetic* properties of the contour tones in question, but it does not necessarily prove that these levels are distinctive *phonological* properties. It is certainly possible to recognize, say, a rising tone as a distinct phonological entity and to identify a number of its phonetic properties, such as 'starting mid', 'ending high', etc., without necessarily implying that these properties are phonological, in the same way that we might recognize, say, a voiceless velar plosive as a phonological entity and identify a number of its phonetic properties—e.g. 'rounded', 'palatalized', etc.—as non-distinctive. Non-distinctive properties may cause assimilation as readily as distinctive ones.

A number of scholars have also voiced dissenting views, and counter-examples have been adduced. Elimelech (1974) claims that in Kru some copying processes treat contours as units, creating a sequence of *rising* tones where each tone begins where the last one left off. Gandour (cited by Fromkin, 1974) presents evidence from the Tai language Lue in which one tone has a level form before rising or falling tones, and a rising form before level tones. This cannot be described satisfactorily in terms of levels, but only in a framework in which contour tones are basic units. A further example is given by Newman (1986a) from Grebo. He notes that in this language the distribution of level and contour tones is such that they belong in the same paradigm, and that contours are therefore independent single units rather than compounds. He concludes that 'none of the theoretical arguments presented against contours as primes has been so compelling as to override the accumulation of descriptive and historical studies on languages of the world that show contours to exist as basic tonemic units on a par with level tones'. Newman supports this conclusion in his description of the tonal features of Hausa (Newman, 1995). Noting that this language has a falling tone but no rise, he points to evidence that rising tones are regularly simplified to level tones. But this argues *for*, rather than *against*, the existence of contour tones as units, since rising tones must presumably exist at some level in order to be simplified. However, since this evidence must be weighed against the considerable body of data from African languages (including Hausa) which points to contours as combinations of levels, Newman has to conclude that 'a proper theory of tone and tonal representation has to be able to capture the ambiguous nature of contours' (p. 769).

It seems that a resolution of this problem is not possible within the terms of this debate, and it may be that we have to settle not only for the ambiguous nature of contours themselves, but also for a typological difference here: though in the majority of languages (mainly African) contour tones can be decomposed into levels, in others (mainly Asian) contours can be unitary.

The terms of the debate have in some respects changed, however, with the development of autosegmental phonology. As we shall see, in autosegmental theory tones are not regarded as part of syllables or other units but are autonomous elements, represented on a separate 'tier' of structure, and they are *associated with* 'tone-bearing units' (TBUs). Some of the difficulties with contour tones can be resolved by multiple associations, i.e. by assuming that more than one tone is associated with a given TBU, especially in those cases where syllables are elided, and their tones are re-attached to other syllables. Though this form of representation removes the need for contour tones in many cases, it is still evident that it caters primarily for tone-languages of the African type, as processes of this sort are rare in Asian languages, and it is notable that autosegmental principles have been far less widely adopted in descriptions of these languages.[20]

The appropriate representation of contour tones has continued to be a matter of theoretical debate in more recent theory, and we shall continue this discussion in the light of further theoretical proposals, below.

4.3.3 DOWNSTEP AND UPSTEP

Another controversial issue in establishing tone-systems is downstep, with its complementary phenomenon of upstep. As we have seen, Welmers (1959) establishes a special kind of tone, a 'drop' tone, to account for downstep. It is pronounced at a lower pitch than the High tone which it follows. A similar approach is adopted by Schachter (1961) in describing Twi; he labels the downstepped tone 'high-change'. The difficulty is that such a tone is not independently definable in phonetic terms, since a 'drop' or 'change' requires reference to a preceding tone. Schachter is therefore prepared to accept two kinds of relationship between

---

[20] For more detailed discussion of autosegmental representations see 4.4.3.

tones: a 'fixed contrast relation', which is the normal paradigmatic contrast between items in a system, and a 'fixed sequential relation' (or 'echo' relation),
where the contrast can only be defined in a sequence. The latter clearly does not
fit comfortably with a phoneme-based approach to tone, since it undermines the
idea of a set of mutually contrasting phonological items.

Winston (1960) discusses the same phenomenon in Efik. In this language there
is again a Low and a High tone, but also a so-called 'Mid' tone, which is, in fact,
a lowered High tone. This tone may occur in different positions in the sentence,
and even more than once in the sentence. However, Winston considers that this
'Mid' tone cannot be regarded as a legitimate tone. In the first place, since the
lowering associated with this tone can take place more than once in the utterance, we would need not just a single Mid tone but several: Mid1, Mid2, Mid3,
and so on, with a different 'Mid' level for each downstep. Additional complications are the fact that the same word would have different tones depending on
where it occurred in the sentence, and the fact that, since downstep is very similar to downdrift, we would have to interpret the latter in a similar way.
Downdrift, which is otherwise relatively straightforward, would therefore become
problematical.

Winston's solution is similar to that proposed by Tucker thirty years earlier.
Instead of recognizing downstepped tones as a separate kind of tone, he introduces a special unit of downstep (marked $^!$), which is inserted before the
downstepped tone to indicate that the pitch of the following tone is lowered.
This downstep is not a tone as such, and therefore does not contrast with the
other tones in the same system; it nevertheless has phonological status. Arnott
(1964) adopts a similar approach to Winston. He points to the fact that, in Tiv,
ka 'it is' always has a High tone and it is followed by a downstep; it can therefore be given the pattern H$^!$. Here, the $^!$ is a property of the word *ka* rather than
of the following syllable, even though it is the latter that is subject to downstep.
Therefore it is inappropriate to recognize a 'drop' or 'high–change' tone, which
attributes the downstep to this following syllable.

Another example is provided by Armstrong's analysis of Ikom Yala (Armstrong, 1968). This language is a terraced-level language (in Welmers's sense) but
with three contrasting tone levels, High, Mid, and Low. Unlike the case of Efik,
'Mid' is here an independent tone which does not arise through downstep.
Downstep itself occurs, affecting not only High tones but also Mid and Low
tones (in the last of these the fall has a wider interval). As before, downstep is
here phonologically distinctive and unpredictable. Armstrong argues that to
regard downstepped tones as a special kind of tone would be difficult and complicated in Ikom Yala, since we would need a downstepped version of all three
tones. He therefore adopts the same solution as Winston and Arnott. Similar
analyses of other languages are given, for example, by Wilson (1968) and Pike
(1970), on Temne and Igbo, respectively.

The problem with this solution, however, is that the status of the $^!$ is somewhat unclear, since it is neither a tone nor a normal phoneme. Armstrong regards it as a *juncture* feature rather than as a phoneme, since, like the 'juncture phonemes' of classical Bloomfieldian theory (see, for example, Trager and Smith, 1951), it has no sound of its own but its presence is evident in its effect on neighbouring phonemes.[21] Pike and Small (1974), in their analysis of Coatzospan Mixtec, identify the downstep as a 'process phoneme' in the sense of Pike (1967). Such a phoneme has no phonetic content but exerts a lowering influence on a following High tone and causes a change of 'key' which persists until the end of the utterance or until the next downstep.

Similar principles apply in the case of the much rarer *upstep*. This is, as the term suggests, the opposite of downstep, since the pitch is *raised*. Pike and Wistrand (1974) note that in Acatlán Mixtec there are 3 tones: High, Mid, and Low, and an additional 'Step-up' tone which can only be found following a High tone or another Step-up tone, and which is higher than the immediately preceding syllable. A High tone following a Step-up tone is level with it, but higher than the High tone which precedes the Step-up tone. Since this phenomenon appears to be analogous to downstep, it can be described in a similar fashion. Those who, like Pike and Wistrand, simply introduce a special tone, can have a 'Step-up' tone instead of a 'Drop' tone. But there is a problem if we try to relate it to intonational features of downdrift, with which it is clearly in conflict. For this reason, Suárez (1983) notes that whereas in a language with down-stepped terraced tones (such as Coatzospan Mixtec) we can regard downstep as a process applying to tones in a sequence, in a language with upstepped terraced tones (such as Acatlán Mixtec), upstep has to be specially accounted for by positing an additional 'Step-up' tone.

4.3.4 TONE FEATURES

4.3.4.1 Preliminaries: The Role of Features

In the paradigmatic dimension, a great deal of attention has been paid to the most satisfactory set of *distinctive features* in terms of which tone-systems can be analysed. It is appropriate to consider first the rationale behind distinctive features in general, and tonal features in particular. Features were originally conceived by Prague School linguists (Trubetzkoy, 1939) as a means of characterizing phonemic oppositions. Jakobson developed them in a number of radical directions (Jakobson, Fant, and Halle, 1952), producing a limited set of auditory and acoustic binary features which were intended to be universal, phonetic and yet relational, in the sense that specific phonetic features are involved, but a particular opposition is a *relative* one along a specific phonetic parameter. In

---

[21] In conformity with the Bloomfieldian tradition, Welmers notes, however, that for him a juncture *is* a phoneme.

their revision of Jakobson's features, Chomsky and Halle (1968) not only revert to more traditional articulatory parameters, but also allow more phonetic realism in the features. They also identify (p. 65) two functions for the features, the 'phonetic function' (concerned with characterizing the phonetic nature of the oppositions), and the 'classificatory function', concerned with the organization of the oppositions in phonological terms.

These considerations are relevant for the distinctive features of tone. A variety of different feature sets have been devised, in which different criteria are given priority over others. The following discussion will consider the nature and relevance of these various criteria, and the systems which result from their application.

4.3.4.2 Systems with Levels

If we restrict ourselves to pitch *levels* in the analysis of tones, then the phonetic characteristics of tones are ranged along a single dimension, that of pitch height. In view of the phonetic homogeneity of this dimension, any subdivisions would appear to be phonetically arbitrary; the crucial question is simply the *number* of levels to be recognized.

Although some earlier writers distinguish more phonetic levels here,[22] most analysts assume that there is a maximum number of *five* levels that need to be distinguished, as a number of languages have been found which purportedly have five distinctive levels.[23] Maddieson (1978) elevates this to a universal principle: 'a language may have up to five levels of tone, but not more'. Not all languages will require all of these, and indeed a system with five levels appears to be rather unusual. For convenience in what follows, we shall refer to them as levels 1 to 5, where 1 is the lowest and 5 the highest. Given the binary nature of distinctive features, however, these five levels need to be assigned to a number of binary distinctions, and there are many different possibilities here. The choice from among these possibilities will depend on both phonetic and classificatory factors, as well as on a number of other principles, such as the frequency and 'markedness' of the different tones, and the kinds of tonal processes that we wish to describe. The assumption here, too, is that features of tone are *universal*. This does not mean that every tone-language has the same set of tones, but rather that they may make use of the same kinds of phonetic contrasts. More or fewer of these features will be used by different languages according to the number of levels required.

From the classificatory point of view, it is usually thought to be necessary for the set of features to be as 'economical' as possible, that is, the smallest number

---

[22] Doke (1926, 1931) notoriously distinguished nine levels for Zulu, but these levels are clearly not phonologically distinct.

[23] The standard example here is Trique (Longacre, 1952), though it has also been argued that this language can be analysed with fewer tones (Wang, 1967). Other languages for which five levels have been claimed include Black Miao and Dan (Anderson, 1978).

of features are used, consistent with phonetic plausibility. The maximum number of tones that can be distinguished by a given number of features is described by the expression 2^n, where n is the number of features. Thus, one feature distinguishes two tones, two features distinguish up to four tones, three features distinguish up to eight tones, and so on. In practice, another criterion, phonetic plausibility, may limit this. For example, if we use the features [±High] and [±Low], then in theory we can distinguish four tones, but in practice only three. A high tone is [+High, –Low], a low tone is [–High, +Low], and a mid tone is [–High, –Low]. The fourth possibility here is [+High, +Low], but this is ruled out on phonetic grounds, since no tone can have incompatible phonetic properties. On the other hand, if we were to use a feature such as [±Mid] in place of [±Low], no such incompatibility need arise, since [High] and [Mid] are not complementary (and therefore incompatible) properties, and we could distinguish four levels with just the two features. The four heights would then be as in Fig. 4.11.

Fig. 4.11   4   [+High, –Mid]
            3   [+High, +Mid]
            2   [–High, +Mid]
            1   [–High, –Mid]

Another solution is put forward by Gruber (1964). He assumes a basic distinction between [+High] and [–High], which allows for a contrast between two tone levels. To cater for more complex systems he proposes a further distinction involving a feature [±High2] ('secondary high'), which provides for a further height distinction *within* each of the categories [+High] and [–High]. Since the properties of pitch height represented by such features can be combined, in Gruber's system four levels would have the feature combinations of Fig. 4.12.

Fig. 4.12   4   [+High, +High2]
            3   [+High, –High2]
            2   [–High, +High2]
            1   [–High, –High2]

Two features allow only four levels, which is generally thought to be insufficient, and for larger systems at least one more feature must be added. However, three features allow up to eight levels, and there are therefore a number of alternative feature combinations that can be used. Wang (1967) describes tones in terms of the features [±High], [±Central], and [±Mid], giving the combinations of Fig. 4.13.

Fig 4.13   5   [+High, –Central]
            4   [+High, +Central]
            3   [–High, +Central, +Mid]
            2   [–High, +Central, –Mid]
            1   [–High, –Central]

Again, phonetic incompatibility comes into play, though in a rather arbitrary fashion, since [+High] and [+Central] can co-occur, but [+High] and [+Mid] cannot; nor can [+Mid] co-occur with [−Central].

Sampson (1969) substitutes [±Low] for Wang's [±Mid], claiming that this is better, because it makes fuller use of all three features, though [−Low] is still redundant for [+High] tones, and [−High] is redundant for [+Low] tones. A tone which is [−High] and [−Low] must be [+Central]. His system is given in Fig. 4.14.

Fig 4.14 5 [+High, −Central, −Low]
      4 [+High, +Central, −Low]
      3 [−High, +Central, −Low]
      2 [−High, +Central, +Low]
      1 [−High, −Central, +Low]

Woo's feature system (Woo, 1969) again caters for five levels with three features. In addition to [±High] and [±Low], she introduces a feature [±Modify] which serves to distinguish high (level 5) from lowered high (level 4), and low (level 1) from raised low (level 2). The resulting features specifications are those given in Fig. 4.15.

Fig. 4.15 5 [+High, −Low, −Modify]
       4 [+High, −Low, +Modify]
       3 [−High, −Low, −Modify]
       2 [−High, +Low, +Modify]
       1 [−High, +Low, −Modify]

Finally, we may note the system given by Maddieson (1972), presented in Fig. 4.16. This system is almost the same as Sampson's, with [±High] renamed [±Raised] and [±Low] renamed [±Lowered]. It replaces Sampson's [±Central] by [±Extreme], in such a way that [+Central] becomes [−Extreme], and [−Central] becomes [+Extreme].

Fig. 4.16 5 [+Raised, −Lowered, +Extreme]
       4 [+Raised, −Lowered, −Extreme]
       3 [−Raised, −Lowered, −Extreme]
       2 [−Raised, +Lowered, −Extreme]
       1 [−Raised, +Lowered, +Extreme]

The impression given by this list of different systems is one of complete arbitrariness, but this is not really the case. Each system is justified by its author in terms of the weight given to specific criteria, over and above the common criteria on which all feature systems are based. Wang, for instance, claims to have selected his features on the basis of an examination of the alternations, both synchronic and diachronic, found in a large number of languages, particularly Asian. Further, since five pitch levels are rare in the languages of the world

(Wang can cite only a handful of these), the feature [±Mid], which is required to distinguish a five-level language from a four-level one, is only marginal in his system. Sampson's system, on the other hand, reflects his belief that features should be more or less equally used.[24] Maddieson's feature [±Extreme] (rather than [±Mid] or [±Central]) aims to reflect another principle: that the overall pitch range used by tone-systems will become wider as the number of tones increases. Labelling a tone [+Extreme] implies that its level is beyond that employed in smaller systems.

One claim made for distinctive features is that they are able to capture the notion of 'natural class'. Items with the same value for a specific feature are assumed to have something in common. Where tones are adjacent in height, this is not a problem; all the systems discussed above regard both the two highest tones as [+High], for example. But this becomes more problematic with non-adjacent tones, as in the case of Woo's [±Modify], or Maddieson's [±Extreme]. The claim of such classifications is that, in Woo's case, levels 2 and 4, and, in Maddieson's case, levels 5 and 1, form natural classes. This is perhaps easier to justify in Maddieson's case, given his claim that both the [+Extreme] tones extend the tone range; Woo's [+Modify] tones appear to be somewhat less of a natural class.

Another way in which different systems reflect assumptions about 'normal' tone-systems is in the use of *markedness*. As we have seen elsewhere, 'marked' features and feature values reflect the principle that some values are more 'normal', more 'expected', or even more 'natural' than others.[25] Most of the scholars cited here assume that the '+' value of a feature is marked and the '−' value is unmarked, so that the feature system should be constructed in such a way that the least marked tone has '−' values for all features, and that the number of '+' values increases as the tones become more marked. For Gruber and Wang the low tone is unmarked, while Woo's and Maddieson's systems make the mid tone unmarked. As Sampson points out, however, it is not necessary for the unmarked values of features to be '−'; he claims that in Hanoi Vietnamese it is the High rather than the Low tone that should be unmarked. Maddieson makes similar claims for high tones in Hausa, among other languages, though conceding the universal principle (Maddieson, 1978) that 'systems in which high tones are marked are more frequent than systems in which low tones are marked'. He notes that languages with the same number of levels may nevertheless differ in 'the arrangement of the tones in a hierarchy of dominance', a test for such dominance being which tone survives in cases of contraction. In Idoma Yala, for example, there is contraction across a word boundary within a Verb + Object construction (Maddieson, 1972). There is a hierarchy of dominance such that

---

[24] Anderson (1978) discounts this argument; for him, 'the substance of this issue is rather obscure'.
[25] The concept of 'naturalness' is, however, problematic, as in some cases it may lead us to conclude that some languages are more natural than others, a claim that is in principle unacceptable.

both High tone and Mid tone dominate Low tone, and High tone dominates Mid tone. This gives a hierarchy High–Mid–Low. In Wukari Jukun and Yoruba, however, both High and Low dominate Mid, so that the hierarchy is High–Low–Mid.

This would suggest that marking should not be universal, but should be different in different languages. However, this violates a fundamental principle, and such a solution is unacceptable to many. Maddieson therefore claims that such differences in markedness are the result of selecting different tones from a universal set. Using his set of features (see Fig. 4.16, above), and assuming that the negative values are unmarked, the five available tones will differ in markedness, with Mid (level 3) being the least marked, High (4) and Low (2) being more marked, and Extra High (5) and Extra Low (1) the most. A two-tone system in which High is dominant therefore uses levels 4 = High and 3 = Low, but one in which Low is dominant has 3 = High and 2 = Low. A hierarchy such as that of Yoruba (High–Low–Mid) can be interpreted as 5 = High, 3 = Mid, and 2 = Low (to have 4 = High would rank High and Low equally).[26]

In spite of these ingenious explanations, and the motivations given for the different systems, the criteria here are so much in conflict that it is difficult to establish the superiority of any one of these systems over the others. Anderson (1978) concludes that 'at present it can only be said that any of the systems surveyed . . . is equally (un)satisfactory'. The fact that such a conclusion must be drawn suggests that the enterprise itself, or some aspect of it, must, at least in the form conducted here, be flawed in some respect.

Given that a major problem here is the phonetic homogeneity of pitch itself, one such flaw in this case might be the insistence on the binarity of feature contrasts. If only one phonetic dimension is involved in tone, then it may be unjustified to seek to identify several binary phonological distinctions along this dimension. Proposals to abandon binarity have, in fact, been made, for example by Ladefoged (1971), and especially by Stahlke (1977), who claims that certain facts of Igede cannot be captured by binary features. However, it is not clear that non-binary features—such as a numerical scale of pitch height—would actually solve the difficulties he describes. Anderson (1978) reserves judgement, suggesting that Stahlke's rejection of binarity is 'somewhat premature'.

4.3.4.3 Systems with Contours

We have seen that the standard view that had developed by the 1970s analyses

---

[26] A principle related to markedness, which is adopted by some scholars, is that of *underspecification*. Instead of merely regarding one feature value as unmarked, frameworks using underspecification only mark certain tones, leaving the others—which are predictable—to be inserted by rule (see especially Pulleyblank, 1986). This has implications for the form of grammars, but it does not affect the set of tone-features themselves, since it is inadmissible to use underspecification as a means of reducing the number of features, as this can lead to features being assigned ternary values, +, –, and unspecified. See Pulleyblank, 1986: 127–30.

contour tones as sequences of levels, so that contour features have not figured in the proposals we have examined so far. Nevertheless, we saw that some scholars have included contours among the tones, and in this case they are also susceptible to analysis in terms of distinctive features. The general issues involved, and the problems encountered, are, however, very similar to those discussed for level tones.

We have noted that Gruber (1964) uses two contour features [±Rising] and [±Falling], while Wang (1967) uses the three features [±Rising], [±Falling], and [±Convex]. There are considerable redundancies in Wang's feature set, since all tones with the feature [+Rising] or [+Falling] must also be [+Contour], and any tone which is [+Convex] must be [+Rising, +Falling, +Contour]. For any tone which is [–Contour], all these other features must have the value '–'. Further, no [+Contour] tone can be [+Central] or [+Mid]. Wang justifies his choice of features in terms of their ability to describe economically alternations between tones in various Chinese dialects. Thus, in Peking Chinese, there is an alternation between a high level and a rising tone; in Chaozhou an alternation between a rise and a fall; and in Canton an alternation between a high level and a fall. He claims that his set of features can describe these alternations by means of a single feature change in each case. The Peking alternation is between [–Contour] and [+Contour] within [–Falling] tones; in Chaozhou it is between [+Rising] and [–Rising] within [+Contour] tones; and in Canton it is between [–Contour] and [+Contour] within [–Rising] tones. Wang can thus also claim that his features capture alternations within *natural classes* (e.g. [–Falling] in Peking, [+Contour] in Chaozhou). However, what constitutes a 'natural class' is not always easy to determine; a fall does not necessarily have anything in common with a rise, and the Chaozhou case, which gives credibility to the feature [±Contour], is not a common one.

In cases where contour tones can be recognized, Maddieson (1978) establishes two implicational universals: first, that 'if a language has contour tones, it also has level tones', and further that 'a language with complex contours also has simple contours'. These principles, if valid, impose some restrictions on contour systems, with consequent implications for what is marked and unmarked.

Both Gruber's and Wang's features for contour tones also raise a further question. Both allow the features [+Falling] and [+Rising] to co-occur in the same matrix, even though they appear to be phonetically incompatible. In such cases they assume that, unlike other co-occurring features, they apply *in sequence* rather than simultaneously, so that the tone is either a fall–rise or a rise–fall. (The feature [±Complex] is used in Wang's system to determine the order of these features, and thus to distinguish the fall–rise from rise–fall; Gruber's system is unable to make this distinction; he claims that no tone-system has both of these complex tones.) The use of features in this way raises a fundamental issue of principle, however, since, contrary to established theory and practice, it introduces a *temporal* element into a single matrix. We shall see below that more recent work has suggested an alternative means of dealing with this problem.

4.3.4.4 Tones and Registers

The feature systems presented so far have been based on the principle that tones can be cross-classified in terms of their membership of intersecting 'natural classes'. As we have seen, many of the problems with such a classification derive from the homogeneity of the phonetic properties of pitch, which provides little or no basis for the establishment of distinctive parameters. Some later systems, particularly within the autosegmental framework, have attempted to provide such a parameter, with a distinction between *tone* and *register*.

So far the term 'register' has been used more or less interchangeably with 'level', following Pike's distinction between 'contour systems' with glides and 'register systems' with levels. However, there is a slightly different usage, derived from musical terminology, which refers to different pitch *ranges* of the voice. In musical terms, a 'register' is a part of the range of an instrument or (especially) a voice which has a particular quality or timbre. Singers, for example, may refer to the 'chest register' or the 'head register', or we may refer to the 'tenor register' of, say, a bassoon. The term has also been employed in discussions of prosodic features in this latter sense, in the case of processes where it is whole ranges of the voice rather than specific levels that are involved.

Let us take as an example a development in a number of Asian languages, to which we shall return in more detail below, where the tone-system has split into two following the loss of contrasts in initial consonants (cf. Haudricourt, 1961; Matisoff, 1973). In Sgaw–Karen, for example, a two-tone system split into two, resulting in four tones; in Cantonese three tones split to give six. In both these cases the resulting pairs of tones differ in overall level: in Sgaw–Karen there is a High Level and a Low Level, and a High Fall and a Low Fall; in Cantonese High Fall, High Rise, and High Level are matched by a Low Fall, Low Rise, and Low Level. In such cases we can speak of the creation of two distinct 'registers', with a parallel set of tones in each.

This concept of register has been taken up by a number of phonologists in relation to the specification of tones, especially in descriptions of Asian languages. Yip (1980) makes a distinction between Register and Tone; the former is specified by means of the feature [±Upper], and the latter by means of the feature [±High]. This gives the feature set shown in Fig. 4.17.

Fig. 4.17

Register	Tone
+Upper	+High
	−High
−Upper	+High
	−High

This set is, of course, very similar to others discussed in 4.3.4.2, above; in fact, apart from the labels, it is identical to Gruber's. However, Yip interprets the system slightly differently, treating the Register feature as *dominant*. While a syllable may have contours combining the Tone features (i.e. H–L and L–H), only one Register feature may occur in a syllable. This means that, since we cannot combine two different registers within a syllable, there are only two rises or falls possible for any syllable, one which is *wholly* [+Upper] and one which is *wholly* [–Upper].

Yip places register features and tone features on separate autosegmental tiers, as in Fig. 4.18. Here, $ represents the syllable; the Register feature [+Upper] is associated with it on one tier; the Tone features H ([+High]) and L ([–High]) are together associated with it on another tier. Yip claims that this system is able to deal with register splits such as that occurring in Cantonese, since it allows the Register feature to be changed without affecting the Tone features. This is also useful in accounting for 'downdrift' and 'downstep' in many languages, where the overall pitch level of the utterance is systematically lowered; this can be regarded as a progressive resetting of the Register feature (see below, 4.5.3). Yip's system is adopted by a number of other scholars, including Pulleyblank (1986), though with the modification[27] that [±Raised] is used instead of [±High] to avoid confusion with vowel height.

Fig. 4.18 [+Upper]
|
$
/\
H   L

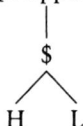

There are, however, some difficulties with this approach. Yip (p. 183) gives the values for the four tones of Mandarin Chinese as in Fig. 4.19. The fourth tone is a fall from high to low (51), yet it must be assigned to the upper register, which implies 53. Yip justifies this with the claim (p. 183) that 'what is important about this tone is that it is high and falling, rather than how far it falls', but it is not clear that its high start is actually any more significant than its low end, and its assignment to the [+Upper] rather than the [–Upper] register appears arbitrary.

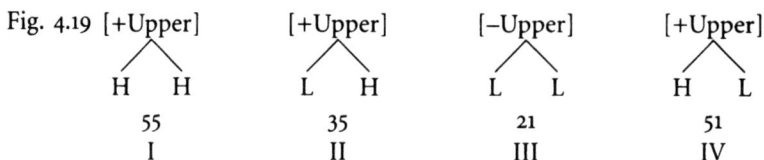

Fig. 4.19 [+Upper]   [+Upper]   [–Upper]   [+Upper]
            /\   /\   /\   /\
           H   H   L   H   L   L   H   L
            55   35   21   51
            I   II   III   IV

In fact, we may question whether this use of the concept of 'register' is actually legitimate. The separation of tone and register implies that they represent not merely different *features* of tones (as, for example, [±High] and [±Mid]) but different *dimensions*. In the specification of Mandarin tones this does not seem

---

[27] According to Pulleyblank (1986: 125), this change was suggested by Morris Halle.

to be the case; [±Upper] is here being used simply as a convenient feature to distinguish different tones, as a way of classifying the tones by isolating one of the several ways in which they can differ. The identification of a distinct 'Register tier' is only justifiable if it represents a discrete dimension of tonal behaviour, for example if there is a systematic morphophonemic relationship between the 'same' tones with a different register. Yip (1992) does, in fact, argue that there is evidence of this kind. She gives examples of neutralization of tonal distinctions in Taiwanese, the Suzhou and Fuzhou dialects, and Cantonese which, she argues, involve loss of Tonal properties while Register properties remain. However, the features identified here as belonging to 'Register' could equally well be regarded as Tonal, and do not in themselves necessitate recognizing a separate Register tier. The case is stronger in the case of downstep, since it is arguable that downstep changes the pitch of tones without affecting their distinctive properties, and thus represents a discrete dimension, distinct from the tonal features. We shall see below (4.5.3) how this can be implemented.

In spite of this serious reservation, Yip's proposal is significant in that it substitutes—in part, at least—a hierarchy of tonal features for the previous cross-classification: Tone is regarded as subordinate to Register. Clements (1983) goes further, explicitly recognizing different layers of features, and, what is more, using the *same* feature on different levels. 'In all cases', he writes, 'we are dealing with subdivisions within an acoustically *homogeneous* phonetic dimension, that of pitch. Hence it is appropriate to describe these oppositions in terms of a unitary pair of features, *h, l* whose correlates are relatively high pitch and relatively low pitch, respectively.' His matrix for an unmarked 4-level system is that of Fig. 4.20(a). Within this framework a 3-level system such as that of Ewe will have the form of Fig. 4.20(b).

Fig. 4.20 (a) row 1: h h   l   l   (b) row 1: h l   l
          row 2: h l   h   l   row 2:   h   l
          Tone: H HM M   L   Tone: H M   L

The first row of these matrices assigns a tone to a 'primary register', while the second row assigns it to a 'subregister' within the primary register. This system represents a break with all previous systems, since differentiation of tones is achieved not by using different features, but by putting the same features on different rows. As we shall see below, this principle can be extended to cases where multiple pitch levels are needed, as in the description of downdrift and downstep.

Other scholars have endorsed the general approach of locating pitch features on different 'tiers'. This approach builds on attempts to establish a 'feature geometry' for segments (Clements, 1985; Sagey, 1986), with different features of segments (representing, for example, place of articulation, manner of articulation, laryngeal features, etc.) arranged hierarchically, as in Fig. 4.21 (taken from Clements, 1985).

Fig. 4.21

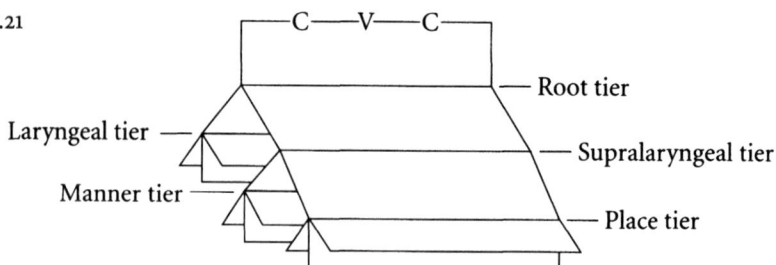

Root tier

Laryngeal tier

Supralaryngeal tier

Manner tier

Place tier

This approach can be applied to tone, and several linguists have devised geometric structures for tones, e.g. Archangeli and Pulleyblank (1986); Hyman (1986, 1992), Hyman and Pulleyblank (1988); Inkelas (1987, 1989); Snider (1988, 1990); Inkelas and Leben (1990); Yip (1989, 1992). For example, Snider (1988) presents a 'three-dimensional' model, in which different tiers of tonal structure are arranged in a geometric configuration as in Fig. 4.22. Here, the Register Tier (h and l) and the Modal (i.e. tonal) Tier (H and L) are united under the Architonal Tier which is linked to the Tone Bearing Units (X).

Fig. 4.22

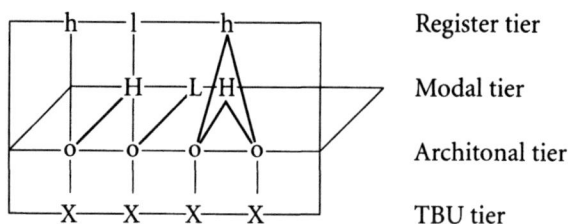

Register tier

Modal tier

Architonal tier

TBU tier

Representations of this sort allow us to resume the discussion of the appropriate analysis of contour tones. As we have just noted, Yip (1980) can accommodate two different values for the same Tone feature on a single syllable, though there is only a single value for the Register feature. In later work (Yip, 1989), she develops this approach, using the principles of feature geometry. The Register feature is now identified with the 'root' node, to which the Tone features are attached. She is able to distinguish cases of *cluster* contours, frequent in African tone-languages, where contours derive from the combination of level tones (see above), from *unit* contours of the Asian type, which are not so derived. The former would be represented as in Fig. 4.23(a), the latter as in Fig. 4.23(b) (the

Fig. 4.23 (a) 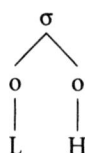   (b)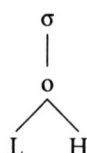

cluster   unit

tonal root node is represented by ° and L and H are abbreviations of [–raised] and [+raised], respectively).

Hyman (1992) adds a further enhancement, in which Tonal features are attached not to the root node itself, but to a Tonal node. He assumes that Tone features cannot be ordered under the Tonal node, but nodes themselves can be ordered. This gives representations such as that of Fig. 4.24 (note that for Hyman the tone-bearing unit is a *mora* rather than a syllable).

Fig. 4.24   Tone-Bearing Unit   (a)   μ   (b)   μ   (c)   μ

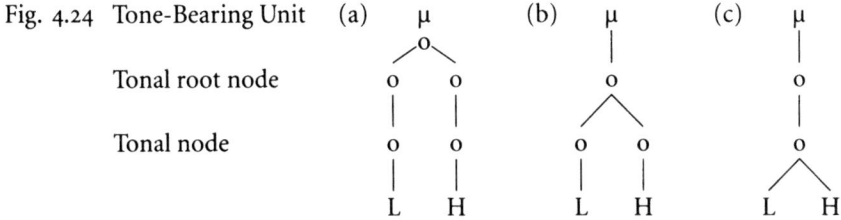

Here, (a) represents a contour with two Tonal root nodes (equivalent to Yip's 'cluster'), (b) is a contour with a single Root node and two Tonal nodes (Yip's 'unit'), and (c), which has only a single Tonal node, represents the simultaneous occurrence of L and H, which produces a Mid tone.

Evidence bearing on this kind of analysis, and particularly the separation of tone and register, has been sought by Bao (1990) in the sandhi processes of various Chinese dialects. If these processes (change of tone in the context of another tone) are regarded as assimilation, then we would expect different configurations of tonal and register features to give different possibilities for such changes, on the assumption that it is the features at the edge which will spread. Bao gives two alternative configurations for tone and register, shown in Fig. 4.25. In Fig. 4.25(a), T (= register) dominates two occurrences of t (= contour tone), as in Yip's 'unit' contour (Fig. 4.23(b)). In Fig. 4.25(b) register and contour tone are sister nodes. In Fig. 4.25(a), either of the two terminal tones of the contour can cause assimilation of a neighbouring tone; in Fig. 4.25(b) the configuration allows for assimilation of register, the contour as a whole, or of the terminal tones.

Fig. 4.25 (a)   T   (=r)   (b)   T   T=tone root
                                                     r =register
                                                     c =contour
                                                     t =terminal elements

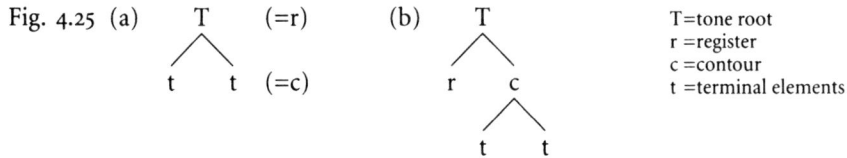

The elaborate representations of Yip, Hyman, and Bao involve a *hierarchical* structure for tonal features, rather than the unordered set generally assumed. This makes available a variety of different structures which can be exploited in distinguishing different types of phenomena. In some cases this variety is certainly achieved at the expense of simplicity; it is a matter of debate whether it is also achieved at the expense of plausibility. In the case of Hyman's representation (Fig. 4.24), (c) could be eliminated by allowing a Mid tone in addition to High and Low; while the distinction between (a) and (b) is necessitated by the elimination of contour tones; their reinstatement would therefore make such representations unnecessary. In the case of Bao's representation, there is some doubt whether the increased possibilities are really required; Chen (1996) concludes that the 'more parsimonious' version, Fig. 4.25(a), is better suited to accounting for the processes involved than the 'enriched variety', Fig. 4.25(b), since many of the possibilities allowed by the latter simply do not occur.

4.3.4.5 Features, Downdrift, and Downstep

Some of the difficulties created by downdrift and downstep have been considered above (4.2.2.3). We must now consider how these phenomena can be handled in terms of distinctive features of tone. In the case of downdrift, this is rarely considered necessary, since the gradual lowering of the pitch is regarded as a low-level phonetic phenomenon, not requiring specification in phonological terms; but downstep is phonologically distinctive, and thus needs to be specified somewhere at the phonological level.

Within most theoretical approaches, however, it has been found possible to avoid giving a feature specification to downstepped tones, since they can be treated as a special instance of downdrift. Welmers (1959) regards downdrift and downstep as different processes, and defines terraced-tone languages in terms of the latter rather than the former. Stewart (1966), however, regards them as the same process, and claims that, contrary to Welmers's classification, Twi (which has downstep) and Hausa (which has downdrift) are actually not typologically different. To this we may add the observation made by a number of scholars that the historical source of downstep is often an original Low tone which is no longer present, usually because the syllable which bore it has been elided. Stevick (1965) speaks of the 'ghost of a low tone' which causes the downstep in Yoruba; Armstrong (1968) refers to 'latent lows' in Ikom Yala. In each case low tones are assumed which are not themselves pronounced but which have an effect on following High tones, causing them to be lowered.

Downdrift and downstep are thus phonetically very similar, indeed identical, processes, since they both involve the lowering of a high tone after a low tone. The only difference between them is that in the case of downdrift the preceding low tone is present, while in the case of downstep it is absent, but nevertheless 'latent'. Given an appropriate descriptive framework, in which such latent tones can be included and then deleted after they have caused the lowering of the following high tone, both downdrift and downstep can be accommodated in a similar fashion. Here, however, we shall consider how downstepped tones may be specified without such a 'latent low'.

As we saw in 4.3.3, there are two ways in which downstepped tones can be described: as special tones in their own right (e.g. as 'drop' tones) or in terms of an inserted 'downstep phoneme' (/'/). The latter approach does not require downstepped tones to be independently specified; they remain high tones, and the lowering effect is produced by the special downstep feature. The former could in principle be assigned a feature specification, though it is not clear what this should be.

One solution is provided by Carrell (1966) in her generative grammar of Igbo; she allocates to downstepped tones a special feature [±echo]. The specification [+echo] indicates that the tone is at the same height as the preceding tone; [−echo] that it is at a lower level. Since Carrell assumes that downstep is the default process in Igbo, [−echo] is taken to be unmarked, and [+echo] introduced where there is no downstep. This approach is essentially a formalization of Welmers's 'drop' tone, though with the reverse value, since [+echo] specifies cases where the tone does not drop. A similar approach is adopted by Larson (1971), who uses the feature [±step], and by Stewart (1992), who analyses Dschang and Ebrié as having, on a separate tonal tier, along with other features, the feature [±stepping].

However, few scholars have used such features, preferring downstep to be specified by processes applying to existing tones rather than by introducing specific tonal features. The arguments here are the same that have been rehearsed in connection with special downstepped tones: first, that the value of the features is only specifiable in relation to the preceding tone, and, second, that the process is a recursive one, and an indefinite number of such features would be required.

Nevertheless, Hyman (1992) provides specific feature representations for downstepped (and also upstepped) tones within his extended feature geometry for tonal features. He separates the 'T(one)-plane' from the 'R(egister)-plane', with separate specifications on each plane. Given three tonal features, H(igh), L(ow), and LH (= Mid), and three register features, L(ow), H(igh) and Ø, he is able to draw up the set of nine distinct tonal representations given in Fig. 4.26, which include downstepped (') and upstepped (↑) High, Low and Mid tones.

Fig. 4.26

T-plane:	H	L	LH	H	L	LH	H	L	LH
R-plane:	Ø	Ø	Ø	L	L	L	H	H	H
TONE:	H	L	M	'H	'L	'M	↑H	↑L	↑M

As can be seen, a downstepped 'H is interpreted as High on the T-plane and Low on the R-plane, while an upstepped Low is Low on the T-plane and High on the R-plane. Downstep and Upstep are therefore achieved by a shift of register. Such a specification does not, of course, of itself provide a mechanism for the lowering of downstepped tones or the raising of upstepped ones, and Hyman therefore has to provide further formal apparatus to achieve this.

4.3.4.6 Tone and Laryngeal Features

We have noted that there is a close connection between tone and other 'laryngeal' features, especially those of voice quality and the voicing of consonants. It is also the case that in some languages there is a relationship between such laryngeal features and tonal register. These relationships raise questions for the feature specification of such tones.

These intimate relationships between tones and other kinds of laryngeal activity inevitably lead to the suggestion that they are different aspects of the same thing. In a system of distinctive features, it may therefore be possible to include several kinds of laryngeal contrasts under a single feature. Halle and Stevens (1971) attempt to account for a wide range of laryngeal phenomena with a set of four laryngeal features: [±spread], [±constricted], [±stiff], and [±slack]. They base this system on physiological models of laryngeal activity which assume two basic dimensions: the narrowing or widening of the glottis, and the tension of the vocal folds. All laryngeal contrasts—including tone—are therefore subsumed under these four features, with tonal features specified by the features [+stiff] (for high tones) and [+slack] (for low tones).

There are, however, several problems with this approach (for a detailed discussion see Anderson, 1978). While it can certainly be argued that similar physiological gestures are involved in all of these cases, this does not necessarily mean that they can be accommodated by the same small set of laryngeal features. In the first place, the features [±stiff] and [±slack] allow for only three pitch levels (the combination [+stiff, +slack] is excluded); furthermore, there is ample evidence that tone and other laryngeal features can have independent significance; finally, the fact that tonal contrasts are in any case *relative* suggests that they cannot be properly accounted for in terms of a specific phonetic opposition based on physiological differences; how do we account, for example, for the fact that high tones may be lowered by downdrift or downstep to a pitch level equal to or lower than that of low tones in the same utterance, if the former are still specified as [+stiff] and the latter as [+slack]?

Ladefoged (1973) presents a more elaborate view of laryngeal features, recognizing eight different kinds of 'glottal stricture', of which Halle and Stevens' 'stiff voice' and 'slack voice' are only two. He offers a physiological explanation for the links between these features and pitch, and suggests that general 'cover features'

Fig. 4.27	Glottal stricture	Pitch	Cover feature
	spread		
	voiceless	high	RAISED
	murmur		
	slack	mid	
	voice		
	stiff		LOWERED
	creaky	low	
	closed		

such as 'RAISED' and 'LOWERED' might be used to express these links, as in Fig. 4.27. He is doubtful, however, about the validity of such cover features, noting that 'pitch and glottal stricture can sometimes covary, but they are often clearly independent features. Most glottal strictures can occur on a wide range of pitches.'

Matisoff (1973) notes similar relationship between laryngeal features. He identifies two contrasting 'laryngeal attitudes', as in Fig. 4.28. As can be seen, each includes not only pitch and voice/voicelessness but also a range of other features, including voice-quality.

Fig. 4.28 TENSE-LARYNX SYNDROME
    higher pitch/rising contour
    association with -ʔ
    voicelessness
    retracted tongue root
    'creaky' voice
    larynx tense/raised

LAX-LARYNX SYNDROME
lower pitch/falling contour
association with -h
voicedness, breathiness
advanced tongue root
'rasping' voice
larynx lax/lowered

More recent work has continued to allow the possibility of accounting for both tone and other laryngeal features, especially voice, with the same limited set of features. Both Bao (1990) and Duanmu (1990) adopt a position similar to that of Halle and Stevens, the former using the single feature [±stiff vocal cords] and the latter the two features [stiff vocal cords] and [slack vocal cords], which allow for three possibilities. However, such an extreme position is unlikely to be sustainable, given the potential independence of voicing and tone. Though Duanmu claims that languages which have a large number of tones, and which therefore use both tone and register features, will also have voice quality distinctions, Yip (1995) points out that this is certainly not true of all such languages; Cantonese, which has different registers, has no such voice quality differences.

Although, from the evidence we have, there is little justification for an attempt to treat tone and voice as manifestations of the same phonological distinction, it would nevertheless be desirable if the close relationship between tonal and other laryngeal features could be accommodated in some way. This might be achieved in terms of feature geometry, in which tone, voicing, and voice quality are subsumed under a common laryngeal node. We shall take up this principle below.

4.4 The Representation of Tone

4.4.1 INTRODUCTION

We have so far examined various proposals for the specification of the paradigmatic aspects of tone by means of tonal and register features. But there are wider issues in the phonological representation of tone, concerned with the relationships between tone and other prosodic features, and the way in which tone relates to prosodic structure as a whole. Unlike the different proposals for feature systems for tone, which depend on selecting appropriate substantive elements within a given formal framework, different views on the role of tone involve different conceptions of the form of phonological structure itself. While we cannot deal adequately with these wider issues within the confines of this chapter, we may nevertheless examine some of the more specific questions raised here, in so far as they affect the representation of tone.

4.4.2 EARLIER REPRESENTATIONS

We have seen that scholars in the first half of the twentieth century applied standard phonemic principles to the representation of tone, establishing a set of distinctive 'tones' or 'tonemes' for each language. These tones accompany the segmental phonemes, but opinions differ as to the relationship between the two. Tones can be assigned to different *domains*; for some scholars, such as Pike, tones are properties of syllables, while for others they are properties of the syllable peak, i.e. the vowel. These two views of the place of tone are represented graphically in Figs. 4.29(a) and (b), respectively. The latter model is adopted by, for example, Schachter and Fromkin (1968) for Akan, and Woo (1969) for Chinese, and by generative phonologists generally, since it allows tone to be specified in terms of distinctive features, tonal features simply being added to the feature matrix of the vowel. The feature representations of tone discussed in 4.3.4 are generally to be understood in this sense. Gandour (1974c) argues that this is essential in the description of Thai, since tone in this language is restricted by the occurrence of certain consonants (see below, 4.6.2.3), and the necessary generalizations cannot be expressed if tone is assigned to the syllable as a whole. Similar claims are made in relation to Xhosa (Leben, 1973b). In Prague School theory, the representation of tone is not completely consistent, but it would appear that tone is typically assigned to moras rather than vowels, with rising and falling tones requiring a bimoraic syllable-nucleus (Trubetzkoy, 1939: 181). This is represented in Fig. 4.29(c).

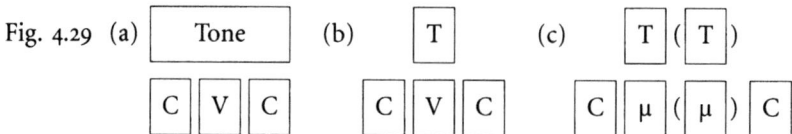

Fig. 4.29   (a) [Tone]   (b) [T]   (c) [T] ([T])

   [C][V][C]   [C][V][C]   [C][μ] ([μ]) [C]

Despite their differences, these different representations take tones to be intimately linked to each successive vowel, syllable, or mora. One approach that takes a somewhat different view is Firthian Prosodic Analysis (Firth, 1948), which avoids a strict separation of segmental and suprasegmental features and prefers to extract much of the phonetic matter of the syllable, word, or other unit, including the tones, as 'prosodies', leaving only a bare skeleton as 'phonematic units'. Fig. 4.30 is an attempt—though a rather inadequate one—to represent this view, showing tone and other prosodies as properties of the whole syllable, and phonematic units (here represented by lower case c and v) as features of individual segmental positions.[28] This diagram fails to do justice to this approach in a number of important respects, since in this framework tone is not necessarily restricted to the syllable; any grammatical or phonological unit may have its prosodies (cf. Sprigg, 1955, 1968).

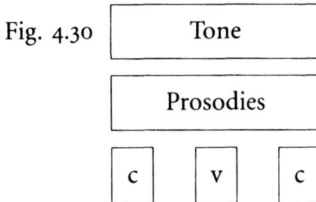

Fig. 4.30

Tone

Prosodies

c	v	c

Though classical generative phonology has generally found it more efficient to regard tone as a segmental feature, evidence has also been presented that this is not always appropriate, and that it may be necessary to regard tones as attached to larger units. Leben (1973a, 1973b) draws attention to the fact, well attested in African languages, that the tone patterns of words in a given tone-class are often constant, regardless of the number of syllables in the word. This phenomenon is illustrated in Fig. 4.31, with examples from Mende. These show that the same tone pattern is present in words of one, two, and three syllables (Leben, 1973b). The monosyllable has a rising–falling tone pattern (represented by ˜); the disyllabic form has a low tone followed by a falling tone, and in the trisyllabic form the syllables have a low, high, and low tone respectively. It will be clear that all three patterns have a L–H–L sequence, which appears as such in the trisyllabic form, but is compressed to L–F in the disyllabic form, and still further to RF in the monosyllable. We can therefore regard all three words as having the pattern LHL, but differently distributed according to the number of syllables. The same is true of the other permissible tone patterns of Mende: H, L, and HL.

Fig. 4.31 mbā   'companion'
nyàhâ 'woman'
nìkílì 'groundnut'

Further evidence for the independence of tones from segmental features is provided by the so-called 'stability' of tones. In some cases, a syllable may be lost through elision or contraction, but its tone is preserved and realized on another syllable. This is illustrated in Fig. 4.32, from Efik (Westermann and Ward, 1933: 149–50). The Efik expression *kûbóm* ('in the canoe') is a contraction

---

[28] For a useful exposition and illustration of Prosodic Analysis see the papers in Palmer (ed.) (1970).

of *ké ùbóm*, with the tone pattern high–low–high, while the expression *kûruà* ('in the market') is a contraction of *ké ùruà*, with the pattern high–low–low. The elision of the vowel *e* permits its tone to be reassigned to the following *u*. It can be seen that the falling tone arises naturally as a combination of High and Low tones on a single syllable. The tone that remains when the syllable is lost in such a case is often called a 'floating' tone.

Fig. 4.32   ké + ùbóm   →   kûbóm
           ké + ùruà   →   kûruà

Another type of floating tone occurs which is not a property of any segment or syllable at all, but must be regarded as present in a particular syntactic construction. In the Babete dialect of Mbam-Nkan, for example (Hyman and Tadadjeu, 1976), when the two words *ŋkùù* ('message') and *pègùù* ('strangers'), which in isolation have only Low tones, are combined to give the meaning 'the message of the strangers' (the so-called 'associative' construction), the first Low tone of the second word is replaced by a High tone (see Fig. 4.33). In this construction, there is evidently a High tone between the two words which is not attached to any segment or syllable, and which replaces the following falling tone.

Fig. 4.33   ŋkùù + pègùù   →   ŋkùù + pégùù

In the related Mbui dialect, the associative construction in one class of nouns is marked by the particle *bɔ́*. When we join the words *bɔ̀kɔ́ɔ* ('crabs') and *bɔ̀ndúm* ('husbands'), both with apparently identical tone patterns and both of this noun-class, to a word such as *sɔ́ŋ* ('bird'), with the meanings 'the crabs of the bird' and 'the husbands of the bird', respectively, the result is different, as we see from Fig. 4.34. We note that the associative particle *bɔ́* is *downstepped*. As we saw in 4.3.4.5, downstep can often be ascribed to a 'latent' Low tone, which causes lowering of the following High, but is not actually pronounced. In this case we could therefore assume that there is such a latent—floating—tone present, but since it applies to only some words (it appears after *bɔ̀ndúm*, for example, but not after *bɔ̀kɔ́ɔ*), we must assume that where this floating tone occurs it is part of the first word. We could therefore represent these two words as *bɔ̀kɔ́ɔ* and *bɔ̀ndúm`*, where the latter is followed by a floating low tone which is not attached to any syllable or segment of the word.

Fig. 4.34   bɔ̀kɔ́ɔ + sɔ́ŋ   →   bɔ̀kɔ́ɔ bɔ́ sɔ́ŋ   'the crabs of the bird'
           bɔ̀ndúm + sɔ́ŋ   →   bɔ̀ndúm ꜜbɔ́ sɔ́ŋ   'the husbands of the bird'

Tadadjeu (1974) reports a similar case from another dialect: Dschang–Bamileke. In this dialect, the associative construction is marked in 'careful' speech in one noun-class by a particle *à* or *è* , with a low tone. However, in 'normal' speech, the particle is omitted. Even without the particle, however, the first syllable of the second word is downstepped, suggesting that there is a floating low tone between the two words, which serves as a marker of the associative

construction. Thus, putting *ǹtsɔ́ŋ* ('thief') together with *sɔ́ŋ* ('bird'), we get *ǹtsɔ́ŋ*
ˈsɔ́ŋ ('thief of bird'). This sort of representation can be employed with many
other cases of downstep, such of those discussed earlier.

On the strength of evidence of this kind, Leben argues that the tone patterns
cannot be a property of individual segments or syllables in languages such as
these; they must belong to the morpheme as a whole, and be represented
suprasegmentally, independently of the segments and syllables. The difficulty is,
however, in determining what this means for the representation of phonological
structure, and how such an approach can be formalized.

4.4.3 THE AUTOSEGMENTAL REPRESENTATION OF TONE

4.4.3.1 Tiers and Tones

Goldsmith's *Autosegmental Phonology* (Goldsmith, 1976) can be seen as an
attempt to provide a solution to the problems of representing tone 'suprasegmentally'. While Leben recognizes that tones cannot necessarily be regarded as
features of segments or syllables, Goldsmith proposes a representation in which
tones are completely separate from these; they constitute autonomous units
—'autosegments'—which are *associated* with segments but not part of them.[29]
The representation thus takes the form of two parallel 'tiers', the segmental tier
and the tonal tier, linked by 'association lines', as in Fig. 4.35, where T = tone,
and t = 'tone-bearing unit' (TBU), i.e. vowel. In Fig. 4.35(a) there is a simple
relationship between tones and vowels, with each vowel having its tone; but the
model also allows for more complex relationships, as in (b) and (c), which show
two tones associated to one vowel, and two vowels sharing one tone, respectively.

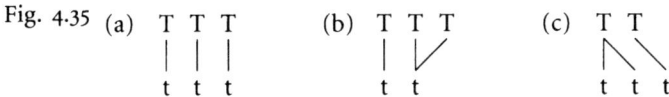

Fig. 4.35 (a) T T T   (b) T T T   (c) T T
               | | | | ⩘   ⩗⩘
               t t t   t t   t t t

This form of representation provides a way of accounting for tone
'suprasegmentally', in Leben's sense, but it goes much further, since it constitutes
a different view of phonological structure as a whole. The latter is no longer
seen as a linear string of feature matrices representing segments, but more in the
nature of a musical score, in which different 'voices' are represented on different
staves. These voices are co-ordinated with one another, but they are in principle
independent.

As noted above, there are significant similarities between this approach and
earlier ones, especially Firth's Prosodic Analysis (Firth, 1948). Goldsmith notes

---

[29] Goldsmith (1976: 20) notes that the term 'autosegmental' is preferable to 'suprasegmental', since
the autosegmental level is actually composed of tonal segments. The point is not, therefore, that
tones are not segmental, but that they are independent of the vocalic and consonantal segments.

the parallel, as also similarities with the 'long component' approach of Harris (1944). Despite the similarities, there are, in fact, considerable differences between Autosegmental Phonology and Prosodic Analysis; the latter is not explicitly formalized, and indeed would reject a consistent formalization, preferring an *ad hoc* treatment for each system. Further, as Palmer (1970) makes clear, not all prosodies are of the 'long component' type, i.e. features extending over longer units; they are seen as much more abstract, including, for example, structural characteristics or features which have no consistent phonetic realization.[30] Most significantly, of course, Autosegmental Phonology differs from Prosodic Analysis in being a *generative* theory, which recognizes underlying and surface representations, with rules to link them. Although they share a non-segmental view of tone, therefore, the two approaches differ in a number of fundamental respects.

Autosegmental representations of tone take the form of a segmental representation of vocalic and consonantal matrices linked by association lines to tonal features. The latter are conventionally labelled H(igh), M(id) and L(ow). These labels are, however, merely abbreviations for tonal matrices, defined by the features [±Highpitch] and [±Lowpitch], where H is [+Highpitch, –Lowpitch], L is [–Highpitch, +Lowpitch], and M is [+Highpitch, +Lowpitch]. The fourth combination, [–Highpitch, –Lowpitch], is excluded (Goldsmith, 1976: 54).[31]

Given such a model, we can account in a consistent way for many of the problems discussed earlier. We may begin with the 'tone melodies' of Mende (see Fig. 4.31, above). We saw that in Mende the same tone pattern (which may be LHL, H, or L) can be said to characterize words with different numbers of syllables. The words of Fig. 4.31 can be represented in autosegmental terms as in Fig. 4.36, with an identical tone pattern differently linked to the tone-bearing units, according to the number of syllables.

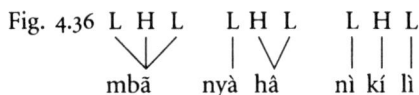

Fig. 4.36 L H L   L H L   L H L
         \|/ | \/ | | |
         mbā   nyà hâ   nì kí lì

Similar principles apply with the 'stability' of tones, illustrated from Efik in Fig. 4.32. Here, a vowel is lost, but its tone is preserved, and re-associated to the neighbouring vowel. This can be represented as in Fig. 4.37.

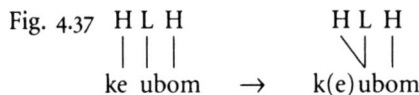

Fig. 4.37 H L H   H L H
           | | | \| |
           ke ubom   →   k(e)ubom

[30] Firth (1948) suggests, for example, that a structure such as CVC might be considered to be a prosody. Interestingly, later developments in autosegmental theory introduce a 'CV tier' on which such structural characteristics are independently represented (Clements and Keyser, 1983).

[31] Note that Goldsmith's use of [+Highpitch, +Lowpitch] for mid tone, and his exclusion of [–Highpitch, –Lowpitch], is the reverse of the usual practice, which would exclude the former and permit the latter. See 4.3.4.2.

The floating tones of Mbam–Nkan, which provide evidence for an inserted H tone which is unattached to a particular segment, are represented in Fig. 4.38. The inserted floating tone, which is encircled, is said to 'dock' onto the following syllable, displacing the existing Low tone, which is deleted.

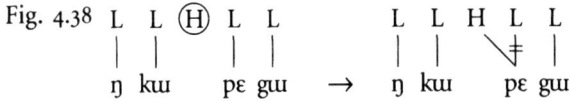

Fig. 4.38
```
L   L  (H)  L   L            L   L   H   L   L
|   |       |   |            |   |    \‡  |
ŋ  kɯ     pɛ  gɯ    →     ŋ  kɯ     pɛ  gɯ
```

Finally, we may examine the case of downstep in Mbui and Dschang–Bamileke. As we saw above, the Mbui associative construction is marked by the particle *bɔ́*, which in some cases is downstepped. We can account for this downstep by including an unpronounced low tone in the representation of the first word in those cases where the downstep occurs. This is illustrated in Fig. 4.39, which shows an unlinked Low tone at the end of *bɔ̀ndúm`*. This causes the following High tone to be lowered, after which the Low tone can be deleted. A similar solution can be offered in the case of Dschang–Bamileke.

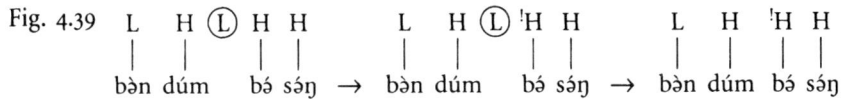

Fig. 4.39
```
L   H  (L)  H  H          L   H  (L) ꜜH  H          L   H  ꜜH  H
|   |       |  |          |   |       |   |          |   |   |   |
bɔ̀n dúm   bɔ́ sɔ́ŋ  →  bɔ̀n dúm   bɔ́ sɔ́ŋ  →  bɔ̀n dúm  bɔ́ sɔ́ŋ
```

4.4.3.2 Association Lines and the Wellformedness Condition

In the autosegmental model, tone is represented separately from the segmental base of the utterance, but tonal features must nevertheless be associated with segments. Since the association is not always the same, the principles determining it are of considerable importance. Goldsmith (1976: 27) establishes the general principles of the *Wellformedness Condition*, which in its original version, runs as follows (cf. above, 2.7.2):

(1)   All vowels are associated with at least one tone.
(2)   All tones are associated with at least one vowel.
(3)   Association lines do not cross.

This means that the representations given in Fig. 4.40(a)–(c) are not permitted; they violate constraints (1) to (3) of the Wellformedness Condition respectively.[32]

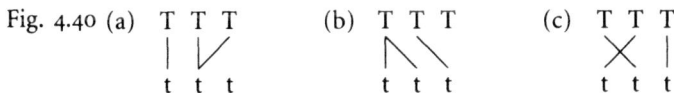

Fig. 4.40 (a)
```
T  T  T          (b)  T  T  T          (c)  T  T  T
|   /                  \  \                  X  |
t  t  t               t  t  t               t  t  t
```

The first two constraints of the Wellformedness Condition ensure that there are

---

[32] Note that the representations of 'floating' tones given in Figs. 4.38 and 4.39 are not regarded as violations of the Condition, even though such tones are unattached, since these are intermediate stages in the derivation of the forms. The Condition applies to the final output of the rules.

no stranded, unpronounceable tones or vowels, and thus exclude many theoretical possibilities. However, there is still considerable latitude in how tones and tone-bearing units are associated with one another. Fig. 4.41 shows a random selection of the possibilities with three tones and three tone-bearing units, none of which violate the Wellformedness Condition.

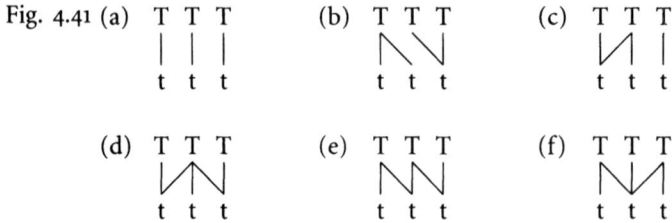

Fig. 4.41 (a) T T T   (b) T T T   (c) T T T
        | | | ⟍⟍   ⟍| |
        t t t   t t t   t t t

     (d) T T T   (e) T T T   (f) T T T
        ⟋⟍   ⟍⟍   ⟍⟋
        t t t   t t t   t t t

In order to limit the possibilities, a number of scholars adopt the principle that tones and tone-bearing units should be associated *from left to right* (Goldsmith, 1976: 117; cf. Williams, 1976; Haraguchi, 1977; Clements and Ford, 1979; Clements and Goldsmith, 1984). With the same number of tones and TBUs, this principle (the *Universal Association Convention*) results in an association such as that of Fig. 4.41(a)—in fact, this is the only possibility out of those given here. If the number of tones and TBUs is not the same, then the principle is implemented by associating any left-over tones or TBUs with the last TBU or tone, respectively, as in Fig. 4.42.[33]

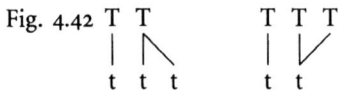

Fig. 4.42 T T   T T T
       | ⟍ | ⟋
      t t t   t t

As an example of the operation of this principle we may take the case of Shona (Kenstowicz, 1994: 331ff.). Shona verbs may be classed as High-tone or Low-tone; in the former case, the High tone of the verb root is associated with all succeeding syllables. Thus, in Fig. 4.43(a), the word *kuténgésérá* ('to sell to') is made up of the High-tone root *téng* preceded by the Low infinitive marker *kù* and followed by a succession of affixes, all of which have a High tone. Another example, this time of the multiple association of tones to a single vowel, was illustrated from Mende in Fig. 4.36; it is presented again in Fig. 4.43(b).

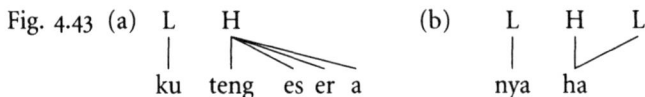

Fig. 4.43 (a) L   H   (b)   L   H   L
        | ⟍⟍⟍ | ⟍⟋
       ku teng es er a   nya ha

Despite these cases, subsequent consideration of the Universal Association Con-

---

[33] The initial association of tones and segments is called 'mapping'; association of left-over tones to the last vowel is 'dumping', while attaching left-over vowels to the last tone is 'spreading'. See Durand (1990: 249).

vention (Clements and Ford, 1979; Halle and Vergnaud, 1982; Ahoua, 1986) has concluded that, while in many languages it is appropriate for several tones to be associated with a final TBU, as in Fig. 4.43(b), this is not always the case. Indeed, the default situation is *not* to have such multiple association. The convention can therefore be reformulated along the following lines (Pulleyblank, 1986: 11):

Map a sequence of tones onto a sequence of tone-bearing units,
   (a) from left to right
   (b) in a one-to-one relation.

Condition (b) precludes multiple association of tones to tone-bearing units. The convention is, however, only the default case; it may be overridden if so stipulated for specific languages.

   Condition (a) is also not always appropriate. In Hausa (Newman, 1986b), it has been claimed[34] that association of tones and segments is best undertaken from right to left. In other cases, it is not possible to associate them automatically in either direction. Here, the links between certain tones and segments are lexically determined (i.e. they are not predictable), and only the remainder will be assigned by rule. Goldsmith introduces a particular formal device for the initial, lexically determined association: the 'star' notation. By marking with '*' the particular tone and tone-bearing unit that are to be associated, and by associating these first, the desired alignment is achieved.

   In Tonga, for example (Goldsmith, 1984a), the basic tone pattern is H L, but words such as *ímákànì* ('news') and *ímúsúnè* ('ox') show that this pattern can be differently aligned with tone-bearing units: the first has H H L L, and the second H H H L, both of which can be seen as instances of the H L pattern. The appropriate alignment can be achieved by marking the L tone of the H L pattern with '*', and likewise the appropriate syllable of the words—in this case the *ka* of *ímákànì* and the *ne* of *ímúsúnè*. These are then associated first, as in Figs. 4.44(a) and 4.44(b), after which the remainder of the association will proceed in a regular fashion (Figs. 4.44(c) and 4.44(d)).

Fig. 4.44 (a)

<hr />

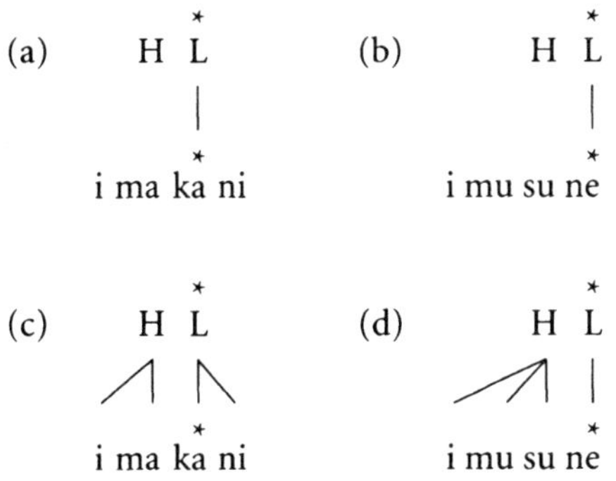

[34] This claim has, however, been rejected by some. See Odden (1995).

This device singles out a particular Tone-Bearing Unit as the centre of the tone pattern, and thus has considerable affinity with the marking of 'accents' in accentual languages. In fact, Goldsmith (1976) applies this notation to English, as a means of specifying the position of the 'nuclear stress' and intonation, while Haraguchi (1977) develops it for Japanese, which has a pitch–accent (see 3.3.4, above). In the case of languages such as Tonga, Goldsmith is able to argue that these languages should also be regarded as accentual rather than tonal. This question will be considered in more detail below (see 4.7.5).

4.4.3.3 The Obligatory Contour Principle

The Tonga case illustrated in Fig. 4.44 involves treating two sequences of tones, HHLL, and HHHL, as instance of the 'same' pattern, H L. It is, in fact, assumed that identical tones in sequence constitute a single occurrence of a tone on the tonal tier; sequences of like tones on this tier are not permitted. This is known as the *Obligatory Contour Principle* (OCP). The principle was put forward by Leben (1973a), and formulated by Goldsmith (1976: 36), as follows:[35]

At the melodic level of the grammar, any two adjacent tonemes must be distinct. Thus HHL is not a possible melodic pattern; it automatically simplifies to HL.

Kenstowicz (1994: 322–3) gives an example from Margi which illustrates the need for such a principle. In this language, definite forms of nouns have the suffix *-árì*, before which a stem-final vowel is lost or becomes non-syllabic. In the example of Fig. 4.45, the word *làgù* ('road'), which is low throughout, could be represented with a sequence of two L tones, as in Fig. 4.45(a), or with a single L linked to both vowels, as in Fig. 4.45(b). In the former case, the loss of the second syllable of *làgù* (*u* becomes *w*) produces a 'floating' tone which will 'dock' on the following syllable, giving—wrongly—a rising tone (LH) on the following vowel. With a single L (in conformity with the OCP), no floating tone is produced, and therefore no rise; this outcome is the correct one.

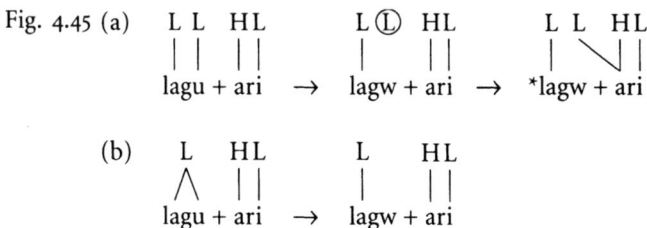

Fig. 4.45 (a)

```
    L L  HL          L Ⓛ HL          L L  HL
    | |  ||           |   ||           |  ＼| |
  lagu + ari   →   lagw + ari   →   *lagw + ari
```

(b)

```
    L   HL            L    HL
    ∧   ||            |    ||
  lagu + ari   →   lagw + ari
```

Though the OCP seems to be justifiable in this case, it is nevertheless a controversial principle, since it not clear to what stretch of speech, or at what level of a phonological derivation, it applies. By 'melodic level', Goldsmith means the

---

[35] Since the labels H and L are actually abbreviations for tonal matrices, the restriction has the effect of prohibiting the occurrence of identical feature specifications for successive tonal segments.

level at which tone melodies can be recognized, for example LHL in Mende, or HL in Tonga, and such melodies will generally apply to morphemes. No morpheme, therefore, will have a pattern with a repeated tone, but there could be such repetition when morphemes are joined together into words; LHL + LHL gives a sequence of two L tones. If the OCP applies *only* at the underlying level, as it appears to do in Shona (Odden, 1986), then this is of no consequence, but if it applies throughout a derivation, then the two L tones will perforce be fused into a single L, associated with both the original TBUs. The evidence in these cases is conflicting; there are cases where adjacent High tones are avoided even in surface forms, but also many languages in which adjacent High tones are common. Odden (1995: 464) concludes that 'the strongest possible version of the OCP at this point is that there may be a dispreference for adjacent identical tones'; this does not amount to a blanket prohibition, however.

4.4.4 CONCLUSION: IMPLICATIONS OF AUTOSEGMENTAL REPRESENTATIONS

Autosegmental representations of tone are widely employed, and most current theoretical discussions of tonal processes in languages use this framework. Of more significance, perhaps, than its use as a descriptive tool are the implications of the model for the place of tone in prosodic structure itself. The separation of tone from other features which the autosegmental framework embodies, at least in its original form,[36] carries the implication that tone is to a considerable degree independent of the rest of phonological structure. Furthermore, although the links between tones and the tone-bearing units of this structure are controlled by a variety of principles—the Wellformedness Condition, the OCP—the validity and universality of these principles is far from established. Autosegmental representations therefore point to the conclusion that tone is less well integrated into prosodic structure than features which are not treated autosegmentally, in the sense that—unlike accent, for example—it is not itself *part* of the prosodic organization, but rather depends on this organization.

4.5 Tonal Processes

4.5.1 INTRODUCTION

In our initial discussion of tone we considered some of the 'mechanical perturbations' which create difficulties for tonal analysis. These perturbations consist of phonological processes which affect tones, changing or modifying them in

---

[36] Since the appearance of the model in the work of Goldsmith in the 1970s, other features besides tone have been subjected to autosegmental treatment, but tone remains the area where the model is most profitably employed.

particular contexts, and thereby obscuring their identity. These processes are of different kinds, and their phonological significance is also different according to whether they can be interpreted as morphotonemic—changing one tone into another—or purely phonetic—changing one variant of a toneme into another.

Though Pike (1948) discusses these processes in some detail, he does not attempt to formalize them, and his toneme-based model does not in any case have any means of doing so. He is more concerned with eliminating the effects of these processes in order to establish the tonal inventories of languages. Later, rule-based models have provided the apparatus—phonological rules—for the formal expression of tonal processes, and it has therefore become possible to consider their nature and role more explicitly.

4.5.2 TYPES OF TONE PROCESSES

Pike (1948: 22ff.) lists a number of different kinds of processes affecting tones, including morphophonemic changes ('change from one toneme to another') and phonetic changes ('change within a toneme'), but his list is neither exhaustive nor systematic. Under the first of these headings we find 'changes in isolated vs. included position', 'morphological changes', 'changes of phrase relationships', 'regular mechanical meaningless changes', 'arbitrary tone sandhi', and 'alternate pronunciations'. He exemplifies some of the well known processes from Mixteco and Mazateco, and cites further examples from standard descriptions. In the case of tone sandhi, where one tone is substituted for another in particular contexts, he quotes extensively from descriptions of Chinese dialects. In Hagu (Amoy), for example, there are complex 'chains' of tone changes, while in Foochow, for which nine tones have been recognized, Pike attempts to systematize the reported changes as in Fig. 4.46 (Pike, 1948: 85).

Fig. 4.46	3, some 4, and 6	are replaced by 1	before 1, 5, or 7
	7	is replaced by 1	before 1 or 7
	5 and 7	are replaced by 2	before 2, 3, 4, 5, or 6
	some 4	are replaced by 2	before 1, 5, or 7
	1, 3, some 4 and 6	are replaced by 5	before 2, 3, 4, or 6
	some 4	are replaced by 7	before 3, 4, or 6
	some 4	are replaced by 8–	before 2
	2	is replaced by 8–	before 2, 3, 4, or 6
	5	is replaced by 9–	before 1 or 7
	1 and 2 remain unchanged		before 1, 5, or 7

Later writers on the subject have attempted to introduce more order and system into the description of tonal process. Unlike Pike, Welmers (1959) does not see them as disruptive factors but as straightforward and regular processes which can be accommodated within the existing theoretical framework. He recognizes different types of phenomena, not only tonemes with their variants, but also morphotonemic alternations and replacive tonal morphemes. Similarly, Spears (1967) attempts to broaden the scope of tonal processes that can be described by incorporating morphophonemic features into his description of Mende, with appropriate rules to interpret the morphophonemes in phonemic and phonetic terms. He notes the existence of such phenomena as 'polarized tones' (where tones take on opposite values from neighbouring ones), and 'tonal extensions' (where the domain of the last tone of a morpheme is extended to the first vowel of the next morpheme). Voorhoeve (1968) also argues for the establishment of a typology of tonal processes, a 'universal grammar of tone', which incorporates 'morphotonological rules' applying to 'base tonemes', and he applies this principle to the comparison of a number of African languages.

The application of the principles of generative phonology to tone, with its underlying (morphophonemic) forms and ordered rules, provides the opportunity for a more formal treatment of tonal processes. George (1970), for example, reinterprets Smith's description of Nupe (Smith, 1967) in generative terms, claiming to be able to simplify the statement by the use of ordered rules. Asongwed and Hyman (1976) demonstrate that the 'bewildering array of tone patterns and tone alternations' in Ngamambo, with five phonetic pitch levels, can be accounted for with two underlying tones, H and L, and a set of morphotonemic rules. An example of the power of this approach is provided by van Spaandonck (1971), who shows how, with suitably abstract underlying forms and ordered rules, the peculiar case of Ciluba, which seems to have reversed the values of the tones found in closely related languages and in Proto–Bantu, can be described. Processes such as 'displacement' (where underlying tones surface on later syllables), 'repetition' (where tones are copied onto later syllables), and 'anticipation' (where tones are regressively displaced), are invoked.

One of the concerns here is to establish *natural* rules for tone. Hyman (1973) explores what he calls 'natural tonal assimilations', which are assimilatory processes in which tones accommodate themselves to other tones. He notes that such assimilations can be *vertical* or *horizontal*, the former involving the raising or lowering of tones in the environment of a higher or lower tone, respectively, and the latter the spreading of tones. Thus, for example, downdrift can be seen as a case of vertical assimilation of a High tone to a preceding Low one, while the change of a High tone to a Rise after a Low tone can be attributed to the spreading of the Low into the High tone to give Low + High. Conversely, the change of a contour to a simple tone (e.g. LH → L, or HL → H) can be interpreted as spreading followed by *absorption*, with the sequence LHH → LLHH (spreading) → L LH (absorption). According to Hyman, both vertical and horizontal assimilations can be *anticipatory* or *perseverative*, i.e. the assimilation can be to a following or a preceding tone, but there are restrictions on the kinds of assimilations that are possible.

Similar goals are pursued by Hyman and Schuh (1972, 1974), who provide a more comprehensive listing of possible 'natural' tone processes. For them, natural synchronic rules affecting tone are not necessarily the same as natural diachronic rules. Among the latter they include 'downdrift', 'low raising', 'spreading', 'absorption', and 'simplification'; among the former are included 'downstep', 'shifting', 'copying', 'polarization', 'dissimilation', 'replacement', and 'displacement'. Examples of some of these can be given here. *Low raising* consists of the raising of a Low tone when it is followed by a non-Low tone, for example in Igbo, where the *ò* of *òké* ('rat') has slightly higher pitch than the *ò* of *òpì* ('horn'); *spreading* is the tendency for the tone of the first syllable of a word to spread to the right, as in Gwari *òkpá* ('length'), which becomes [òkpǎ] (the Low tone of the first syllable spreads onto the High tone of the second, producing a rise). *Absorption*, a sub-type of spreading, results in the change of a contour tone to a level tone when it is followed by a level tone at the same height as its end point, so that a Rise becomes Low before a High tone, and a Fall becomes High before a Low tone. The process here involves the spreading of the second part of the contour (High in the case of a Rise, and Low in the case of a Fall) onto the next syllable, where it is absorbed by the existing tone, leaving only the first part of the contour on the first syllable. Among the synchronic processes, *shifting* involves the movement of a tone onto the following syllable, for example in Mbui–Bamileke, where an imperative followed by an object, for example /lɔ́ɔ́/ + /bòsə́ŋ/ ('look for the birds'), becomes [lɔ̀ɔ̀ bə́sə́ŋ], with the High tone of the first word shifting to the first syllable of the second; *copying* occurs when a syllable with no underlying tone acquires a tone from a neighbouring syllable, as in the case of Mbui, where /lɔ́ɔ́/ + wa / ('me') becomes [lɔ̀ɔ̀ wá], with a High tone on *wá*; *polarization* describes the process whereby a toneless morpheme acquires a tone with the opposite value to what follows, as in the case of the Igbo prefix *a*, which becomes High before a Low tone (*ázà* = 'sweeping') but Low before a High tone (*àgá* = 'going'); *displacement* is the realization of a tone at a distance, for example in Sukuma, where the expression *ǹ-kòlò*, which is ambiguous in isolation, meaning 'sheep' or 'heart', is disambiguated when followed by an adjective, with a different tone on the final syllable of the latter: *ǹ-kòlò ǹ-tàalè* ('big sheep') vs. *ǹ-kòlò ǹ-tàalé* ('big heart').

Given the wide range of different tonal processes here, it is natural to ask to what extent they can be generalized. Several of the processes just described, such as spreading, absorption, shifting, and copying, involve the influence of one tone on an adjacent tone, and it might therefore be possible to identify a common principle here. Schuh (1978) groups together spreading, absorption, and copying as types of influence from an adjacent syllable, and adds tone displacement, since he considers that 'it must have developed from spreading which has become limited to certain morphological environments'. Thus, most of these processes can be regarded as different forms of spreading. It can also be observed that these processes appear to apply almost exclusively from left to right. Schuh elevates this to a general principle claiming that spreading *always* operates from left to right.

Spreading is contrasted with *assimilation*, which may apply in either direction, either as *anticipatory* ('the first tone becomes more like the second') or as *perseverative* ('the second tone becomes more like the first'). As an example of the former Schuh cites data from Ewe (see Fig. 4.47), where Low tones becomes Mid before High.

Fig. 4.47 /ɸù lá/ → [ɸū lá] ('the sea')
/nyì lá/ → [nyī lá] ('the cow')

As a case of perseverative assimilation Schuh cites downdrift. Since downdrift tends to affect high tones rather more than low ones, Schuh considers that it should be seen not as a result of the superimposition of an overall falling intonation onto the utterance but rather as the assimilation of High tones to Low tones.[37]

Although many types of rule can be assigned to the 'spreading' or 'assimilation' category, there are others which do not fall into either of these two, including *dissimilation* and *polarization*, both of which entail adjacent tones having opposite values. Though some cases of these may be regarded as the synchronic outcome of diachronic spreading processes, Schuh concedes that this is not always the case, and we must recognize the possibility of this category as an independent type.

As a final type of process we may note the existence of *paradigmatic replacement*. This label covers many cases of tone sandhi, particularly in East Asian languages, which cannot be regarded as either spreading or assimilation. The principle here is that one of the tones in the tonal inventory of the language is replaced by another. This was illustrated above in Fig. 4.46 from Foochow Chinese. Some cases of this kind can be interpreted as assimilatory, for example the replacement of a 1st tone by a 2nd tone in Mandarin Chinese when followed by a 1st or 4th tone. (This was illustrated in Fig. 4.10, above.) However, the sandhi rule in the same language which replaces a 3rd tone by a 2nd tone before another 3rd tone is clearly *dis*similatory. If paradigmatic replacement is recognized as a genuine rule type, it creates theoretical problems for some frameworks, since it acknowledges the existence of a system of surface tonal contrasts which is at odds with the classical generative view.[38] Schuh recognizes this type of rule, but restricts it to East Asian tone-languages. For him, this is part of a general typological difference between the rule types of African and Asian tone-languages. Whereas the former 'operate syntagmatically as typical feature-

[37] Schuh notes that this interpretation should also require Low tones to be assimilated to High tones, resulting in the gradual raising of Low tones as well as the lowering of High tones. That this does not generally take place is obviously a weakness of this theory.
[38] There is, in fact, some dispute about whether the last-mentioned Mandarin sandhi rule is actually a case of paradigmatic replacement, since a number of writers, from Hockett (1947) onwards, have claimed that the resulting tone is distinct from the 3rd tone. However, perceptual tests have shown that Mandarin speakers are unable to distinguish them, and that *mái mǎ* ('bury a horse') is indistinguishable from *mǎi mǎ* ('buy a horse') (Wang and Li, 1967; Norman, 1988: 147).

changing rules of assimilation, etc.', the latter 'involve relatively simple replacements from a fixed inventory of tones'.

4.5.3 AGAIN: DOWNDRIFT AND DOWNSTEP

As a postscript to the discussion of tonal processes we may return to downdrift and downstep. We have examined a number of aspects of these processes at various points in this chapter, including the specification of downstepped tones with a 'drop' feature on the downstepped syllable or with a downstep 'phoneme' (/!/) before it, the use of tonal 'registers' to distinguish downstepped, upstepped, and normal tones, and the insertion of a latent or floating Low tone. We shall now consider some aspects of the processes themselves.

The use of a Low tone to provide the context for downstep naturally makes this process identical with downdrift, and the two can then be seen as a single process, the only difference between them being the necessity in the case of downstep of inserting a Low in the appropriate places if it is not otherwise present, and of deleting all Lows after the downstep rules have applied. There are some difficulties with amalgamating the processes, however, since downstep has phonological consequences, and must therefore apply at an earlier stage in a derivation than downdrift, which is generally seen as a low-level phonetic rule. Nevertheless, the majority of writers on this subject attempt to cater for both with the same set of processes.

An important consideration is that neither of these processes should affect the distinctiveness of the tones themselves. Downdrift is clearly phonetic and with no phonological consequences, and downstep, despite its phonological status, similarly leaves the distinction between tones intact for what follows. The rules must therefore affect properties of the tones that are not part of their distinctive values. One solution, offered by Peters (1973), is to provide an algorithm for adjusting the pitch levels of successive tones. Thus, if all syllables in the utterance are initially given the pitch value o ([o pi]), then (with the convention that higher numbers mean lower pitch) we can apply the rules of Fig. 4.48, which progressively lower the pitch level of High tones by one point, and the pitch level of Low tones by 3 points whenever there is a step up or down.

Fig. 4.48   [+Hi] → [1 Pi] #___
            [−Hi] → [3 Pi] #___

An alternative approach is adopted by Hombert (1974), who interprets downdrift as an intonational feature which applies to the whole phrase, and which operates only in those cases where the distinctiveness of the tones is not endangered. It will therefore not apply to two High tones in sequence, but will apply to a High tone following a Low.

A more radical solution is proposed by Clements (1983), which utilizes the metrical scheme of Liberman and Prince (1977). Clements uses the hierarchical feature framework presented in Fig. 4.20, above, with the two features h and l on different rows, and combines this with a metrical tree in which the nodes are labelled with these two features. A string of tones such as H L L | H L | H H L L L | H H (where downdrift occurs with each H following a L, i.e. at the points marked |) will convert into the tree of Fig. 4.49.

Fig. 4.49

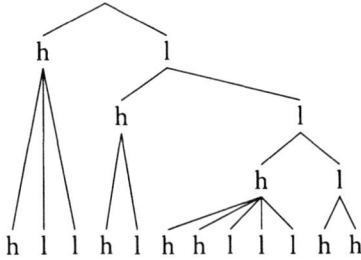

This scheme provides a hierarchy of pitch features, with each successive h after a l representing a drop in pitch, and therefore a shift of register. Though Clements considers the possibility of interpreting this hierarchy in terms of numerical pitch levels, he rejects this in favour of a 'pitch comparator' which determines the relative pitch of adjacent tones.

Huang (1985) adopts a similar approach, though he introduces a level of 'tonal feet' into the tree, where each such foot corresponds to a node dominating the lowest level in Clements's tree. We thus obtain the tree given in Fig. 4.50.

Fig. 4.50

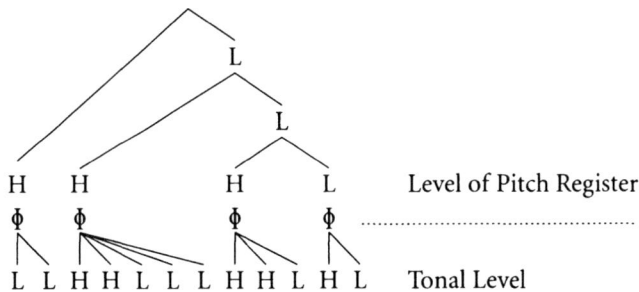

Though clearly different in detail, the approaches of Clements and Huang are evidently similar in spirit; both invoke higher levels of prosodic organization as a means of specifying downdrift. In both cases, too, the framework can be extended to cover downstep, by the use of floating Low tones.

4.6 Tone and the Syllable

4.6.1 INTRODUCTION

The definition of a tone-language given by Pike (1948: 3) requires there to be 'lexically significant, contrastive, but relative pitch on each syllable', and we have tacitly assumed in most of our discussion that tones are, indeed, assigned to syllables. Pike is by no means alone in holding this view; nineteenth century writers, from Christaller (1875) onwards, made a similar assumption, as did earlier twentieth century scholars. In Jones and Plaatje (1916), for example, we read that 'a tone is defined as the pitch of the voice with which a syllable is pronounced'.

However, as we saw in 4.4.2, not all scholars have accepted this principle; many scholars, including Schachter and Fromkin (1968), Woo (1969), and others who describe tones in terms of classical generative phonology, regard tone as a property of *segments*, almost always vowels. The same view is held in autosegmental phonology, where the tone-bearing units to which tones are associated are generally considered to be vowels. On the other hand, Sapir (1931), and Trubetzkoy (1939), among others, associate tones with the *mora*, arguing on the basis of the relationship between tonal complexity and vowel length or syllable quantity.

We shall consider here a number of factors bearing on this issue, and in particular we will examine the relationship between tones and the various segmental and prosodic features of the syllable. In the first place, there are possibilities of a relationship between tones and the vocalic nucleus of the syllable; more significantly, there are relationships between tones and the consonants of the syllable margin. Tones can normally only be realized on *voiced* segments,[39] and hence the nucleus, which is in the overwhelming majority of cases a voiced vowel, is appropriate as the bearer of tone. The consonantal margin may, however, be voiced or voiceless, and in the latter case it is arguably incapable of functioning in this capacity. We shall see, however, that there are nevertheless close relationships between consonants and tone. We have already noted that tone is related to other laryngeal activity, and this includes different types of phonation.

4.6.2 TONES AND SEGMENTS

4.6.2.1 Vowel Quality

Experimental studies (Ladefoged, 1964; Hombert, 1977, 1978) have shown that there is a connection between vowel height and fundamental frequency: the higher the vowel, the higher the pitch. There are various theories which attempt to account for this; some assume a transfer of muscular tension from tongue to larynx; others invoke various muscular and/or aerodynamic factors. Ladefoged (1964) and Lehiste (1970) adopt a 'tongue-pull' theory according to which the high tongue position exerts a pull on the laryngeal muscles.

---

[39] Nevertheless, several investigators (Jensen, 1958; Hadding-Koch, 1962) report that tones are still distinct in whispered speech, when no voicing is present. This may be the result of accompanying laryngeal features, which allow the tones to be recognized even without voice.

Whatever the phonetic explanation, however, the phonological implications of this connection are probably negligible in the majority of cases, and very little evidence is available which would point to a systematic phonological exploitation of this phenomenon. Suggestions have sometimes been made that the development of Chinese tones may have depended on vowel quality (Hombert, 1977), while Pilszczikowa-Chodak (1972) attempts to demonstrate a correlation between tone and vowel height in the verb and noun plurals of Hausa. Newman (1975) shows, however, that, despite initial plausibility, this claim is unfounded. Dimmendaal and Breedveld (1986) also present evidence for tonal influence on vowel quality in Turkana. But in spite of these examples, it appears that tone and vowel height are in principle independent features, and it is to the consonants that we must turn for evidence of a relationship between tone and segments, especially in so far as they contribute to the historical development of tones. Matisoff (1970) remarks that 'the point of tonogenetic tension in the syllable seems never to be the vocalic nucleus. Rather it is the initial and/or final consonants which trigger the development of tones and which are themselves the most susceptible of change or loss due to tonal phenomena they have engendered.' We must therefore turn to the relationships between tones and consonants.

4.6.2.2 Initial Consonants

Much of the evidence for the close relationship between tones and consonants comes from the historical development of tones in South East Asian languages. This evidence is not limited to any particular language group; indeed, the fact that similar phenomena are encountered in a number of different language families lends greater force to the arguments, indicating a universal tendency rather than a phenomenon restricted to a particular time and place.

We may note first of all that there is evidence from a range of languages, including non-tone languages such as English, that the pitch of the vocalic part of the syllable is influenced by the nature of the *preceding* consonant. Experimental results reported by a number of scholars, such as Lehiste and Peterson (1961), Lea (1973), Ohala (1973, 1978), and Hombert (1978) confirm that in English and other languages the pitch of vowels following voiceless consonants is higher than that following voiced consonants. A possible phonetic explanation for this phenomenon, at least in the case of plosive consonants, is the rate of air-flow through the larynx during the articulation of the consonant (Ohala, 1973). If the consonant is a voiceless plosive, there will initially be high pressure on the release of the consonant, producing high pitch; if the consonant is a voiced plosive, however, air will continue to flow into the mouth during the closure and the pressure-drop across the larynx on release of the consonant will be small, producing a lowered pitch. Different manners of articulation, such as sonorants and obstruents, aspirated and glottalized plosives, and different places of articulation (Ladefoged, 1964: 42) may also produce different effects.

Such differences are, of course, small, and they are generally of no phonological significance. However, they may acquire such significance in a number of ways. One consequence of these different effects, which appears in a number of tone-languages, is the occurrence of different forms of certain tones after specific consonant types. Ladefoged (1964: 42) reports, for example, on evidence that Ewe tones have lower allophones (allotones) in syllables beginning with some voiced consonants. More significant are cases where different tones (and not merely allotones) occur only after certain consonants. Li (1948), for example, notes that in Sui, a Tai language spoken in Guizhou province, syllables containing initial unaspirated stops, simple nasals, laterals, and fricatives occur with all six of the tones found in this language, while in syllables beginning with voiceless nasals, pre-glottalized consonants, voiced stops, and the glottal stop, only three of these tones occur. Gandour (1974d) also observes that in Thai no high or rising tone occurs on a syllable that begins with an unaspirated stop consonant.

Such phenomena are not restricted to East Asian languages. Hyman (1973) describes an assimilation rule in Ewe (from Stahlke) which raises a Low tone to Mid before a following High tone unless the initial consonant of the Low tone syllable is a voiced obstruent; similar features are found in the Bassa and Nupe languages of West Africa (Meussen, 1970). Such processes are particularly widespread in the Nguni languages of Southern Africa, where certain voiced consonants ('depressor' consonants) have the effect of lowering tones. In Zulu, for example (Cope, 1970; Laughren, 1984), Low tones become Extra-low when adjacent to such consonants, e.g. in ìzìhlâlò ('seats')—the depressor consonant is underlined.

Perhaps the most persuasive evidence for a close link between tone and initial consonants, however, is provided by historical developments in several South East Asian tone-languages, which in many cases result in the extension of the tone-system, or even the development of tones in originally non-tone languages (tonogenesis). These developments have come about through regular processes of phonemic split, in which the non-phonological pitch differences induced by different consonant types have become phonologically distinctive through the loss of the conditioning environment.

Though these developments are noted by Jakobson (1931), the most influential discussion of the phenomenon is that of Haudricourt (1954, 1961), who shows that Vietnamese, which had previously been considered a Tai language because of its tones, is in fact a Mon–Khmer language, despite the fact that the Mon–Khmer languages are otherwise non-tonal. He demonstrates that the tones of Vietnamese are secondary developments arising from the loss of consonantal distinctions. Three tones developed through the loss of final consonants (see below), and each tone subsequently split into two through the loss of the initial voiced/voiceless distinction. Similar developments can be demonstrated for other languages (cf. Haudricourt, 1961). In Sgaw–Karen, a two-tone system, with a Level and a Falling tone, split into a four-tone system, with high and low level tones and high and low falling tones. The high tones developed after voiceless and glottalized plosives (k, pʰ, tʰ, bˀ, dˀ) and voiceless or aspirated nasals and laterals (hm, hn, hl), while the low tones developed after voiced plosives (b, d, g) and voiced nasals and laterals (m, n, l). At this stage the different variants of the tones were merely allotones, but the subsequent merger of voiced and voiceless plosives (b, d, g > p, t, k) and of the voiced and voiceless nasals and laterals (hm, hn, hl > m, n, l) produced a phonological distinction between them. Similar developments are found in Thai languages, in Miao–Yao (Chang, 1973), in Austronesian languages (Bradshaw, 1979), and in various Chinese dialects. Many of the latter, such as Cantonese, doubled their tonal inventory when initial voiced plosives merged with voiceless ones, leaving the non-distinctive variants of the tones that had developed after them as distinct phonological tones.

The situation following such splits is not always as straightforward as this, however. A two-way split has occurred, according to Henderson (1979), in Bwe Karen, but there appears to be a three-way tonal contrast in this language, with lexical contrasts such as lɛ¹ ('moon'), lɛ² ('leaf'), and lɛ³ ('to keep') (1 is high, 3 is low). Henderson argues that the two-way contrast can nevertheless still be retrieved from synchronic data since, if we exclude certain categories of syllables, such as those occurring in loan-words, some particles, and certain disyllabic words, then we find that voiced initials occur only with mid or low pitch, while syllables with initial [ʔ], voiceless unaspirated plosives, implosives, and voiceless aspirated plosives, occur only with high and mid pitch. This gives the skewed distribution given in Fig. 4.51, with consonant contrasts only in syllables with a mid pitch, and only two pitch levels exploited by any one set of initials.

Fig. 4.51 *Pitch*:

1	2	3
	/hm/	
/hm/	/m/	/m/
/hn/	/hn/	
	/n/	/n/
/hl/	/hl/	
	/l/	/l/

According to Haudricourt (1961), complexities of a different kind are found in Tung and Mak, where a three-way split occurs following the merger of voiced, aspirated, and glottalized initial consonants. Thus, the three original tones of Tung became nine. Similar processes in other languages, such as Thai and Lao, did not lead to such complex tone-systems, as mergers took place (Haudricourt, 1961; Brown, 1965; Gandour, 1974b; Chamberlain, 1979). In Standard Thai, for example, three original categories of consonants—aspirated stops and nasals, glottalized and voiceless plosives, and voiced plosives and nasals—which developed variants of the three original tones after them, merged, but the result was five tones rather than nine, as in Fig. 4.52, following tonal mergers.[40]

Fig. 4.52 *Original consonants*   *Original tones*

	A	B	C
hm-, hn-, ph-, th-, kh-	Rise	Low	Fall
bˀ-, dˀ-, p-, t-, k-			
b-, d-, g-, m-, n-, l-	Mid	Fall	High

In the majority of cases, however, the loss of initial consonant distinctions results in a two-way split in the tonal system. This is the main justification for the recognition of a *register* system in languages of this kind (cf. 4.3.4.4, above), distinct from a *tone*-system, since we may get a parallel set of tones in the different registers. For example, the tones of Modern Chinese dialects can generally be traced back to the Middle Chinese tonal system, which had four tones, traditionally known as *píng* ('level'), *shǎng* ('rising'), *qù* ('departing'), and *rù* ('entering'). But the tonal splits that occurred with the loss of distinctions in the initial consonants produced two 'registers', designated *yīn* and *yáng*. This gives eight tones, *yīn-píng, yīn-shǎng, yīn-qù, yīn-rù*; and *yáng-píng, yáng-shǎng, yáng-qù, yáng-rù*, where tonal and register categories are combined (Karlgren, 1926; Norman, 1988).

As we have noted above, although the recognition of 'registers' as opposed to 'tones' in these cases has a sound historical and phonetic basis, its synchronic phonological justification is more doubtful. There is not necessarily any difference, as far as the current system is concerned, between 'register' features and 'tonal' features, and no necessary systematic relationship between the 'same' tones on different registers. The use of the concept of 'register' merely as a dimension of tone-systems does not seem to be justified.

4.6.2.3 Final Consonants

Analogous, but not identical, phenomena are found with *final* consonants. Here, however, the effects do not appear to depend on features such as voicing and aspiration, but are generally restricted to consonants with a laryngeal articulation: [h] and [ʔ]. As we have already noted, it is common to find limitations on the occurrence of certain tones before final plosives, and especially the glottal plosive [ʔ]. It is already observed by Jones (1913), for example, that Nanking Chinese has five tones, but the fifth tone differs from the third only in being followed by a glottal stop; similarly, Taylor (1920) notes that a particular variety of one of the tones of Thai occurs only in syllables which end in a short vowel

---

[40] These three categories of consonants are reflected in the Thai writing system, which was devised before the mergers occurred, and consequently represents tonal distinctions in an indirect way, through a mixture of consonant letters and tone markers. Consonants are described as 'high', 'mid', and 'low', according to their relationship to the tones.

followed by a glottal stop, or by a glottalized consonant, while the limited tonal distinctions in Burmese depend on whether the syllables are 'checked' or not. Chiu (1930) makes similar remarks about Amoy Chinese: two of its eight tones only occur in syllables closed by voiceless plosives or [-ʔ], while in Sui, according to Li (1948), one of the three tones occurs in syllables closed by [-p], [-t], or [-k]. Likewise Thai restricts certain tones to occurrence before (glottalized) plosives or the glottal stop (Gandour, 1974a, 1974d). In general, therefore, we can identify as one of the effects of final glottal consonants the fact that they restrict the kinds of tones that can occur in the syllable concerned, usually allowing only level tones and shortening the vowel (Yip, 1995).

As with initial consonants, final consonants can produce tonal splits when distinctions are lost, 'phonologizing' the pitch differences that have developed before them. Matisoff (1973) traces the development of tones in Mon–Khmer languages. The proto-language had three types of syllable ending: a vowel or nasal, an -s which developed into [h], and a stop which became [ʔ]. By the sixth century the final [-h] and [-ʔ] had been lost, but their effects were felt on the pitch of the syllable: a *fall* had developed before [-h] and a *rise* before [-ʔ], giving a three-way system of level, falling, and rising tones.

The effects of final consonants are, however, more limited than those of initial consonants. Though Maran (1973) asserts that the loss of a voice distinction in final consonants led to the tonal system of Jinghpaw (Jingpho), Hombert (1978) and Hombert, Ohala, and Ewan (1979) claim that there is no evidence that the loss of a voice distinction in final consonants can lead to tonal distinctions; they do accept, however, that the loss of the glottal stop has significant effects, producing a high–rising tone in Vietnamese, a high tone in Burmese, and the rising (*shǎng*) tone in Middle Chinese. According to them, the loss of final [-h] may be responsible for the falling (*qù*) tone in both Middle Chinese and Vietnamese. However, they seek explanations for the 'well-attested pattern' of 'tone originating from the effect of prevocalic stop consonants or postvocalic glottal consonants, and tone rarely or never originating from the influence of postvocalic non-glottal consonants or from vowel height'.

In some cases, developments depend on a combination of initial and final consonants. Matisoff (1970) claims that the high–rising tone of Lahu arose only in syllables which both began and ended with a 'glottal incident', such as a glottal stop. Similarly, Maran (1973) claims that the tonal system of Tibeto–Burman languages arose through the combined effects of initial and final consonants. According to Egerod (1971), in Chinese, 'tones developed from final features are pre-Ancient and tones developed from initial features are post-Ancient'.

One claim made by Hyman (1973) is that 'consonants affect tone, but tone does not affect consonants'. Although this claim appears to hold for the majority of cases, it is certainly not without exceptions, and a number of cases of tonal influence on final consonants have been adduced. In the first place, syllable final pitch movements may lead to the development of glottal constrictions: a falling tone may fall so low as to end in 'creak', which, with devoicing, may produce [h], as in Jinghpaw (Jingpho) (Hombert, 1978). Similarly, a rising pitch may lead to a final glottal closure. Maddieson (1974) suggest that this is the source of the Danish *stød*; he regards it as the reflex of the original tonal distinctions found in Norwegian and Swedish (see below), where the tensing of the vocal cords required for the rising pitch was overdone, resulting in a glottal closure.

Influence of tones on existing consonants is also attested, though it is rare; Maddieson (1974) reports that in Jinghpaw (Jinghpo) consonants may be voiced following low tones, while in Thai breathy voiced stops occur after high-pitched tones. He also asserts, though less plausibly, that cases of 'tone-spreading' might be interpreted as the spread of the pitch of the tone to the following consonant, and thence to the following vowel.

4.6.3 TONES AND VOICE QUALITY

Voice quality differences are exhibited by many languages. They are noted, for example, by Sapir (1931) for Gweabo,[41] and in several East Asian languages, such as Burmese, Vietnamese, and some dialects of Chinese. In Cambodian, a systematic distinction of two voice qualities is found (Henderson, 1952), which can be labelled Register I and Register II. The first of these has a 'head voice', with relatively high pitch; the second has a deep, breathy and 'sepulchral' quality, with lowered larynx and a lower pitch, and it is even 'frequently accompanied by a certain dilation of the nostrils'. However, as Henderson points out, 'the Cambodian "registers" differ from tones in that pitch is not the primary relevant feature'. In Burmese, a four-way system of 'phonation registers' can be established for the older language: 'level' (laryngeally unmarked), 'creaky' (glottal stricture), 'heavy' (high), and glottal stop (Egerod, 1971).

In tone-languages, such voice quality differences are often linked to particular tones or tonal registers. Weidert (1987: 26off.) identifies four tones in Tamang, two of which have 'clear' phonation and two have 'breathy' phonation. In Shanghai Chinese (Zee and Maddieson, 1980; Yip, 1980, 1992) there are five tones, two of which can be assigned to low register and which are accompanied by breathy voice, or 'murmur'. Similarly, in Tibetan (Yip, 1992) a high and a low register can be distinguished, which, according to Yip, are accompanied by a 'phonation register' difference; the high register can be labelled 'tense', and it is accompanied by a variety of laryngeal features, including aspiration and the glottal stop; the low register may again be accompanied by breathy voice.

Duanmu (1990) claims that large tone-systems, such as those found in many South East Asian languages, will always use voice quality as well as pitch, but, as pointed out by Yip (1995), this is not necessarily the case; Cantonese, for

---

[41] Trubetzkoy (1939) reinterprets Sapir's data, suggesting that his four registers can be reduced to three if we include a voice quality correlation (*Trübungskorrelation*).

example, has a large system of tones, but does not use voice quality distinctions.

4.6.4 TONES, QUANTITY, AND THE MORA

Another property of the syllable with which tones interact is *quantity* or *weight*. We have already observed that tones (or rather the syllables on which they occur) may differ in length; in Mandarin Chinese, for example, a syllable bearing a third (falling–rising) tone is longer than, say, one bearing a fourth (falling tone). The quantity of syllables is also dependent on the tone in Otomí (Sinclair and Pike, 1948) and in Thai (Abramson, 1962: 108). According to Upson (1968), there is a mutual dependence between tone and length in Chatino, with allophones of length conditioned by tone, and allotones of tones conditioned by length: tones are lower if long.

'Long' tones, like 'long' vowels, may be analysed as a sequence of two units. Indeed, the two analyses are likely to coincide, with 'long' vowels being assigned two tones. Thus, by eliminating 'long' vowels from Yoruba, Siertsema (1959a) is able simultaneously to reduce the tone inventory, since 'long' tones become sequences of short ones. This approach is particularly relevant for contour tones, which, as we have seen, are regularly regarded as sequences of levels; it was already adopted by Christaller (1875), who noted that syllables in Twi with a long vowel or diphthong may have two tones.

Leben (1973b) gives arguments along these lines for regarding tone as a segmental feature. In Thai compounds, long vowels may be shortened, and in such cases the tone is simplified from a contour in the 'isolative' form to a mid level tone in the 'combinative' form (see Fig. 4.53). This suggests that, if a long vowel is analysed as a geminate (VV), then each component vowel bears a tone; when the vowel is shortened, only one tone occurs.

Fig. 4.53	*Isolative*		*Combinative*		
	thiː	nai	thiˑ	nai	'where'
	HL	LH	M	LH	
	siː	khaːu	siˑ	khaːu	'white'
	HL	LH	M	LH	

The arguments can, however, be reversed. Gandour (1977) uses evidence from the development of Thai dialects to justify regarding contours as units. He notes that, historically, in Northern Thai dialects syllables with low rising and mid rising tones were lengthened, while in Southern Thai dialects it was syllables with low rising, mid level and low level tones that were lengthened. Other syllables were shortened. Gandour concludes that these developments can only be understood and generalized if we regard both level tones and contours as single units.

If 'long' tones are divided up into sequences, then it is naturally possible to assign them to *moras* rather than syllables (see 2.5.4). This approach is adopted by Sapir (1931) in his analysis of Gweabo. Observing that, in two-mora syllables in this language, each mora 'keeps its dynamic individuality', Sapir assigns separate tones to each mora. A rather similar approach is adopted by Trubetzkoy (1939). In his discussion of the 'register correlation' he states first of all that all languages with such a correlation are mora-counting, but notes that registers are not, in fact, required in Northern Chinese, because its four tones can be analysed as a system with two tones, each of which may consist of either one mora or two. A further application of the mora in tone analysis is found in work by Stevick on the African languages Yoruba (1965) and Ganda (1969b). We have already observed Stevick's solution to the problems of tonal combinations in the former case: he analyses long vowels as bimoraic, and assigns tones to moras rather than syllables.

Despite a very different theoretical framework, recent work demonstrates a similar preoccupation with this problem. Odden (1995) shows that in Kikuria tones should be assigned to moras rather than syllables. A High tone is assigned to a specific mora of the verb stem, depending on the tense/aspect; in the perfective, for example, it is assigned to the fourth mora, and a long vowel counts as two moras, as in Fig. 4.54.

Fig. 4.54 n-[tɛrɛk-eré   'I have cooked'
          n-[ga-tɛrɛk-ére   'I have cooked them'
          n-[karaang-ére   'I have fried'
          n-[ga-karaáng-ére   'I have fried them'

However, the flexibility provided by autosegmental phonology in relating tones to other tiers means that there is some indeterminacy with regard to how the tones are associated to moras. Fig. 4.55 represents the five different ways in which, according to Odden (1995: 450), this could be achieved.

Fig. 4.55

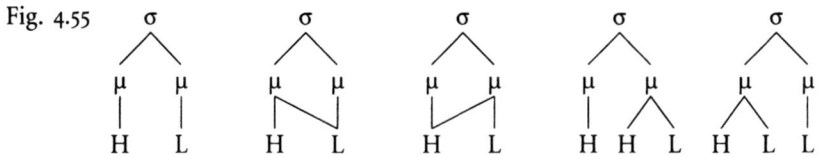

On the other hand, assigning the tones to the syllable as a whole solves this problem, as in Fig. 4.56, since there is only one possibility here. (It does not allow for mora-counting in Kikuria, however.)

Fig. 4.56

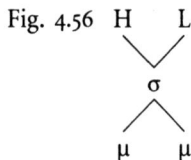

The same debate is pursued by Yip (1995) in relation to East Asian tone-languages. She notes, as we have already seen, that in Chinese languages it is often the case that only a subset of tones—usually level ones—occurs in syllables closed by a voiceless plosive, and that such syllables are generally shorter than the others. One approach to this phenomenon is to assume that the *mora* is the tone-bearing unit, and that obstruent final consonants are *not moraic*. Syllables with such finals will therefore be short. Since, in this approach, contour tones require two moras, they cannot occur in such syllables.

Though he does not make use of the mora as such, Duanmu (1990: 151) assumes that 'all Chinese syllables are bimoraic', and explains the non-occurrence of contour tones on syllables closed by voiceless plosives by a phonetic limitation on the realization of tones on these segments. Either way, contour tones are assigned to *two* tonal root nodes, as shown in Fig. 4.23(a), above. We have seen, however, that for Yip contours are units in Asian tone-languages, and therefore are assigned to a single root node, as in Fig. 4.23(b). We therefore do not need the mora as a tone-bearing unit in these cases.

4.6.5 CONCLUSION: TONE AND THE SYLLABLE

We have seen evidence that the features associated with tones are related in various ways to different parts of the syllable: to the segments—the vowel quality, the initial, and the final consonant—and also to other syllable features such as voice quality and quantity. These relations are not always straightforward, and they are clearly by no means consistent; they do not amount to the total dependence of tone on these other features, still less the dependence of other features on tone, but they are significant, and demand some sort of explanation.

For some scholars, the relationships between tone and segmental features suggest that tone itself should be regarded as segmental. While advocating—as we have seen in 4.4.2—a 'suprasegmental' approach to tone, Leben (1971, 1973a) nevertheless allows tone to be segmental in those languages, such as Thai, where a dependence on segmental features is demonstrable (cf. also Gandour, 1974c). In Thai, as in other South East Asian languages, the distribution of tones is restricted by the structure of the syllable: while all five tones may occur in 'live' syllables (those ending in a vowel or sonorant consonant), only a limited set can occur in 'dead' syllables (those ending in a plosive consonant). The argument for a segmental treatment of tone in Thai is that if tone rules require reference to segments (as they do in Thai), then tone itself must be a property of segments. As Kenstowicz and Kisseberth (1979: 273) put it, 'if tones were fundamentally separated from segments, then one would not expect tones to be affected by anything other than tones. The fact that segments which do not inherently bear the tone may affect tone suggests that tone is located on segments.' However, the dichotomy here is clearly false, since it leaves out the possibility that tone is neither completely independent nor segmental; it could be associated with a prosodic unit such as the syllable. For this reason, and leaving aside the linear formalisms on which the segmental interpretation is based, it is possible to draw quite different conclusions from the relationships between tones, segments, and syllabic features: that the various features display a degree of mutual dependence which suggests that they form a composite whole.

How this whole can be represented formally is a more controversial matter, however. One approach, adopted by Firthian scholars, is to take an integrated view of the syllable, resisting the temptation to divide it up into a sequence of segmental units, even where features are ostensibly restricted to particular syllable positions. This can be exemplified by Henderson's description of Thai (Henderson, 1949). In Thai, the characteristics of syllable initial consonants are rather different from those of syllable final ones; the latter are restricted to nasals and unreleased plosives, while the former include the full range of voiceless, voiced, and aspirated plosives, affricates, fricatives, nasals, r, l, and j. Henderson recognizes three kinds of syllable prosodies: (a) prosodies of syllable-beginning, (b) prosodies of syllable-end, and (c) prosodies of the syllable as a whole. Thus, (a) includes one or more of the following properties: 'plosion, aspiration, voice (except with nasality) affrication, friction, lateralisation, rhotacisation, and labialization (except with velarity)'; (b) consists primarily of 'closure without plosion'; and (c) includes 'tone, quantity, labialization, labiovelarization, and yotization'. *All* of these properties are ultimately features of the syllable.

Henderson represents Thai utterances phonologically in a hierarchical fashion, as in Fig. 4.57 (the levels have been numbered for reference). Tone is here treated primarily as a syllable prosody (Level 4) though some aspects of it, such as sandhi phenomena arising as a result of the juxtaposition of syllables, and the occurrence of the neutral tone, are described at Level 3. Relations are established between tone and stress, and tone and quantity, by their co-occurrence on the different levels: stress (or lack of it) is represented at Level 3, while quantity appears at both Level 3 and Level 4. Segmental features such as aspiration, plosion, voice, etc., are operative at Level 5.

Fig. 4.57 1 Prosodies of Sentence
2 Prosodies of Sentence Parts
3 Prosodies of Polysyllables and Sentence Pieces
4 Prosodies of Syllables
5 Prosodies of Syllable Parts
6 Consonant and Vowel Units

One characteristic of this form of representation—which may be construed as a weakness or as a strength depending on the point of view—is that the prosodies are not necessarily phonetically explicit or consistent. We observed this in the prosodic treatment of length (3.5.3.3), where the 'exponents' of a particular prosody could include a range of different phonetic properties, and the prosody could therefore be used to account for vowel and consonant length simultaneously. In the case of tone a similar flexibility is employed, for example in the case of the pitch of final sentence particles, which, according to Henderson, carry a 'sentence tone', which is regarded as a sentence prosody, and is 'a complex of the syllable prosodies of tone and quantity, and is usually realized as one of the five tones proper to monosyllables, combined with either shortness or length'.

Non-linear formalizations of the relationships between tone and other syllable features have certain things in common with the Firthian approach. Instead of recognizing 'prosodies' as abstractions from the syllable or from larger units they place different features on different tiers. Thus, Odden's representation of the tonal and moraic tiers, given as Fig. 4.56, above, shows that tone and quantity can be represented as independent properties of the syllable, linked via the syllable node (Odden, 1995). In a similar way, Yip (1995), using more elaborate feature geometry, relates register and glottal aperture features to the syllable via a laryngeal node (see Fig. 4.58). On the other hand, the features represented autosegmentally in this approach are specific *phonetic* properties rather than the *abstract* properties of prosodic analysis. From the perspective of prosodic analysis, what is represented in the autosegmental approach is not the phonological properties comparable to prosodies but their phonetic *exponents*.

Fig. 4.58

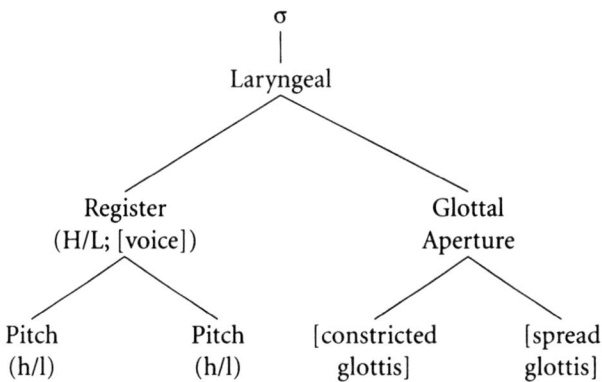

What these different approaches have in common, however, is that they take the *syllable* (and in some cases larger units) to be the focus of tonal, laryngeal, and in some cases segmental, features; they differ in the particular way in which the features are related to one another and to the syllable, and in how these relationships are represented.

4.7 Tone and Accent

4.7.1 INTRODUCTION

We saw in Chapter 3 that accentuation may take several forms, and can be manifested through a variety of phonetic features, though these may be grouped under two cover terms, *stress–accent* and *pitch–accent*. Both of these may involve pitch features; pitch is a major component of stress (3.2.4), and is the defining feature of pitch–accent (3.3.4), but both are distinct from tone, although the latter, too, is primarily a matter of pitch.

Functionally speaking, a distinction can be made, using terminology which derives from Prague School theory, between the *culminative* function of accent and the *distinctive* function of tone. The culminative function is that of indicating a contrastive position, while the distinctive function involves an opposition at a particular point. In Saussurean terminology, accent is syntagmatic; tone is paradigmatic.[42] The distinction can also be characterized in other ways. Voorhoeve (1968) remarks that tone-languages mark every syllable; stress languages mark one syllable within a larger unit; Hyman (1978) suggests that the paradigmatic relations of tones serve to *identify* them, while the syntagmatic relations of stress serve to *locate* it.[43]

Neither tone nor accent is a universal phenomenon in languages; we therefore find tone-languages without accent, accent-languages without tone, languages with neither tone nor accent, and languages with both. Given that the two are not necessarily phonetically completely distinct, interactions between the two are to be expected. These interactions may differ according to whether accent is a matter of stress or of pitch–accent.

4.7.2 INTERACTIONS OF STRESS AND TONE

In experiments on both non-tone and tone-languages, Lea (1973) found that the fundamental frequency tends to be higher in stressed syllables than in unstressed ones. This is likely to be the source of the different varieties of tones that are widely reported to occur in stressed and unstressed syllables in tone-languages. Pike and Oram (1976) note that 'each word in Diuxi Mixtec has a stressed syllable which is marked by a long vowel. In addition to this stress, some words have a second stress. This second stress occurs only on the last syllable of the word and is marked by intensity and by allotones of both High and Low tones. There is a contrast of High versus Low tone, and there are allotones which occur in relation to the presence versus absence of word-final stress.' In Mandarin Chinese, 'toneless' syllables are found in unstressed positions; their pitch range is very narrow, and the length of the syllable is relatively short. The pitch of these syllables depends on the preceding tone; they are 'half-low' after the High Level

---

[42] Prague terminology consistently distinguishes between a *contrast* (which is syntagmatic) and an *opposition* (which is paradigmatic). See footnote 17 to Ch. 2.

[43] Meinhof (1915) offers an 'explanation' for the occurrence of 'stress–accent' or 'pitch–accent' (i.e. tone). He observes that stress characterizes the languages of white races, and pitch–accent those of black and yellow races, and concludes that while white races do not necessarily excel in manual dexterity or acuteness of observation, they do so in matters of will and judgement—'in the qualities expressed by the stress–accent' (p. 33). Clearly, these curious prejudices are both ridiculous and unacceptable.

tone, mid after the High Rise, 'half-high' after the Low Fall–Rise, and low after the High Fall (Chao, 1968). Similarly, Hiranburana (1972) notes that in Thai the tones of unstressed syllables are effectively reduced to short, mid and level.

However, such is the interdependence of tone and stress in such cases that the relationship can be interpreted the other way round: while Chao considers that the tonelessness of syllables depends on their lack of stress, Yip (1995) claims that lack of stress may follow from being toneless. The difference between Mandarin and Taiwanese dialects on the one hand and that of Shanghai on the other is, she claims, that in the former toneless syllables cannot bear stress, whereas in the latter, where stress is initial, and non-initial syllables lose their tones altogether, lack of tone follows from being unstressed. 'In any case, there is a clear connection between the inability of toneless syllables to bear stress in Mandarin, and the inability of stressless syllables to bear tone in Shanghai.' This position is, however, very questionable. Apart from a few particles which are never stressed and which can be seen as lexically toneless, all Mandarin syllables can have tone in suitable contexts, and loss of tone in unstressed position is optional, depending on speech style. It is therefore perverse to regard lack of stress as a consequence of lack of tone.

Another language where stress and tone have been claimed to interact is Yoruba. In this language, according to Siertsema (1959b), 'both in isolated words and in the sentence, there are clearly audible stresses, and certain close syntactic groups are characterized by a definite rhythmic pattern which may even affect the original lexical tones of the words.' Siertsema claims that the seven tonal classes of Yoruba nouns recognized by Ward (1952) can be reduced to three if we take stress into account. She classifies nouns in terms of the co-occurrence of stress with different tones: those that have stress on the High tone, the Mid tone, and the Low tone, though whether this actually simplifies the description is doubtful, since subclasses are still recognized according to the position of the stressed syllable in the word.

According to some scholars, the close relationship between stress and tone may result in one replacing the other. Taylor (1920) had already noted the difficulty of analysing Burmese tone because of the uncertainty as to whether it is stress or tone that is involved: some speakers seem to use one and some the other. E. V. Pike (1974) also notes the difficulty for the linguist in analysing some systems where high pitch could be interpreted as tone or as part of the stress system, though she concludes that the difference may be apparent because stress tends to affect the length or quality of the vowel, the realizations of the consonants, and the pitch of the other syllables, while tone does not. The confusion of tone and stress may also provide a mechanism for tone loss, which has happened in, for example, some Bantu languages, notably Swahili. Johnson (1976) shows this loss in progress in the closely related languages Low Runyankore, High Runyankore, and Haya. Penultimate stress is found in Low Runyankore in cases where Haya and High Runyankore have either a High tone or a Falling tone—these tones cannot occur on the final syllable in these languages. Thus, the pitch prominence associated with the High or Falling tones is converted into stress, but only in penultimate position, resulting in a fixed accent.

Further evidence for the relationship is provided by the way loan-words from languages with stress systems, notably English, are interpreted tonally. This is discussed for Hausa by Greenberg (1941) and more recently by Leben (1996). The basic principle is plain: stress is interpreted as involving a High tone, though the details are complex, as Leben makes clear. Hausa has, as we have observed above, High, Low, and Falling tones but no stress as such. The syllable bearing the stress in English is usually given a High or Falling tone, for example in *soojà* ('soldier'), *ràsît* ('receipt'), *ràkoodàa* ('recorder') (ˆ indicates a Fall and ˋ a Low tone; High tone is here unmarked). But the fact that longer words are given *two* High tones, as, for example, in *hedìmastàa* ('headmaster'), or *kirsìmatì* ('Christmas'), suggests that English stress is not interpreted by Hausa speakers in purely 'accentual' terms, as a culminative feature marking one syllable in the word, but rather in purely 'tonal' terms, as a HL tonal sequence. Leben provides rules for 'tonal foot formation', where each foot is such a sequence. Thus, representing the boundaries of tonal feet with [ ], [soojà] has one tonal foot, [hedì][mastàa] and [kirsì][matì] have two, while the second syllable of rà[sît], with a Falling tone, also constitutes a foot, this word being equivalent in its tonal structure to rà[koodàa]. But the fact that the equivalence of stress and a [HL] tonal foot is not always maintained is evidence that stress and tone are still independent. Some words, such as *baasukùr* ('bicycle'), or *kaabeejì* ('cabbage') have two High tones in succession, suggesting a further type of tonal foot [HH].

The interactions are of several different kinds. In considering the interactions between tone and stress–accent, van der Hulst and Smith (1988c) identify two types of phenomenon: (1) cases where tone is dependent on stress, and (2) cases where stress is dependent on tone. The former is well attested and will be discussed further below. The latter is more problematic; it has been claimed (Pankratz and Pike, 1967) that stress in Ayutla Mixtec is attracted to syllables with High tone, and similar claims have been made for a number of other languages. However, this phenomenon is clearly not common, and it may well be susceptible to alternative interpretations. In what follows, we shall consider primarily the nature of so-called 'tonal accent' systems, and the possible role of tone as an accentual feature.

4.7.3 TONAL ACCENT

The cases discussed so far involve the interaction of tone and stress as independent prosodic features, though usually with stress in the dominant position. In some languages, tone is even more subordinate, since tonal contrasts appear *only* in stressed syllables. These languages include the so-called *tonal accent* languages of the European type, such as Norwegian and Swedish, and, with additional complications, Serbo–Croat, Lithuanian and Latvian, together with a few others. Outside Europe, similar phenomena have been described for Somali (Armstrong, 1934) and Punjabi. In such languages the subordination of tone to accentuation is such that they are often not considered to be tone-languages at all, but merely languages with different kinds of accents.

Norwegian and Swedish

In both Norwegian and Swedish there is a stress-timed rhythm comparable to that found in other Germanic languages, but the stressed syllables are associated with two different pitch patterns, traditionally known as Accent I and Accent II. In Standard East Norwegian, for example, Accent I has a rising pitch; the stressed syllable starts low and rises, as in Fig. 4.59(a), the rise being spread over the following syllables in the case of a polysyllabic foot (Fig. 4.59(b)). Accent II, on the other hand, which occurs only in polysyllabic words, commences slightly higher, and falls before rising, as in Figs. 4.59(c) and 4.59(d) (Popperwell, 1963).

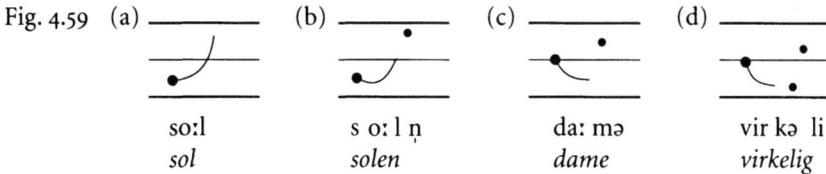

Fig. 4.59 (a) so:l / sol   (b) s o: l n̩ / solen   (c) da: mə / dame   (d) vir kə li / virkelig

In Swedish the situation is entirely comparable, though the phonetic features are different. Here, the pattern of both accents is *falling*, as in Fig. 4.60 (Björkhagen, 1944; Gårding, 1977). Accent I is represented in Figs. 4.60(a) and 4.60(b), Accent II in Figs. 4.60(c) and 4.60(d).

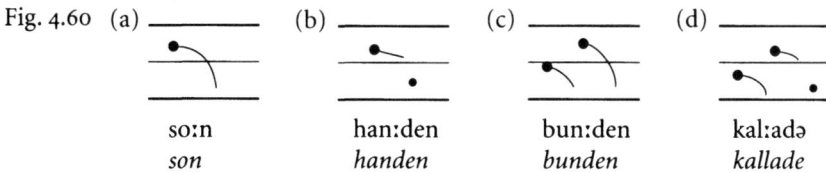

Fig. 4.60 (a) so:n / son   (b) han:den / handen   (c) bun:den / bunden   (d) kal:adə / kallade

In both these languages minimal pairs are encountered which are distinguished solely by the accents.[44] Examples are given in Fig. 4.61.

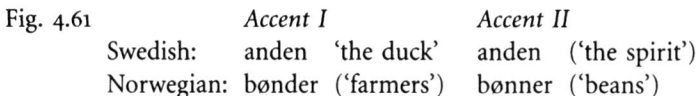

Fig. 4.61

		Accent I	Accent II
Swedish:		anden 'the duck'	anden ('the spirit')
Norwegian:		bønder ('farmers')	bønner ('beans')

---

[44] Jensen (1961) cites a large number of minimal pairs in Norwegian. Haugen (1967) and others point out, however, that not all of the pairs are really minimal, as the words are morphologically different and generally belong to different word classes. The occurrence of the different accents is, in fact, predictable in more than half the cases.

The interpretation of these phenomena poses a number of problems. From the phonetic point of view, the two accents of Norwegian and Swedish do not differ from each other in such features as stress or length; the difference lies primarily in the pitch.[45] However, the precise nature of the pitch differences is rather variable; the phonetic realization varies greatly from dialect to dialect (see Haugen and Joos, 1952). In Standard East Norwegian and Southern Swedish, a significant point is that the pitch of the first syllable of Accent I is generally very similar to that of the second syllable of Accent II. In Norwegian both syllables are rising; in Swedish both are falling. This means that it is possible to see both accents as involving the same phonetic pitch features but differing in their *timing*; the pitch features of the accent—particularly the 'crest' of the intonation (in East Norwegian its lowest point, in Southern Swedish its highest)—occur on the stressed syllable in the case of Accent I but are displaced onto the following syllable in the case of Accent II. However, this should not be interpreted as the displacement of the accent itself, since the stress element of the accent is on the same syllable in both cases. It does mean, however, that we can only interpret the pitch features as Accent I or Accent II if we know the location of the stressed syllable. As Haugen and Joos (1952) express it, 'the melody is not in itself distinctive, but acquires distinctive value when it is associated with stress in a particular way'.

Though traditionally called 'word-tones', the pitch patterns associated with these two accents are not restricted to words as such in their realization, but apply to the whole foot. A number of complications have been identified here, however. Vanvik (1961) suggests that Norwegian has a third accent, occurring only in polysyllabic feet, giving a three-way distinction, e.g. *landet* /'lanə/ ('the land') with Accent I, *lande* /'lanə/ ('to land') with Accent II, and *land er* /'lan ə/ ('land is'), which has a pitch pattern differing slightly from the other two. But, since this last pattern occurs only where there is a word-division after the stressed syllable, Borgstrøm (1962) and Haugen (1963) reject this analysis, and derive the third pattern from the presence of a juncture. Haugen and Joos (1952) are also able to accommodate further 'perturbations' associated with intonation, by dividing the patterns into a 'nucleus' and a 'contour' (or 'satellite'). The former includes only the first part of the pattern, which in Norwegian is low in Accent I and falling in Accent II; this is the significant part. The satellite portion is non-distinctive and is subject to intonational variations.

A further complication is the fact that Accent II is much more restricted in its distribution than Accent I. The former occurs only in polysyllabic words; the latter may occur in either monosyllabic or polysyllabic forms. This being so, both Rischel (1960, 1963) and Vanvik (1961, 1963) conclude that we cannot speak of Accent I in monosyllables, since there is no possibility of contrast here.

---

[45] Hadding-Koch (1962) suggests that there may also be differences in the intensity profile of the two accents.

Rischel (1960) goes further, arguing that, since there is no contrast in monosyllables, the distinction must be located in the second syllable of polysyllabic feet. Thus, in a contrast such as *huset* 'hʉːsə ('the house'), with Accent I, vs. *huse* 'hʉːsə ('to house'), with Accent II, the distinction is in the final suffix (/ə/); and since the phonetic difference is one of timing, he proposes to represent these as /hʉːsˈə/ and /hʉːsəˈ/, respectively, where /ˈ/ represents the accent, located before and after the vowel of the suffix, respectively.

Other scholars, such as Haugen (1963) and Jasanoff (1966), reject this analysis, but nevertheless attempt to accommodate the asymmetry between the two accents in terms of *markedness*: according to Haugen (1963), Accent II, which is more restricted in its distribution, is phonetically more complex, and 'can most naturally be described as a displacement of the tonal curve of Accent I', is marked. Furthermore, since Accent I can be said to coincide with the stressed syllable and it is used in loan-words, where it corresponds to the stress of the source language, it is regarded as simply *stressed*, and having no tone; Accent II can then be said to have not only stress but also tone.

Haugen integrates this view of tonal accent with other aspects of Norwegian prosody, and proposes a hierarchy of features. Since Tone can only occur in conjunction with Stress, and the latter is restricted to long syllables, the hierarchy is as in Fig. 4.62.

Fig. 4.62

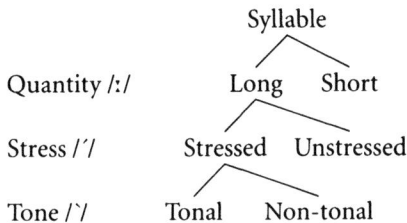

Syllable

Quantity /ː/   Long   Short

Stress /ˈ/   Stressed   Unstressed

Tone /ˋ/   Tonal   Non-tonal

This solution does create a number of problems, however. If Tone is restricted to Accent II, then the contrast between the two accents becomes a matter of the presence vs. the absence of tone, rather than a distinctive opposition between two tones; the marked tone cannot contrast with the unmarked one, since the latter is non-distinctive.[46] This effectively makes tone comparable to accent, but this 'accent' is different from, and additional to, the stress–accent that also occurs in Norwegian and Swedish; indeed, the two kinds of 'accent' are assumed to co-occur in the case of Accent II.

Given these differing analyses, it is clearly difficult to generalize. Nevertheless, what is clear from virtually all analyses of these phenomena, and particularly from Haugen's hierarchical tree given in Fig. 4.62, is that tone is here completely

---

[46] This approach is comparable to Trubetzkoy's treatment of length (cf. Ch. 3), which similarly regards the unmarked value as non-distinctive, and creates the difficulty that the marked value cannot be distinctive either, since it cannot be opposed to a non-distinctive property.

subordinate to stress. What we have in the case of these languages is a stress-based system involving a culminative accent. But overlaid on this essentially syntagmatic phenomenon is a paradigmatic pitch contrast of a rather limited sort. The pitch distinction is limited to the accented syllables, or more accurately the foot, and is further restricted distributionally, since contrasts are limited to polysyllabic feet. Nevertheless, the tonal distinction still remains, however restricted it may be; we may therefore regard these languages as having a *tonal accent*, i.e. a (culminative, syntagmatic) accent which is itself subject to further (distinctive, paradigmatic) differentiation through tone.

That the analysis of accent in these languages continues to be a controversial matter, and that the same problems and solutions are still under discussion, is evident from some more recent work, carried out in a non-linear framework. Lorentz (1984) contrasts the 'toneme' hypothesis, according to which there are two phonologically distinct tones associated with the accented syllable, with the 'accent' hypothesis, which recognizes only a single pitch pattern, differently aligned. These reflect the approaches discussed above. However, Lorentz reinterprets the accent hypothesis in autosegmental terms, recognizing a single pattern—which may differ from dialect to dialect—which is differently associated to the syllables. For Stockholm Swedish, this pattern will—according to Lorentz —be H *L H, and for Bergen Norwegian L *H L, where the tone marked '*' is associated with the accented syllable. In order to achieve the correct association, a syllable with Accent I is similarly marked with '*', while a syllable with Accent II is marked '→', following a convention suggested by Goldsmith (1982), which signifies that the pattern is shifted one syllable to the right (for discussion of this approach to accent, see 4.7.5, below).

Using an analogous non-linear framework, but adopting (in Lorentz's terms) the alternative 'toneme' hypothesis, Withgott and Halvorsen (1988) assign L(ow) and H(igh) tones to Accent I and Accent II words respectively, in Eastern Norwegian. Treating Accent I as unmarked and therefore predictable, the L tone here is introduced by rule, but the H of an Accent II word is lexically specified. These are linked with the stressed syllable of the word. Other tonal specifications are carried out by rule, assuming an overall pattern (M)L(H) for Accent I and (M)HL(H) for Accent II. Withgott and Halvorsen thus reverse Lorentz's approach, which recognizes a single pattern and two kinds of accent, substituting two different patterns with a single kind of accent. They reject 'the reductionist analysis of the two tone accents as one melody with two rules of time alignment, which we would like to avoid because of both phonological and phonetic facts'.

These analyses in no way undermine our conclusion regarding the relative status of tone and stress in Norwegian and Swedish. Both the 'accent' and the 'toneme' approaches of Lorentz require prior identification of the accented syllable—whether lexically or by default rule—and the subsequent assignment of tone patterns—whether different patterns or the same pattern differently aligned—

with these accented syllables. Again, therefore, we see a pitch distinction overlaid on, and subordinate to, a culminative accent.

Serbo–Croat

The tonal phenomena of Serbo–Croat are in many respects similar to those of Norwegian and Swedish, though the phonetic details are different, and there are additional complications. Traditional descriptions recognize four accents, differing not only in pitch but also in length. They are usually marked with the diacritics given in Fig. 4.63 (Corbett, 1990). The differences between the patterns are usually only clear if a further syllable follows: with both 'falling' and 'rising' accents the accented syllable itself is relatively high, but with the 'falling' accents the following syllable is low, while with the 'rising' accents it is high. With the 'short' accents, there is little or no difference in the pitch of the accented syllable itself, but with the 'long' accents there is a higher pitch at the beginning of the syllable in the case of the 'falling' accent and at the end of the syllable in the case of the 'rising' accent (Matešić, 1970; Lehiste and Ivić, 1978).

Fig. 4.63   *Long   Short*
        Falling   ˆ   ``
        Rising   ´   `

As with Norwegian and Swedish, there are restrictions on the occurrence of the accents. The rising accents cannot occur on final syllables; they can therefore occur only in polysyllabic forms. The falling accents can only occur on initial syllables, though they are also retracted onto a preceding proclitic syllable: *vȅdi* ('took out') vs. *nȅ vadi* ('did not take out'). Rising and falling accents therefore only contrast on the initial syllable of polysyllabic words, as the minimal pairs of Fig. 4.64(i) show; long and short accents can contrast in other positions (cf. Fig. 4.64(ii)) (Matešić, 1970).[47]

Fig. 4.64   (i) pàra ('steam') vs. pàra ('money'); Lûka ('Luke') vs. lúka
                                                                        ('harbour')
            (ii) pèro ('pen') vs. Péro ('Peter'); lȕk ('onion') vs. lûk ('bow').

The addition of the further factor of quantity here makes the situation in Serbo–Croat somewhat more complex than that of Norwegian or Swedish, since accent, tone, and length intersect and may restrict one another, and it also provides opportunities for a wider range of theoretical interpretations. From a functional perspective, not all of these features are of equal phonological significance,

---

[47] As with the Scandinavian languages, the origin of the tonal distinctions is a matter of dispute. However, some of the restrictions on their occurrence have a clear historical explanation. During the 15th century, the accent was moved back one syllable, and the shifted accent received a rising tone. This explains the non-occurrence of final accent in polysyllabic words (since the accent moved to the previous syllable) and the restriction of falling accents to initial syllables (they could not move back and become rising). Cf. Matešić (1970); Lehiste and Ivić (1978).

but there is some difficulty in deciding which is the determining feature, and which the determined.

As we have noted, quantity is traditionally an intrinsic part of the Serbo–Croat accents. According to classical Prague School theory, quantity distinctions are a prerequisite for tonal features of this kind, since they allow the accent to fall on either of the two moras of a long syllable, resulting in a difference of pitch pattern (*Tonverlaufkorrelation*). It is indeed possible to interpret the distinction between the two 'long' accents in this way, since in the falling accent the pitch is initially high and falls, and in the rising accent it is initially low and rises. However, there is a difficulty, inasmuch as there is also a distinction between the two short accents, where a 'polytonic' interpretation is not possible. In the latter case, the presence of a following syllable is required to identify the accent concerned, but this cannot be accommodated within the theory, either.

Despite the traditional analysis, quantity does not need to be included as part of the accents in Serbo–Croat, however. Length distinctions are not confined to the accented syllable; they can also occur in the syllables following (though not in those preceding) the accent. It is therefore possible to extract or 'filter out' (Browne and McCawley, 1965) quantity from the accents, leaving only a distinction between 'falling' and 'rising' types. According to Trager (1940), quantity is in any case subordinate to accent, because the latter affects the former.

The status of the falling and rising accents themselves is not equal, however. The falling accent is, as we have noted, restricted to the initial syllable of the word, and is retractable onto a proclitic syllable, while the rise can occur everywhere, except on a final syllable (which may be seen as following from the fact that it needs two syllables for its realization). For this reason, Trubetzkoy (1939) regards the rise as the only genuinely 'free' accent; the fall is denied any distinctive function, though it is accorded a 'demarcative' role, indicating the beginning of the word. Since there is therefore only one accent (the rising accent), its pitch pattern cannot be regarded as distinctive either. The 'falling' accent is regarded as a non-distinctive variant of lack of accent. Trubetzkoy also notes phonetic differences between the falling and rising accents which justify his approach. Whereas the rising accent is largely a matter of pitch, the falling accent has a strong dynamic component. This means that there are two different kinds of accent in the system simultaneously, and these do not necessarily coincide. The implications of this for the theory of prosody are not clear, and Trubetzkoy is himself puzzled by it.[48]

Trager (1940) is also able to eliminate the tonal features from the accents, but on a different basis. For him, the falling and rising accents differ in both stress and pitch, where 'stress' is here interpreted in the standard Bloomfieldian man-

---

[48] Trubetzkoy notes (1939: 193–4) that, if this interpretation is correct, Serbo–Croat is the only language known which has both a free accent and a non-culminative intensity correlation.

ner as a matter of loudness. Thus, the falling accent begins loud and becomes weak, while the rising accent begins loud and increases in loudness, this loudness continuing into the following syllable. The pitch differences here are considered to be automatic consequences of the differences in the stress contours, and therefore non-distinctive: in the falling accents the pitch falls as the stress weakens; in the rising accents the pitch also rises with the increase in loudness.

Another interpretation focuses on the representation of the rising accent. Since this accent extends over two syllables, the accented syllable and the immediately following one, it is possible to distinguish it from the falling accent by marking the second, rather than the first, syllable as accented. This approach is adopted by Hodge (1958), and others, and goes back to the last century. The two accents remain unambiguous, because the falling accent is always initial. We then merely need to interpret them phonetically in an appropriate manner: an accent on an initial syllable is interpreted as falling, an accent on another syllable is interpreted as a rising accent on the preceding syllable (Browne and McCawley, 1965). In order to specify the pitch features, Browne and McCawley assume a classical generative model, though they do not formalize their rules in any way.

Not all linguists regard pitch as phonologically irrelevant, however, and more recent studies, e.g. Matešić (1970) and Babić (1988), adopt versions of the traditional approach, with distinct tonal accents. Babić, for example, describes the accentual features of Croatian dialects in terms of autosegmental theory, recognizing different tonal classes of words. High and Low tones are assigned to these words, by associating them with accented and unaccented syllables, as appropriate. In so far as either the position of the accent or the tonal features are predictable (depending on the dialect), they do not need to be specified lexically, but are introduced by rule. Quantity differences can also be accommodated, by associating tones with either mora of a heavy syllable.

As in the case of Norwegian and Swedish, therefore, there are different approaches to the phonological interpretation of the pitch features of Serbo–Croat, some of which accord phonological status to pitch, and others which do not. This suggests two conclusions: first, that pitch forms a part of the accentual complex in the language, but also that its role is a subordinate one. It is the precise nature of this subordination that appears to be at issue in the various theoretical proposals that have been made.

4.7.4 TONE AND THE FOOT

We have seen that in languages with accentuation the occurrence of an accented syllable defines an accentual unit. Where accentuation is realized by 'stress' (in the sense of this term presented in Chapter 2), there may also be 'stress-timing' (cf. also 3.9.3.1). The presence of stress in a tone-language means that tone itself may be seen in terms of an accentual structure, so that the accentual unit is also a unit of tone.

In languages such as Norwegian and Swedish, which have a stress-timed accentual structure comparable to that of English, and where the tonal features are dependent on the occurrence of the stress, the tonal features may be regarded as having the accentual unit—the foot—as their domain. For this reason it does not make sense to treat the tonal accents as properties of the syllable, with juncture features to locate the pitch pattern on a different syllable according to whether it is Accent I or Accent II. The pitch patterns associated with these accents are essentially *foot-patterns*; hence their association with stressed syllables.

A superficially similar situation is found in a number of tone-languages of a very different type, including Mandarin Chinese and other East Asian languages. Though some Chinese languages, such as Cantonese, as well as other languages such as Vietnamese, are syllable-timed and have no stress, Mandarin has both a syllable–tone system and a stress-timed rhythm. The interaction between tone and stress is here not limited to the production of specific variants of the tones in unstressed syllables; in many cases the tones of unstressed syllables may be lost altogether, as we have seen. This does not mean, of course, that they are spoken with no pitch at all, but rather that the pitch of such syllables is predictable from that of the stressed syllable, which retains its inherent tone; they are said to have the 'neutral' tone. According to Chao (1968), the tone range of neutral syllables is flattened to practically zero and the duration is relatively short. The pitch is described as 'half-low' after tone 1, as 'middle' after tone 2, as 'half-high' after tone 3, and as 'low' after tone 4.

Since in this case, too, the tone pattern is determined by the stressed syllable, we could regard it as a 'tonal accent'; since it is carried by the foot as a whole, we may again see the tone as a property of the foot. The overall situation might therefore be compared with that of Norwegian or Swedish. Chiu (1930) describes the Amoy dialect of Chinese in precisely these terms, noting that 'in every group of syllables there is one with a "tone-accent", that is to say retaining its normal value'.

However, there are clearly differences between the tonal features of Mandarin on the one hand and Norwegian or Swedish on the other. Apart from a few grammatical morphemes which have inherently 'neutral' tones, every syllable in Mandarin Chinese has a potential, or underlying, tone, and it is legitimate to consider that it loses its tone when in an unstressed position. In Norwegian and Swedish, however, the different accents are associated with the word as a whole, and there are no 'underlying' tones for unstressed syllables. Despite a superficial similarity in the phonetic realization of tone in the two languages, therefore, they are typologically quite different.

4.7.5 TONE AND PITCH–ACCENT

In the interactions between tone and accent that we have considered so far, we have limited the discussion of accent to matters of stress, but, as we observed in

Chapter 2, accent may also be realized as pitch, and there are also relationships between this pitch–accent and tone. The issue in this case is not that of *interaction* as such, but rather of *demarcation*; since the realization of both pitch–accent and tone involve the same phonetic parameter, the question raised is the means of distinguishing them. Under what circumstances are pitch features to be interpreted as tone, and when are they to be regarded as pitch–accent? Since accent is *culminative*, in the sense that it singles out one item within a unit, what is crucial is its *location* rather than the specific features of its manifestation, as the latter are predictable, once the location is determined. These characteristics also mean that accent has a structural role in the prosody of the language, and is subject to a range of rules and principles which affect this structure.

Tone has a rather different set of attributes, but in some cases it is possible to interpret apparently tonal features in more or less accentual terms. This possibility is evident in a number of proposals made from the 1960s onwards, particularly with regard to the Bantu languages. These proposals treat tone not as an opposition between equivalent entities—High and Low—but as an asymmetrical relationship between a dominant and a subordinate item. Meussen (1963), for example, notes the lack of correlation between underlying High and Low tones in Tonga and surface High and Low tones; this suggests to him that we should not regard the underlying tones as High and Low at all but rather as *Determinant* and *Neutral*, where the former, but not the latter, has an active role in the derivation. Stevick (1969a) proposes recognizing not two equivalent and contrasting tones—High and Low—in Proto–Bantu, but rather a single High tone, Low tone syllables being regarded as 'toneless'. Such proposals imply that tone may have a culminative function, and therefore have some characteristics of accentuation. Thus McCawley (1973), in analysing Tonga in terms of Meussen's categories, notes similarities between this approach and the analysis of Japanese, in which pitch can be assigned only to certain syllables which are regarded as accented.

In several publications, McCawley (1964, 1970, 1978) attempts to clarify these matters by drawing a distinction between tone and pitch–accent languages in terms of underlying specifications and phonological rules; a language is regarded as a pitch–accent language if it requires at most the specification of the *location* of pitch phenomena in its underlying forms, rather than the pitch features themselves, and if the rules affecting the pitch patterns are in the nature of accent reduction rules, comparable to those involving stress in a language like English. (McCawley's approach to the typology of tone and accent languages will be discussed further in 4.7.6, below.)

These ideas receive a more formal treatment in an autosegmental framework, especially in the work of Goldsmith (1976, 1982, 1983, 1984a). It will be recalled that in this approach tones are represented on a separate tier, independent of the segmental or syllabic base, and tones and tone-bearing units must then be associated with one another. As discussed in 4.4.3.2, above, Goldsmith's Wellformedness Condition, though imposing some constraints on possible associations, still allows considerable latitude, and other principles, such as the Universal Association Convention, have been introduced to reduce the possibilities. This convention assumes a left-to-right association of tones and tone-bearing units and as far as possible a one-to-one relation between the two.

We have also seen that the possibility of alternative associations must still be reckoned with, however, and to this end Goldsmith (1976) introduces the 'star' convention, which provides an initial association of the tone pattern and the tone-bearing units. This is illustrated for Tonga in Fig. 4.44, reproduced here as Fig. 4.65. As we see, the tonal distinctions can be interpreted as differences in the alignment of the tone pattern (the Basic Tone Melody) with the tone-bearing units of the utterance. In Fig. 4.65, this pattern is H L, and Goldsmith achieves the appropriate association of this pattern to words by marking a particular syllable and the Low tone of the pattern with '*', and associating the two. In other languages the pattern and the marked tone may be different; in Ruri it is L H L, with the H tone starred. Following the initial association, subsequent application of general principles of association links the remaining tones and tone-bearing units.

Fig. 4.65 (a)   H L̊   (b)   H L̊
                  | |
              i ma kå ni   i mu su ně

         (c)   H̊ L   (d)   H̊ L
              ∧ ∧   ∕ |
              i ma kå ni   i mu su ně

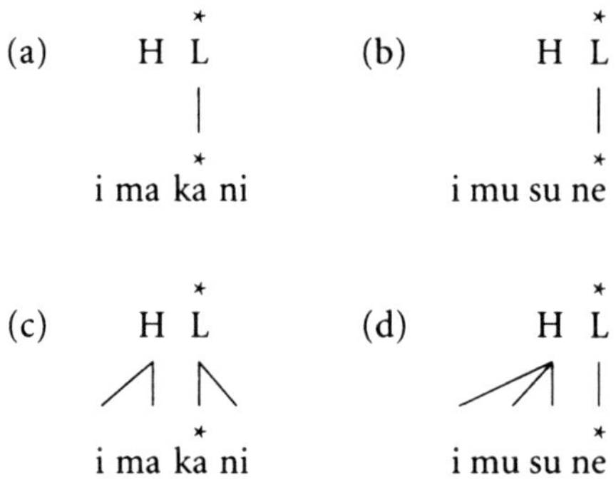

This device is also used by Goldsmith (1981) in aligning intonation patterns to nuclear accents in English, by Haraguchi (1977) in specifying pitch–accents in Japanese (see 3.3.4, above), and by Halle and Vergnaud (1987a) in assigning tonal accents in Lithuanian. We have also seen its use in Norwegian and Swedish (4.7.3). Its use in languages such as Tonga implies that the phenomena involved are analogous, and, indeed, Goldsmith has interpreted Ruri, Tonga, and other languages as *accent* languages rather than tone-languages. Several arguments are put forward in defence of this interpretation. First, there is a single tone pattern—the Basic Tone Melody—which recurs on each relevant unit. Thus 'the tonal representations consist strictly of an integral number of copies of a fixed, language specific Basic Tone Melody' (Goldsmith, 1982). This means that there is effectively no choice of tone, but merely a choice of how to align the pattern with the syllables, in the same way that the pitch features are aligned with a particular syllable or mora in the case of pitch–accent. Second, in such languages only one pattern is usually allowed for each unit, in the same way that there is generally only one accent per unit in an accent language. In all these cases, therefore, the languages can be regarded as accentual in their underlying structure, with tonal features being inserted at some point in the derivation to replace the underlying accents. This means that there may be rules in the grammar which are accentual in nature, and which apply before the insertion of tonal features, as well as tonal rules, which apply to the pitch features themselves.

Goldsmith (1983, 1984a) also adds a diachronic perspective to this analysis. Proto–Bantu is commonly agreed to have been a tone-language, with two tones (High and Low) and a free choice of tone on each syllable. Thus, a two-syllable stem could have the four possible tone patterns HH, HL, LH, and LL. However, the HH pattern appears to have become HL by 'Meussen's Rule' (Goldsmith, 1984b), a process that, by eliminating the occurrence of two adjacent High tones, suggests an embryonic accentual system, with High-toned syllables interpreted as accented. In Tonga, where, according to Goldsmith's analysis, Low tone can be considered accented, there has been a further change, with the accent shifting from High to Low. The Tonga Low tone continues to be associated with syllables which bore the original High ('accented') tone in Proto–Bantu.

This approach has been applied to a number of other languages, such as Haya (Byarushengo, Hyman, and Tenenbaum, 1976), Somali (Hyman, 1981), Luganda (Hyman, 1982), and Kimatuumbi (Pulleyblank, 1983; Odden, 1982, 1985). In Haya (Byarushengo, Hyman, and Tenenbaum, 1976), no morpheme has more than one High tone, and its function can thus be regarded as culminative. There are also rules in the language which 'reduce' High tones to Low, in the manner of stress reduction rules. It is therefore possible to interpret the High vs. Low distinction as 'accented' vs. 'unaccented', marking the former with '*' and leaving the latter unmarked. In Kimatuumbi (Pulleyblank, 1983; Odden, 1985), nouns can be similarly analysed in terms of one High tone per word, so that the basic tone melody is High, and there is a rule mapping the High tone onto the 'accented' syllable. Similar analyses are given for other languages.

As a further enhancement of the 'accent' proposal, Goldsmith (1982) allows for the possibility of using '→' and '←' in place of '*' in those cases where tones are displaced to the right and left, respectively. The effect of these is to place an accent on the next tone-bearing unit to the right or left, as in Fig. 4.66.

Fig. 4.66 (a) $\vec{V}$ C V → V C $\overset{*}{V}$

       (b) V C $\overset{\leftarrow}{V}$ → $\overset{*}{V}$ C V

There is, however, some lack of clarity about how all these phenomena should be analysed and interpreted. In the case of Kimatuumbi, Odden (1985) does not assert that all apparently tonal phenomena must be analysed accentually, nor does he claim that the underlying forms are accentual and that they are converted to tonal representations in the course of the derivation. Rather he claims that Kimatuumbi has *both* tonal *and* accentual phenomena, and that these have different formal characteristics; they must co-exist in certain derivations, and some rules refer to both. The language thus distinguishes non-accentual High tone, accentual High tone, and non-accentual Low tone. Furthermore, the accentual analysis only applies to nouns and adjectives; verbs have no such accentual characteristics and are assigned tones directly. Thus we cannot claim that accent is changed into tone, or that the use of 'accent' is simply a way of saying that tone is restricted in its underlying occurrence.

Furthermore, if a language is to be analysed as accentual, we might expect to find other properties, typical of accentual languages, associated with these tone patterns, for example an elaborate system of accent subordination or a metrical structure, such as we have observed in Chapter 3. However, Goldsmith asserts that such properties are not necessary for an accentual interpretation of tone patterns. As far as Ruri and Tonga are concerned, he claims that both are accentual languages 'yet neither display such characteristics as "accent subordination" or vowel-stress as one might have, wrongly, expected to find in an accent system', and 'the notion of accent appears to have no influence on syllabic loudness, or, more significantly, syllable length, or rhythm, in the broadest sense'. Furthermore, 'the accentual and tonal systems of Ci-Ruri and Ci-Tonga support a view according to which accent is not a local property of a segment, nor a relational property of relative prominence; it is, rather, a simple formal device for relating parallel autosegmental tiers' (Goldsmith, 1982). Thus, having identified properties of these languages which appear analogous to accent, and having interpreted them in autosegmental terms, Goldsmith then identifies accent itself with the formal devices of autosegmental phonology which are used to represent these properties: accent is simply the asterisk used in autosegmental representations, and has no other properties.

The lack of typical 'accentual' properties in these languages casts doubt on the appropriateness of this analysis, and not all scholars have accepted it. Hyman and Byarushengo (1984) revise their earlier description of Haya (Byarushengo, Hyman, and Tenenbaum, 1976), reverting to a 'tonal' analysis. In their new framework, the fact that not all syllables have a distinctive tone is accommodated by initially leaving them unspecified, and specifying only the High tones; the remaining tones are specified in the course of the derivation by means of 'tonification' rules. (This is essentially the same position as that of Stevick, 1969a—see above.) Thus, the stage with only High tones specified corresponds to the earlier 'accentual' level, and the fully specified stage corresponds to the earlier 'tonal' level. The difference between languages which can be analysed 'accentually' and those which can be analysed 'tonally' is regarded as a matter of how early in the derivation 'complete tonification' is achieved.

Pulleyblank (1986) adopts a similar approach, arguing that an accentual analysis is inappropriate for tonal phenomena and should in principle be ruled out altogether. Though Goldsmith's approach captures the culminative nature of the tonal pattern—only one asterisk per unit is allowed—this 'accent' is not comparable to stress, since, unlike stress, it does not reflect a hierarchical metrical structure. The asterisk is also used, in true accentual languages, to mark the heads of feet, but it has no such function in this case; nor does it, unlike stress, have any relationship to such factors as syllable weight. Another of Goldsmith's arguments in favour of his approach is that it captures the asymmetry of the tones in a tone melody, with one (marked with the asterisk) having special status; according to Pulleyblank, however, this does not necessitate or justify an accentual analysis, since a pure tone-system may also have such asymmetries (in many tone-systems, one of the tones can be regarded as 'neutral' or 'unmarked'). Pulleyblank also suggests that a derivation which replaces an 'accent' by tones is in any case ruled out by a general constraint on phonological rules put forward by Chomsky and Halle (1968). Goldsmith's argument that the representation consists of an integral number of occurrences of a 'basic tone melody' is also dismissed, since this involves recognizing a level of structure where such a pattern is found. According to Pulleyblank, there is no such consistent level of phonological structure; the underlying forms do not necessarily have these properties, since some of the patterns are introduced by rule, while further rules may apply to such patterns, and they may therefore not appear in surface forms, either.

Pulleyblank's alternative is the underspecification of tones at the underlying level, with specific 'prelinking' of unpredictable associations of tones and syllables in the lexicon. Predictable (default) tones are inserted later. Since there is evidence that the default tone in Tonga is Low, it is the High tones that will need to be prelinked in this case. This is evidently quite different from Goldsmith's approach, according to which it is the syllables which bear the Low tones that would need to be lexically marked, since these are associated with the 'accent'.

There is thus considerable doubt about the appropriateness of an accentual interpretation of these languages. Even in cases where this interpretation has been claimed to be appropriate, not all tonal features can be shown to be accentual in nature, so that we cannot regard these languages as unambiguously 'tonal' or 'accentual'. It is, furthermore, not entirely clear what criteria are to be used to assign pitch features to tone or accent, other than the stipulation that accent involves 'one per morpheme'. Accent proper, as discussed in Chapter 3, must involve more than this. Nevertheless, it must be acknowledged that languages of this kind, where much of the tonal pattern is predictable, do differ from 'full' tone-languages in a number of important respects, and suitable provision must be made for them in any typological framework. If they are to be interpreted as tone-languages, then it is evident that tone is here much more constrained than in 'full' tone-languages. For this reason, it may be appropriate to follow the terminological lead set by Voorhoeve (1973) on Safwa, and Schadeberg (1973) on Kinga, and describe them as 'restricted tone-languages', or, following Odden (1988), as having 'predictable tone'.

The same interpretation may perhaps be given to other cases where tone and accent interact. In current theory, stress is generally specified metrically, i.e. in terms of a metrical tree or grid, constituting a 'metrical tier' (see Ch. 3), whereas tone is represented on an autosegmental 'tonal tier'. The co-occurrence of stress and tone therefore becomes, formally speaking, the co-occurrence of a metrical and a tonal tier. While some scholars have rejected such co-occurrence, assuming that a language has one or the other, the fact that languages may have both tone and accent suggests that both tiers may be required. Furthermore, if tone tends to be subordinate to stress, rather than the reverse, we might expect this to be evident in how these tiers interact.

Some suggestions to this effect have been made. Goldsmith (1987b) establishes the following *Tone–Accent Attraction Condition*, which stipulates that if a syllable bears a tone, all metrically stronger syllables must also bear one. A stronger form of this—which is assumed in discussions of this question—requires that no syllable with a High tone should have a lower level of accent than a syllable with a Low tone.

Tone–Accent Attraction Condition
A tone-to grid structure is wellformed if and only if there is no tone-bearing syllable which has a lower level of accent than a toneless syllable.

Hyman and Katamba (1993) illustrate this principle in Luganda, accounting for accent by designating certain moras as metrically strong (and hence capable of attracting tone). Bickmore (1995a) similarly applies Goldsmith's condition to Lamba, which, he argues, is a transitional type between pure tone-languages and toneless Bantu languages such as Swahili. It would therefore appear to be a 'restricted' tone-language which has both an accentual structure and tonal features which depend on them. In Bickmore's analysis, Lamba has an alternating pattern of prominence which can be metrically assigned, and exhibits 'tone to stress attraction', as lexically-specified High tones shift onto metrically prominent syllables. The remaining syllables receive low tone by default. Bickmore argues, therefore, that for this language we need both a metrical tier to determine the positions of prominence and a tonal tier to provide the lexical tones which are attracted to these positions.

Bickmore's description does not make it clear whether the 'stresses' that are assigned here are real or merely place-holders for High tone. If the latter, then this analysis of Lamba would fall under Goldsmith's 'accentual' interpretation of tone, with a 'star' to mark the tone-bearing unit to be associated with High tone. If, on the other hand, the 'stress' is here genuinely accentual, then the 'tone attraction' condition provides more evidence for the subordination of tone to stress in such restricted tone-systems.

4.7.6 TONE AND ACCENT: TYPOLOGICAL CONCLUSIONS

As we have seen, the relationship between tone and accentuation raises a number of important questions, not only about the nature of their interaction, but also about the typology of tone and accent, and ultimately about the definition of a 'tone-language'. Languages where tone is in some way limited by accentuation or does not exercise a fully distinctive role create difficulties here, and not all scholars are willing to recognize them as fully tonal. Pike (1948) is quite strict about the criteria which are to be applied in order to identify a tone-language; he includes only those languages in which every syllable has a separate tone. His main typological criterion *within* tone-languages is based on the kinds of tone found, giving 'register' and 'contour' types.

There is, however, another type of language within Pike's categorization: languages with 'word–pitch systems' (Pike, 1948: 14–15). These include languages of the type discussed in this section, such as Swedish and Norwegian, but also Japanese. According to Pike, these are not tone-languages, even though pitch is acknowledged to play a distinctive lexical role, since its distinctiveness is restricted 'to certain types of syllables or to specific places in the word'. This exclusion is unfortunate, as the distinctions in Swedish and Norwegian are clearly tonal, if on a restricted scale. Furthermore, Pike's grouping of these languages with Japanese is misguided, since pitch in this language has a purely accentual function.

Hockett (1955: 65–72) ignores the differences between tone and stress and treats them both as 'accentual systems'. His typology is based on the nature of the system: whether it is 'linear' or 'non-linear', and whether it is 'with zero' or 'without zero'. In the case of *linear* systems, the contrasts are along a single dimension, i.e. two or more different pitches or degrees of stress; in *non-linear* systems, contrasts 'cannot be lined up along some single scale of articulatory or acoustic property'. An 'accentual' system which includes both tone and stress— such as that of Norwegian or Swedish—is therefore likely to be non-linear, since it operates in two dimensions. Systems have zero if, in Hockett's terms, one of the contrasting items is *isolable*, i.e. it can occur without the others. In practice this means that the system opposes a particular feature to its absence, or one of the contrasting items can be seen as unmarked. In these terms, therefore, Norwegian and Swedish are 'non-linear systems with zero', since, in addition to having a stress system like that of English, 'loud stresses are of two types, differing in tonal contour', and the 'simple' contour (Accent I) is isolable and unmarked. These two languages are opposed to Apache, Mazateco, and Mixteco, which in Pike's terms are register–tone languages, and which in Hockett's scheme are 'linear systems without zero', and to Vietnamese and various dialects of Chinese, including Cantonese, which are 'non-linear systems without zero'.

Hockett treats both Norwegian and Swedish on the one hand and Mandarin on the other as belonging to the same type, viz. as 'non-linear systems with zero', but on quite different grounds: Swedish and Norwegian have a non-linear *stress* system, because stressed syllables have two different tonal forms (unstressed syllables constitute 'zero stress'). Mandarin has a non-linear *tone* system, because the tones are contours rather than levels; here it is toneless syllables which constitute 'zero'. This allows us to distinguish these two types, despite their apparent similarity in effectively assigning tones to the foot (see 4.6.4, above). Similarly, Hyman (1978) describes Mandarin as having *accent superimposed on tone*, since although unaccented syllables are toneless, all four underlying tones occur on all syllables. Languages like Serbo–Croat, on the other hand, have *tone superimposed on accent*, since each phonological word has one obligatory accented syllable, which may have a High or Low tone.

In an unpublished but influential paper, McCawley (1964)[49] recognizes four language types, according to the presence of tone and accent. The types are listed as follows.

(1) bound accent (English), where the tone features are totally predictable
(2) partially free accent (Serbo–Croat, Bambara), where the tonal behaviour is of one of two types
(3) free accent (Japanese), where the tonal behaviour is determined by the location of the accent
(4) tone-languages, where each syllable is specified for pitch.

This classification is useful in its separation of pitch–accent from tone, but it is weakened by its failure to distinguish pitch from tone (presumably in an effort to avoid the notion of 'surface contrast' which is implied by this distinction, and which was repudiated in classical generative phonology). McCawley's type (1) does not involve tone at all, his type (3) involves pitch–accent but not tone, and his type (4) involves tone but not accent. It is only his type (2) which involves interaction between tone and accent, but it seems insufficiently differentiated, since it includes both Serbo–Croat and Bambara, which have rather different prosodic systems. In Bambara, each word is either High or Low-toned, giving a superficial similarity to Serbo–Croat, but it is clear from the descriptions we have that the language still retains many characteristics of a syllable-tone language. A two-syllable 'high' noun, for example, has the tone pattern HH, while a three-syllable 'high' noun has the pattern HLH. Although there is stress in Bambara, its relationship to tone is quite different from that found in tonal accent languages, since stress falls on the last High-toned syllable of a sequence, e.g. *mángóró yí'rí* ('mango tree'), *mángóró nyí'mán* ('the

---

[49] Since this talk was not published, information about its contents is derived from the discussion in e.g. Wang (1967), Woo (1969), Fromkin (1974), and McCawley (1978).

good mango').[50] Stress assignment must therefore follow tone assignment (cf. Woo, 1969). This is the reverse of the situation in Norwegian or Swedish, and it also conflicts with McCawley's principle (1964, 1970, 1978), established for a genuine pitch–accent language like Japanese, that accent rules always apply before tone rules.

However, McCawley (1970, 1978) argues that the distinction between tone and pitch–accent is not an absolute one. If they are to be distinguished at all then it must be in terms not of their phonetic characteristics—both involve pitch—but on the kinds of phonological rules that apply and the manner of their application. He argues that accentual phenomena are subject to accent reduction rules of the kind that have been described for English (e.g. by Chomsky and Halle, 1968), whereas tones are subject to tonal rules of pitch assimilation. The difference between a pitch–accent language and a tone-language may, he claims, lie in the point in the grammar where the tonal rules take over from accent rules. Tone-languages proper, such as Chinese or Kikuyu, make reference to tonal rules throughout the phonology; pitch–accent languages, such as Japanese, have rules of an accentual type, comparable to those of English; Ganda appears to be an intermediate type, where accentual rules apply to assign tone patterns, but the rules are then of the tonal type. Thus, 'Ganda can be described as having a pitch–accent system in its deep phonology and a tonal system in its surface phonology'.

Woo (1969) takes issue with McCawley's classification. She argues that, since neutral tones in Mandarin are derived from [−stress] rather than the reverse, full tone-languages such as Chinese are subject to the same kinds of reduction rules as non-tone languages, contrary to McCawley's claim. She also argues that although Japanese is unlike Chinese in its prosodic system, it should nevertheless *not* be grouped typologically with English. She follows the suggestion that accent languages might have diacritics (accent marks) associated with morphemes, which are later interpreted as pitch. However, though this might be appropriate for Japanese, it would be unsatisfactory for English, where accent—according to Chomsky and Halle (1968)—is predictable.

If each morpheme in tonal accent languages is be assigned a diacritic specifying its tonal characteristics, this is, according to Woo, comparable to the assignment of a feature to specify harmony characteristics in vowel harmony languages. She therefore proposes that such languages should be called 'tone harmony' languages. Her typology thus includes the following types.

(A) lexical tone-languages, where the pitch contour of a lexical formative is specified for pitch on every vowel (Mandarin, Cantonese, Igbo)

---

[50] It will be noted that the 'High' word *mangoro* has High tones throughout in this construction. In isolation, it has the pattern HLH, as mentioned above.

(B) tone harmony languages, where a diacritic is associated with each lexical formative, and where the diacritic is later interpreted to give the pitch contour of the formative (Japanese, Bambara)

(C) non-tone languages, where the lexicon contains no prosodic features associated in any way with formatives (English, Northern Tepehuan).

According to Woo, we could combine types A and B as 'tone-languages', as distinct from type C, though this would have no great significance. What is more important is the fact that in A and B accent can exist independently of pitch, and therefore needs separate specification.

Woo's categories are still not entirely satisfactory, however. The different types are defined according to the lexical specification of prosodic features rather than according to the nature of the features involved, and she groups together under the label 'tone harmony' such diverse languages as Japanese, Mende and Serbo–Croat, whose prosodic characteristics are rather different.

The fact that such a variety of different typological groupings have been devised for languages which have both tone and accent clearly indicates that there is no single typology that can adequately reflect both the similarities and the differences between the languages involved. McCawley (1978) notes that 'for each of the languages discussed in this section, one can ask the question, "Is it a pitch–accent language or a tone language?" However, I think that that is a stupid question to ask, since the material covered in this section makes clear that the various characteristics of pitch–accent systems and of tonal systems are to a fair extent independent of one another and that there is no reason for squeezing the diversity of phonological systems discussed here into a simple dichotomy.' In view of this conclusion, it would appear to be more profitable to identify typological *parameters* than to try to classify languages themselves.

As far as accent and tone are concerned, McCawley draws the distinction between them in terms of rule types and stages in phonological derivations. A more traditional approach would characterize the difference in *functional* terms: accent is culminative and syntagmatic; tone is distinctive and paradigmatic. There are also phonetic differences, since accentuation may be achieved by several means, including stress (a cover term for a range of features, including pitch, which may be associated with the accent) or pitch alone; tone, on the other hand, is almost exclusively pitch, though a number of other features, such as laryngeal differences, may also accompany the pitch contrasts. Finally, accent and tone may have different *domains*. As a *culminative* feature, accent does not apply to every syllable, but merely to some, and it may be involved in rhythm and timing; as a *distinctive* feature, tone may serve to distinguish domains of different sizes, though its primary domain is the syllable.

It will be clear that no single one of these criteria by itself can distinguish the two phenomena, but, taken together, they do enable us to do so. Since they are distinct, they can operate independently and can interact, though not always in the same way. Thus, just as full tone-languages are by no means uniform in the way in which they use pitch, so languages in which both tone and accent occur simultaneously do not necessarily show the same interactions, and may present different results.

Any typology of languages based on the relationship between tone and accent is therefore likely to prove unsatisfactory and, to a certain extent, arbitrary. Nevertheless, it is difficult to discuss these phenomena without establishing some kind of classification, however inadequate. We may begin, therefore, by distinguishing languages on the basis of the presence of tonal and accentual features, giving the four categories of Fig. 4.67.

Fig. 4.67	[±tone]	[±accent]	*Examples*
	+	+	Mandarin, Zulu, Swedish
	+	−	Cantonese, Hausa
	−	+	English, Spanish, Japanese
	−	−	French

However, although this scheme adequately reflects the use of tone and accent in different languages, it produces rather meaningless groupings, treating Mandarin and Cantonese as different types, but Zulu and Swedish as the same.

A more elaborate and more differentiated scheme is presented in Fig. 4.68. (Full) tone-languages (types I and II) are those in which tone is independent of accentuation, though there may be interactions with a stress system, should one be present. Cantonese and Hausa have no stress system, and can be called *non-accentual* tone languages; Mandarin and Zulu are *accentual* tone languages, since they have a stress system as well as tone, and the two may interact; in Mandarin tonal distinctions may be lost in unstressed syllables. Tonal accent languages (III), such as Swedish or Serbo–Croat, are those in which there is a stress-based accent and a tonal system, but the tonal system is dependent on the stressed syllables. In pitch–accent languages (IV), such as Japanese, there is an accentual system but no tonal system, and the accentual system is predominantly based

Fig. 4.68	Language Type	Tone	Accent	Accent Type	Examples
	I. Non-accentual tone-languages	Yes	No	—	Cantonese, Hausa
	II. Accentual tone-languages	Yes	Yes	Stress	Mandarin, Zulu
	III. Tonal accent languages	Yes	Yes	Stress	Swedish, Serbo–Croat
	IV. Pitch–accent languages	No	Yes	Pitch	Japanese
	V. Stress–accent languages	No	Yes	Stress	English, Spanish
	VI. Non-accentual languages	No	No	—	French

on pitch. In *stress–accent* languages (V), such as English, there is a stress-based accentual system, but no tone. Languages such as French, which have neither tone nor word-stress,[51] may be called *non-accentual* languages (VI).

Such a classification is, as already acknowledged, of limited value, as the typological parameters are really more important than the language types. Furthermore, it could still be argued that it is underdifferentiated, since it fails to distinguish languages which have different prosodic characteristics. Although English and Spanish are both stress–accent languages without tone, the role of stress is different in each case, since English is stress-timed, but Spanish is not. Similarly, although Norwegian, Swedish and Serbo–Croat are all tonal accent languages, Serbo–Croat differs in incorporating a quantity distinction. Types II and III, Accentual Tone languages (Mandarin, Zulu) and Tonal Accent languages (Norwegian, Swedish, Serbo–Croat) are also not differentiated by the criteria given here, since they have both a tonal system and a stress-based accentual system. The difference between them lies in the fact that tone is subordinated to accent in the latter, but not in the former, and this is also reflected in differences in the *domain* of the tonal contrast, which is the syllable in the former case, but the foot in the latter, since the tonal domain is here dependent on the accentual domain. An overall prosodic typology would therefore need to include further typological parameters, such as rhythmical and quantitative types. Fig. 4.68 cannot aspire to being such an overall typology, but merely indicates the basic language types which result from accentual and tonal parameters.

This scheme is concerned with the interactions between tone and accent, and it does not, therefore, attempt to establish a typology for 'pure' tone-languages

Fig. 4.69   TONAL SYSTEMS

Free Tone	Restricted Tone, including tonal pitch–accent
Chinese	Mende
Ewe	Japanese
	Tonga
	Haya

METRICAL ACCENT SYSTEMS

Stress–Accent	Metrical Pitch–Accent
English	Vedic Sanskrit
Latin	Ancient Greek
Modern Greek	Malayalam
Chinese	

[51] French does, however, have a phrasal stress. See Ch. 3, footnote 69.

themselves. For the same reason, it does not specifically identify the 'accentual tone languages' of Goldsmith, such as Tonga, as a separate type, since these languages are here considered to be *non-accentual* tone languages. They would figure as a separate category *within* such a type, as 'restricted tone languages'. Clark (1988) distinguishes 'free' from 'restricted' tone-languages in this way, and includes Zulu, which she analyses accentually, in the latter category. However, since this category also includes Japanese, her scheme evidently differs from the one adopted here. She does nevertheless recognize that languages may have two prosodic systems simultaneously, one tonal and one metrical, and Zulu is considered to be one of these. Her system is given in Fig. 4.69.

4.8 Conclusion: Tone and Prosodic Structure

In this chapter we have surveyed a wide range of tonal phenomena and examined a variety of theoretical proposals to account for them. These have included the nature of tonal systems and the distinctive features that are needed to order these systems paradigmatically, the appropriate representation of tonal features in the syntagmatic dimension, and the interactions between tone and other prosodic features, especially accentuation. We have also considered how, and to what extent, the interactions between tone and accent can be used as a criterion for the typological classification of languages.

In the course of this discussion a variety of pointers have been identified to the place of tone in prosodic structure, though this matter has not been discussed explicitly. One aspect of this is the establishment of the appropriate *domain* of tone; in spite of claims that tone is, in some cases as least, a *segmental* feature, evidence has been presented for regarding its domain as the *syllable* though, in cases where tone is dependent on accentual features, it may also be the *foot*. Larger units may also be involved in cases of tonal interaction, i.e. in tone sandhi.

A further indicator of the prosodic role of tone is found in its interactions with other prosodic features, especially accent. What is especially noticeable in these interactions is that tone almost always appears to have a subordinate position with respect to accent: cases of the dependence of tone on accent are far more numerous—and more clear-cut—than cases of the dependence of accent on tone, if, indeed, the latter occurs at all. This also appears to be true, though perhaps less obviously, of the relations between tone and quantity. Though there are some instances of length being determined by tone, with 'long' and 'short' tones, in the majority of cases tonal structure tends to be subordinate to length, with the number of tones determined by the quantity or weight of syllables.

In sum, therefore, a preliminary finding here is that tone *reflects* prosodic structure, but does not *determine* it. In this it contrasts markedly with other prosodic features, especially accentuation, which, as we saw in Chapter 2, is a major determinant of prosodic structure. Thus Beckman (1986: 2), in contrasting the roles of accent and tone, notes that the former 'seems to function less as a distinctive feature than as an organizational feature'. These ideas will be developed further in the final chapter of this book.

5

Intonation

5.1 Introduction

5.1.1 THE STATUS OF INTONATION

Intonation has traditionally been regarded as a problem. Scholars have frequently drawn attention to the difficulties and uncertainties surrounding its analysis, its systematic description, and its incorporation into linguistic models and theories. These difficulties have doubtless contributed to its relative neglect; it is often treated as an optional element, which may be effectively disregarded, or at best assigned to the periphery of the subject. In monographs on the phonology of individual languages it is frequently relegated—in so far as it is mentioned at all—to the final pages, as an inessential appendix to the description proper.[1]

The difficulties posed by intonation are of several kinds. There is no doubt that a particular skill is required of the investigator in perceiving and notating intonation patterns accurately. It is also the case that reliable instruments capable of extracting the fundamental frequency—the major phonetic component of intonation—from the speech signal were not available until just before the second world war (Grützmacher, 1939; Meyer-Eppler, 1948). However, neither of these circumstances really accounts for the difficulties; the practical skills can be learnt, and much can be achieved auditorily, without instrumental means. Besides, the lack of appropriate instruments hardly applies to recent work.[2] This suggests that the problems of intonation are more of a theoretical than a practical kind, and relate to its nature and role rather than to its phonetic properties.

Intonation certainly has a number of characteristics which set it apart from other prosodic features. In the first place, it is *meaningful*. Other features, both prosodic and non-prosodic, do not in themselves *have* meaning, but merely

---

[1] That intonation is the last of the prosodic features to be discussed in this book is not to be construed as an endorsement of this practice; it is a matter of practical convenience, since discussion of intonation and its structure presupposes consideration of other features such as accentuation and tone.

[2] There is considerable reliance on instrumental analysis of pitch patterns in some recent work. But although a concern for an accurate factual basis is laudable, overreliance on such data can also be unsatisfactory, since it cannot of itself provide a phonological analysis, and, by obscuring the difference between relevant and irrelevant features, may even impede it. Thus, though one might hesitate to endorse expressions such as 'laboratory fetishism' (van Dooren and van den Eynde, 1982), one can nevertheless support the view that auditory analysis is usually a better basis for the phonological analysis of intonation.

serve to distinguish meaningfully different linguistic items. Thus, features such as stress and tone may have a variety of phonological functions (in Prague School terms, as we saw in Chapter 3, they may be distinctive, culminative, or demarcative), but they share with segmental features the fact that they are not inherently meaningful. But intonation is different; a falling intonation, for example, is often assigned meanings such as 'statement' or 'complete', while a rising intonation may be given meanings such as 'question' or 'incomplete'. Whether the labels given to such meanings are accurate is beside the point here (they are generally far too specific); what is significant is the fact that intonation, unlike other prosodic features, actually has meanings.

Though the precise meanings of intonation patterns may be elusive, it nevertheless appears that they are of a kind which is more relevant for the broader discourse functions of sentences than for their propositional content. Patterns are therefore often described in terms of the 'attitudes' or 'emotions' of the speaker rather than grammatical functions or categories. This leads many scholars to conclude that they are 'natural' and universal rather than arbitrary and language-specific.

A further characteristic that sets intonation off from other prosodic features— and indeed from other linguistic features in general—is that the distinctions it makes are often not discrete, but constitute a *gradient*. A falling intonation, for example, may fall from different heights and to different extents, with no discrete divisions and no clear boundaries between the forms. Furthermore, these differences reflect a parallel gradience of meaning. Since for many scholars linguistic distinctions are in principle discrete, and do not permit such gradience, the status of intonation as a genuinely 'linguistic' phenomenon is thereby placed in doubt.

All this might suggest the conclusion that neither in its phonetic nor its functional characteristics is intonation really a linguistic phenomenon at all, and that it belongs—as suggested by the title of an article by Bolinger—'around the edge of language'. According to this view, it therefore has affinities with *paralinguistic* features such as cries and exclamations, as well as with such non-linguistic phenomena as gesture. Indeed, Martinet (1964: 95–6) considers it to lie outside the definition of language proper, since it fails to comply with what for him is a defining principle of language: 'double articulation'. According to this principle, meaning is mediated through phonological form, and since intonation is claimed to express meaning *directly*, it cannot be included in the definition of language.[3] Such a conclusion would, of course, explain and justify the marginalization of intonation in linguistics.

However, this conclusion is not necessarily valid. First, not all intonational distinctions are matters of gradience; there are categorical distinctions such as high vs. low pitch, or rise vs. fall, and even gradual phonetic distinctions can in

---

[3] Martinet does grudgingly concede, however, that 'intonation cannot be denied some sort of linguistic value', since speakers can use it 'for certain purposes of differentiation' (p. 96).

principle be reduced to discrete phonological choices. Further, not all intonational meanings necessarily relate to 'emotions' and 'attitudes'; a variety of more narrowly linguistic functions have been ascribed to intonation patterns. The pitch features associated with these functions are also by no means always 'natural' and universal, but differ from language to language, and hence reflect an arbitrariness characteristic of linguistic, rather than non-linguistic, phenomena. Thus, though some aspects of intonation and its meaning may perhaps be legitimately treated as lying outside language, this certainly does not apply to all of it.

The conceptual difficulties here are reflected in the terminology, including the definition of the term 'intonation' itself. For many scholars, 'intonation' covers, as we have noted, both 'linguistic' and 'paralinguistic' features; others are more selective, however, and include only the 'linguistic' aspects under this heading. In his discussion of 'pitch fluctuation', Abercrombie (1967: 103–4) distinguishes *vocal gesture* (a term which he attributes to Ogden and Bloomfield) from *speech melody*. The former has an 'indexical', non-linguistic role; it is (probably) universal and instinctive, and is 'not susceptible of phonological treatment'. The latter, on the other hand, is 'pitch fluctuation, in its linguistic function', and is 'not only part of a language, it is a highly distinctive part'. However, for Abercrombie, speech melody includes tone as well as intonation, since both are linguistically significant manifestations of 'pitch fluctuation'.

Whatever the terminology used, however, there is a general assumption here that we need to distinguish between the 'linguistic' and the 'non-linguistic' aspects of intonation. Unfortunately, it appears that the distinction cannot necessarily be made in a consistent and non-arbitrary way, and different scholars draw the boundaries at different points. Nor is it necessarily the case that we can automatically regard the discrete, categorical distinctions of intonation as 'linguistic' and its gradual, gradient differences as 'paralinguistic'. If this is so, then it raises important questions about the nature of phonological distinctions in general (see especially Bolinger, 1961, for discussion of gradient phenomena in language). However, this matter will not be pursued further here; the present chapter has the more modest goal of considering the ways in which intonation patterns can be analysed phonologically, and how their structure relates to prosodic structure in general.

5.1.2 BACKGROUND TO THE STUDY OF INTONATION

Intonation, like tone, is not an area of language to which much attention was paid before the twentieth century. That the pitch of the voice varies during speech had certainly long been known,[4] and we find general, though unsystem-

---

[4] In a celebrated late 18th century controversy, the Scottish Lord Monboddo asserted that speech is delivered on a monotone, provoking a response from Joshua Steele (see below), who succeeded in convincing him of the contrary.

atic, observations on these rises and falls very much earlier. In the case of English, one of the earliest of these commentaries was that of John Hart, who devotes some of his *Orthographie* of 1569 to a discussion of the use of intonation, particularly in relation to punctuation. Several later orthoëpists followed him in this. The most noteworthy early contribution, however, is that of Joshua Steele (1775), who provides an elaborate notation system for indicating accent, rhythm, pause, and intonation.[5]

Much general discussion of the use of different intonation patterns is found in works on rhetoric and elocution, especially from the late eighteenth century. These generally identify a number of different 'tones'—rising, falling, level, and so on—with indications as to the kinds of sentences that are appropriate to their use. Walker (1787), for example, provides symbols for rising, falling, and level pitches, as well as rising–falling and falling–rising ones, with extensive illustrations of how they are to be used. Much the same approach is still found a hundred years later in the elocutionary works of Bell (1886). He identifies five basic types of 'inflexions': fall, rise, fall–rise, rise–fall and the 'double compound inflection' rise–fall–rise, as well as some others, and associates meanings with each. His general, and insightful, conclusions as to these meanings are given in Fig. 5.1.

Fig. 5.1   (1)   A rising tone is prospective, or anticipatory of meaning
          (2)   A falling tone is retrospective, or completive of meaning
          (3)   A mixed or undulating tone is suggestive, or inferential of
                meaning
          (4)   An approximately level tone is reflective, or suspensive of
                meaning

Though we are accustomed to finding a new impetus to the study of prosodic features in the work of Sweet, in the case of intonation he is able to add little to this rhetorical tradition, pleading the inadequacy of his own skills and training (Sweet, 1877: x). Following Bell, he distinguishes three 'primary forms' of intonation, 'level', 'rising', and 'falling', the last two of which can be either *leaps* or *glides*, as well as 'compound rising' (falling–rising) and 'compound falling' (rising–falling) tones, and, like Bell, a rising–falling–rising tone. He also recognizes three different *keys*, 'high', 'middle' and 'low', which involve different overall pitch levels for the utterance or its parts (Sweet, 1906: 68–71).

With their attempt at classification of the different intonational possibilities, the studies of Bell and Sweet at least make a start in determining the role of intonation in utterances. But what is lacking here is any clear conception of the *structure* of intonation, and an understanding of how the pitch pattern of the utterance is *organized*. Although Bell notes that these tones can be preceded by a 'preparatory tone', and he refers to the 'unity of inflexion throughout every

---

[5] For discussion of Steele's work, see Abercrombie (1965); Alkon (1959). For an overview of the development of intonation studies see Pike (1945: ch. 2), Crystal (1969: ch. 2), Gibbon (1976).

accentual phrase' (1886: 44), no criteria are given for establishing such phrases.

The application of experimental techniques, which we find from the last decade of the nineteenth century in the study of other prosodic features, was handicapped in the case of pitch, as noted above, by the absence of an adequate means of extracting pitch from the speech signal, and phoneticians had to rely entirely on auditory analysis, supplemented by only rudimentary aids. Jones (1909), for example, produced detailed auditory transcriptions of 'intonation curves' by using the gramophone, repeatedly lifting the needle in order to determine the precise pitch at each point. A similarly detailed analysis was done for the final 'cadence' of German utterances by Pollak (1911). But, again, the usefulness of these analyses is severely limited by the lack of understanding of the larger structures involved.

An initial step in analysing the nature of these structures is made by Coleman (1914). He devises a musical notation system in which either numbers or a continuous line can be placed on a stave, representing the pitch level. More significantly, he relates intonation to accentual features in a more explicit way than Bell, concluding that it is the chief factor in the indication of 'emphasis', the latter being either contrastive prominence or non-contrastive intensity. This insight paves the way for the analysis of the structure of intonation patterns in a language such as English, in which, as we saw in Chapter 3, there is a focal point coinciding with the so-called 'sentence accent' or 'tonic stress'. This principle is exploited especially in the works of the so-called 'British School' of intonation analysis, which will be considered in more detail shortly. Apart from this, however, it must be concluded that there was little understanding of the nature and structure of intonation before the rise of the major structuralist schools of linguistics in the second quarter of the twentieth century.

5.2 Preliminaries to the Phonology of Intonation

5.2.1 THE PHONETIC BASIS

Intonation shares its phonetic basis with both tone and pitch–accent; in each case it is primarily the fundamental frequency of the voice that is involved, though, as we have seen in earlier chapters, the close relationship between pitch and other laryngeal features means that these other features may also participate. At the extremes of the pitch range, for example, differences of voice quality may also accompany the intonation pattern. Such additional features are, however, automatic phonetic consequences of the pitch features and are of no phonological significance. The situation is somewhat different in the case of the relationship between intonation and accentuation, however, in those (many) languages where these two co-occur. Here, the relationship is not necessarily determined by phonetic constraints but may be phonological. Whether we consider the accentual features to be part of intonation (as in the British tradition) or as a separate phonological parameter (as in Bloomfieldian practice) is, however, in part a matter of definition or even merely of terminology. In practice the two are clearly linked and must be treated together at some stage of the description.

There is no doubt, however, that the most important phonetic parameter involved in intonation is pitch. Phonetically, therefore, we can regard the intonation of an utterance as a continuous—and continuously varying—pitch pattern. There are, strictly speaking, breaks in this pattern for voiceless consonants, since there can be no pitch without voice, but these are not generally perceived as such; to the ear the pattern is uninterrupted (Laver, 1994: 484). Since the pitch is continually changing—sustained level pitch is not common—the issue in the phonological analysis of intonation is usually a matter of identifying phonologically significant falls and rises in pitch, and determining the structure of the patterns produced.

We shall not need to consider here the details of the physiological mechanisms involved in the production of the pitch features of intonation, the acoustic properties of the fundamental frequency produced, or the perception of these features, important though they are in a wider context. For consideration of these matters, which are also relevant for tone and pitch–accent, see Lehiste (1970: 54–83), 't Hart, Collier, and Cohen (1990: 10–37), and Laver (1994: 450–62).

5.2.2 PROBLEMS WITH THE PHONOLOGY OF INTONATION

In the case of the prosodic features discussed so far in this book, it has been remarked that the systematic analysis of the feature concerned only became possible with the introduction of a phonological perspective, enabling the ordering of observations according to their linguistic relevance. With intonation the situation is not quite so clear, for the reasons touched on briefly above. In the first place, as Ladd (1996: 20) points out, the fact that intonation patterns have meanings leads to an assumption that there is no need for a phonology of intonation. Studies are conducted which seek to relate assumed meanings directly to intonational features, without establishing a phonological structure or a set of features as an intermediary. 'For the most part', he writes, 'the authors of such studies make no attempt to identify phonological categories. Instead, they simply take a set of intonational functions for granted, and assume that the most appropriate description of how these functions are expressed is in terms of the continuously varying parameters of speech—in particular the suprasegmental parameters of F_o, duration, and intensity'. Such studies can be exemplified by the work of Fairbanks and Pronovost (1939), who investigate the phonetic features involved in the expression of different emotions: contempt, anger, fear, grief, and indifference. They find that anger involves a wide pitch range, with rapid movement; grief, on the other hand, is expressed using a narrow range with slow pitch changes and vibrato; similar characterization is given for other emotions. Similarly, Fónagy and Magdics (1963) analyse the intonation patterns expressing ten 'emotions': joy, tenderness, longing, coquetry, surprise, fear, complaint, scorn, anger, and sarcasm. They find similar means of expression used in a variety of different languages, and also relate the intonations to typical musical forms which are used for these emotions. The implication is that the intonation patterns are a direct reflection of universal human vocal responses to the emotions in question, an approach which appears to make the recognition of a phonological system for intonation completely unnecessary.

A second factor which has impeded the establishment of a phonology of intonation is, as noted above, that the principles and procedures of conventional segmental phonology, which envisage the reduction of phonetic differences to categorical phonological distinctions, cannot readily be applied. Thus, an utterance might be given a rising, falling, falling–rising, etc. intonation, each of which is phonetically and semantically different, and which we might consider to be phonologically distinct (how these patterns should be *represented* phonologically is a different issue). *Within* each of these categories, however, we find a range of variation; the fall might begin and end at various heights, and fall slowly or quickly. Here, there are no discrete phonetic categories, and each of these parameters of variation is a continuum. We might simply choose to regard the varieties of fall or rise as phonologically irrelevant, and comparable to allophones or phonemes, but the difficulty is that they are also meaningfully different; the continuous phonetic scale is reflected in a parallel continuous scale of meaning.[6] It is therefore difficult to identify, on the basis of the criterion of distinctiveness of meaning, a restricted number of phonologically distinct entities which underlie the very large number of occurring phonetic manifestations.

There are a number of strategies open to us in attempting to overcome these difficulties. Most modern scholars would certainly wish to establish a phonology of intonation, which is comparable with that of other prosodic features, in which abstract phonological categories can be said to underlie a wide range of phonetic manifestations. On the other hand, the special character of intonational distinctions, and in particular their gradient nature, cannot be ignored. Hence, we cannot necessarily treat the phonology of intonation in exactly the same terms as that of other prosodic features.

5.2.3 INTONATION AND PROSODIC TYPES

If we are to provide an adequate phonological framework for intonation, this framework must take account of the intonational features not only of languages such as English, which has been thoroughly described from the early decades of the twentieth century onwards, but also of languages of different prosodic types, including languages with tone, tonal accent, and pitch–accent. Indeed, it must be applicable to *all* languages, since intonation is found, in one form or another,

---

[6] For a discussion of such 'matched continua' see Trim (1969).

in every language that has been investigated (Bolinger, 1964). Not all scholars have accepted this principle; in discussing intonation, Pike (1945: 25) notes that 'tone-languages may have various types of pitches superimposed upon them', but considers that 'these types tend to be vocal reflections of physiological states, or general pitch characteristics, rather than specific pitch contours organised into an intricately interwoven structural pattern'. Similarly, in considering tone (Pike, 1948: 16–17), he claims that while 'all tone-languages have intonation of the emotional type, with the general height of the voice affected, and so on', they do not have 'a highly organised contrastive system with a limited number of relative levels controlling the formation of intonations that carry shades of meaning'. He thus justifies a distinction between 'tone-languages' on the one hand, and 'intonation languages' on the other, as incompatible alternatives. Cruttenden (1997: 9) is less absolute, acknowledging that 'tone and intonation are not completely mutually exclusive in languages', but he nevertheless speaks of a 'limited amount of superimposed intonation', and notes (p. 12) the 'reduced, though still present, potential for intonation' in tone-languages and pitch–accent languages.

It would indeed be surprising if the pitch features of intonation were to take the same form in languages where pitch has tonal or accentual functions and those where it does not, for the obvious reason that pitch features may be pre-empted for these latter functions which, from a linguistic perspective, may be considered primary. But this does not mean that the pitch features associated with tone and intonation are mutually exclusive; rather it means that they must accommodate themselves to one another in appropriate ways. Intonation may therefore have different kinds of organization in tonal, tonal accent, and pitch–accent languages on the one hand, and in languages without these features on the other. What is needed, therefore, is a framework which is not merely adapted to languages of the last type, but is flexible enough to accommodate manifestations of intonation in tone and pitch–accent languages.

Most of the models of intonation that have been devised are specifically based on English and languages with similar prosodic characteristics.[7] Some of the basic concepts presented in these models do not appear, in fact, to be universal, while they also fail to include features present in other languages. In the former category come the 'nuclear tones' of the British school and the 'pitch–accents' of Pierrehumbert's model, which, being dependent on accentuation, are certainly not found in some languages; in the latter come the pitch features associated with final particles in tone-languages such as Cantonese, for which no provision is made in most models.

The phonological framework for intonation must therefore ultimately be

---

[7] The Swedish model of Gårding (see below) is exceptional, in that it incorporates the tonal accents of Scandinavian languages, and it has also been applied to Chinese (Gårding, 1984). However, as noted below, this is not really a phonological model of intonation but rather a strategy for generating artificial intonation contours.

rather broader than the models currently proposed. Since most discussions of intonation have focused on English and other European languages with similar prosodic structures, however, it is with this narrower framework that we shall be concerned in the first instance. We shall return to a broader view in 5.8, below, where intonation will be considered in a wider context.

5.3 Models of Intonation

5.3.1 INTRODUCTION

In spite of the difficulties of intonation analysis outlined above, considerable progress has been made by a number of scholars from the 1920s onwards in establishing the basis for a descriptive framework. These developments have not been exclusively, or even primarily, the work of theoretical linguists; a major contribution has also been made by more pedagogically oriented scholars, for whom the theoretical framework has not been the prime concern.

As far as the theoretical approaches are concerned, the major European school of phonology, the Prague School, does not provide an explicit model for the description of intonation. An early discussion by Karcevskij (1931) is in very general terms and remains inconclusive, while Trubetzkoy (1939) devotes only a couple of pages to the topic, and most of his discussion is concerned with the demarcation of sentence intonation from the 'word tone' of tonal accent languages (see 4.7.3). He notes, however, that most (non-tone) European languages have a distinction between a falling and a rising intonation, used for indicating finality and continuation, respectively, with in some cases a further 'listing' intonation. He also distinguishes intonation proper from register differences, the latter being used in some languages to distinguish 'yes/no' questions (*Entscheidungsfragen*) from other kinds of question, or to set off parenthetical expressions, though such differences are always accompanied by intonational differences proper. In what way intonation and register are to be distinguished phonetically or phonologically is not clarified, however. Furthermore, there is no consideration of the structure of intonation patterns. For more useful discussion of intonation and its structure we must therefore turn to other schools and traditions of analysis.

5.3.2 THE BRITISH SCHOOL

For the earliest systematic contribution to the analysis of intonation we need to look not at theoretical schools but at more practically-minded scholars, chief among whom are those of the 'British School'. This tradition of analysis does not explicitly espouse any particular theoretical precepts, but provides a descriptive framework for intonation, often with a pedagogical orientation. This does not mean, however, that there is no phonological basis to the analysis; in many cases it is clear that phonological criteria are applied in establishing the distinctive elements of the description, but there is generally no overt discussion of these criteria, nor any attempt to invoke theoretical principles to support them, still less to justify theoretical principles themselves. Nevertheless, this tradition provides a consistent set of descriptive categories and has been extremely influential.

The origin of the British approach lies, paradoxically, in the work of the German scholar Hermann Klinghardt—see, for example, Klinghardt and Fourmestraux (1911), Klinghardt and Klemm (1920), and Klinghardt (1927)—in which he presents an analysis of French, English, and German intonation, respectively. He establishes an intonation unit (the *sprechtakt*[8]) and recognizes a number of different intonation patterns, represented by a string of dots of different heights, one for each syllable. In the descriptions of English and German, the dependence of the pattern on the accented syllables is particularly noted, with larger dots used for accented than for unaccented syllables. The unstressed syllables before the first stress are called the *auftakt*; those after the last stress the *abtakt*. Klinghardt also makes (accurate) observations on the differences between English and German intonation patterns and usages. His approach is illustrated in Fig. 5.2, in this case from German (Klinghardt, 1927: 7–8).[9]

Fig. 5.2

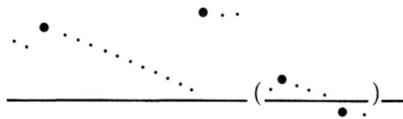

daß die 'liebe in solchen tagen ihre eigenen
'wege ging, (wird 'niemanden ver'wundern)

This approach was taken up by British scholars, who refined and developed it. As we have seen above, a characteristic of the British school is the incorporation of accentual features—specifically the phrasal accent (what we have called Level 2 accent)—into the intonation. This approach begins with Coleman (1914), but it is developed particularly by Palmer (1922), who identifies the syllable on which the main accent falls as the *nucleus*, and this enables him to introduce a tripartite structure for the unit (called the *tone-group*), consisting of *head, nucleus*, and *tail*, where the first and the last do not necessarily occur. Thus, the utterance *I don't like that sort of thing*, with the nucleus on *like*, can be analysed as in Fig. 5.3.

Fig. 5.3 *Head   Nucleus   Tail*
       I don't   like   that sort of thing

---

[8] The *sprechtakt* does not correspond to the musical *Takt* (= 'bar' or 'measure'), but to a whole phrase. Note that Klinghardt does not adopt the standard German orthographic convention of capitalizing nouns.

[9] A slight adjustment has been made in the layout of Klinghardt's example in order to correct a printing error.

Other scholars in the same tradition, however, notably Armstrong and Ward (1926) and Schubiger (1935) on English, Barker (1925) on German, and Coustenoble and Armstrong (1934) on French, follow Klinghardt rather than Palmer in not dividing up the unit; they simply represent the intonation pattern within each unit as a string of dots, with, in the case of English and German, bigger dots or lines for the accented syllables. In fact, in his later work (1933), Palmer, too, reverts to this approach, re-analysing his combinations of heads and nuclei as a limited number of fixed patterns.[10] On the other hand, Kingdon (1958b) and Schubiger (1958) recognize more divisions than Palmer, with a *pre-head* (the unstressed syllables before the first stress, equivalent to Klinghardt's *auftakt*), *head* (the first stressed syllable together with following unstressed syllables), *body* (the part between the head and the nucleus), *nucleus*, and *tail* (the last two are the same as Palmer's). Some examples from Kingdon's work are given as Fig. 5.4; the wedges represent the stressed syllables, and the dots the unstressed ones. Such displays are tied in with Kingdon's 'tonetic stress marks' (Kingdon, 1939); the syllables *can* and *force* are marked in the transcription with a mark indicating a low fall and a low rise, respectively.

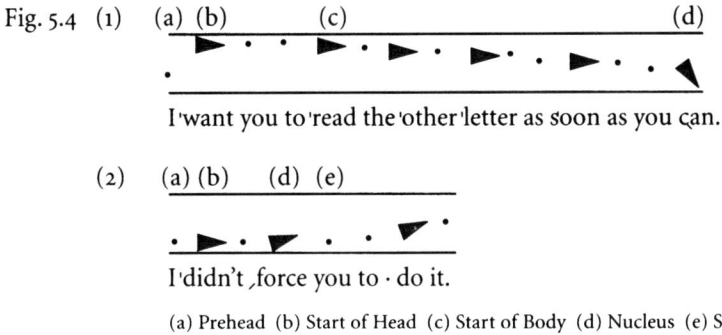

Fig. 5.4 (1)   (a) (b)   (c)   (d)

I'want you to'read the'other'letter as soon as you can.

(2)   (a) (b)   (d) (e)

I'didn't ,force you to · do it.

(a) Prehead (b) Start of Head (c) Start of Body (d) Nucleus (e) Start of Tail

The same tradition is followed by O'Connor and Arnold (1961), in a widely-used textbook. They similarly recognize Preheads, Heads, Nuclear Tones, and Tails (the Body is not given independent status), and list ten possible combinations of these as the major patterns of English intonation. Their Tone Group 6, for example, has an optional low Prehead, an optional low Head, an obligatory low–rising Nuclear Tone, and an optional Tail; Tone Group 4 has a high–falling Nuclear Tone, preceded by a stepping or high falling Head, or else by a high Prehead, and so on. Fig. 5.5 illustrates one possibility for this latter tone-group (large dots are accented syllables, and small dots unaccented ones; filled dots are obligatory for this pattern, and unfilled dots optional).

[10] Palmer's pedagogical aim is reflected in the picturesque mnemonic labels—he describes them as 'fanciful'—that he gives to these patterns: Cascade, Dive, Ski-jump, Wave, Snake, and Swan. More puzzlingly, he justifies his reversion to unified patterns on the grounds of adequacy, since it is the result of 'new facts about intonation that have since come to light' (Palmer, 1933: 1).

Fig. 5.5

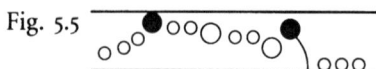

Whatever their pedagogical utility, a major weakness of these descriptions from a phonological perspective is that no clear distinction is made between phonological segmentation of the pattern into independent distinctive parts on the one hand, and phonetic segmentation into convenient descriptive segments on the other. Neither Kingdon nor Schubiger considers this question explicitly, as discussion of such theoretical matters lies outside their pedagogical aims.

As far as the actual patterns themselves are concerned, Klinghardt and Klemm (1920) and Armstrong and Ward (1926) are mainly concerned with the difference between falling and rising patterns (Armstrong and Ward describe these as Tune I and Tune II respectively, and Kingdon reverses the numbers), but Palmer (1922) identifies four different 'nucleus tones' (high fall, low fall, rise and rise–fall) and three different heads (inferior, superior, and scandent), and notes ten different combinations (the rise–fall nucleus occurs only with the scandent head). O'Connor and Arnold (1961) recognize two preheads, four heads, and six nuclear tones, but these are grouped, as we saw above, into ten combinations.

The British approach received a more theoretical treatment by being incorporated into the 'Scale and Category' (later 'Systemic') framework of Halliday. Halliday's work on intonation (Halliday, 1963a, 1963b, 1967, 1970) has been extremely influential, not least because, in addition to being explicitly phonological, providing a set of categories for the phonological description of intonation, it also places these categories within an overall model of language structure and meaning.[11] Halliday's descriptive categories are entirely compatible with the British tradition; in fact, they are the same as those of Palmer, the latter's 'head' and 'nucleus' being renamed 'pretonic' and 'tonic'. But Halliday goes further, identifying the phonological choices that speakers make in using intonation, and the grammatical choices that underlie them. These choices, to which Halliday gives the names 'tonality', 'tonicity', and 'tone', relate to the division of an utterance into tone-groups, the location of the intonational nucleus ('tonic') within the tone-group, and the choice of intonation pattern, respectively.

5.3.3 AMERICAN STRUCTURALIST ANALYSES

Bloomfield (1935) interprets intonation in terms of 'secondary phonemes' (phonemes which characterize larger combinations), in this case phonemes of pitch. For English, he recognizes five such phonemes: fall [.], rise [?], lesser rise [¿],

---

[11] Halliday might be said to have been unfortunate, inasmuch as the development of his own Systemic model coincided with the irresistible rise of transformational-generative grammar in the 1960s, by which it was largely eclipsed. Since the standard theory of generative grammar provided no viable model of intonation, however (see below), Halliday's framework has remained popular even among scholars who have rejected his Systemic model.

exclamatory pitch [!], and suspension [,], the first three of which occur at the end of the sentence, while the last two occur either in combination with these or in a non-final position, respectively. Harris (1944) attempts to apply more rigorous procedures, giving numerical values to the pitch levels of individual syllables (for example 1221130—3 is highest, 0 is lowest—for *I don't know where he's going*), but systematically reducing these on distributional grounds, so that pitch 2 is 'an allophone of pitch 1 in stressed position', while pitch 4 always occurs with contrastive stress and can also be regarded as an allophone of pitch 1. In this way, Harris is able to reduce the number of possible pitch sequences to a relatively small number. However, he concludes that, unlike the situation with segmental phonemes, 'each of these pitch sequences is a single component whose length is that of the whole utterance or phrase. This is permissible since the successive parts of the sequence are not independent of each other (e.g. before 30, only 1's occur) and may all be considered parts of one element.' Thus Harris does not ultimately recognize any phonological structure for the intonation pattern.

By far the most important American contribution, however, is that of Pike (1945), which, together with that of Wells (1945), creates the basis for the 'phonemic' analysis of intonation. Both conveniently come to the same conclusion: that four distinctive ('phonemic'), relative, pitch levels[12] can be established for American English, and that these can be grouped together into patterns, or *contours*. According to Pike, these pitch levels constitute *contour points* in the pattern. The most important contours, usually occurring at the end of the utterance, are called *primary contours*. The first contour point in a primary contour (the *beginning point*) occurs on a 'heavily stressed syllable'; the contour ends with an *ending point*, while some contours also have a *direction-change point* in between. The primary contour may be preceded by an unstressed *precontour*, the two together forming a *total contour*. Unlike Harris, therefore, Pike recognizes a *structure* for the intonation pattern. His analysis is illustrated in Fig. 5.6, which contains two such total contours. The contour points in each contour are joined by hyphens, and the beginning point of the primary contour is preceded by °.

Fig. 5.6 *The doctor bought a car*
  3–   °2–4–3 4–   °2–4

The approach of Wells (1945) is quite similar to that of Pike, though the theoretical framework is more apparent; Wells calls his analysis the application to pitch of 'all the principles and methods of segmental phonemics'. Pitch phonemes are grouped into sequences which constitute morphemes; this means that the contour as a whole has no *phonological* status. The usual American English

---

[12] Pike numbers these levels from the top down, with 1 = extra-high and 4 = low. Wells adopts the reverse numbering. The latter convention has prevailed.

contour is given as 231, with pitch 3 occurring on the main stress. Trager and Smith (1951) follow the lead of Wells, recognizing four pitches, each of which can have allophones which are slightly higher or lower. At the end of each contour various modifications occur which can be attributed to one of three *terminal junctures*: 'single-bar' /|/, 'double-bar' /||/, and 'double cross' /#/. The unit which is characterized by the contour is a *phonemic clause*. A representation of the utterance 'How do they study?' in these terms is given as Fig. 5.7.

Fig. 5.7 /²hǽw+də+ðèy+³stɔ́diyʼ#/

Though devised for English, this approach has been applied to a number of other languages, for example Spanish (Stockwell, Bowen, and Silva-Fuertalida, 1956), German (Moulton, 1962), and Italian (Agard and Pietro, 1965). In all cases, a number of pitch phonemes are recognized , as well as terminal junctures.

5.3.4 INTONATION IN GENERATIVE GRAMMAR

Intonation does not figure prominently in the classical framework of generative phonology. Stockwell (1960) tries to reconcile the Trager/Smith analysis with the formal framework of Chomsky's early transformational model (Chomsky, 1957), with the help of five additional rules (see Fig. 5.8). To provide for the fact that each sentence has an intonation pattern, Chomsky's initial rule (S → NP + VP) is modified to Rule 1 in Fig. 5.8; the syntactic structure of the sentence is represented by Nuc which is rewritten as NP + VP as before. The Intonation Pattern (IP) can then be generated by Rules 2 to 5, which spell out the possibilities. The pattern consists of a Contour (C) and a Juncture Point (JP); the Contour can represent either a Discontinuity or a Continuity; the former results in a falling pitch with a terminal fade, the latter in a final non-low pitch with a terminal fade, or a terminal rise.

Fig. 5.8 1. S   → Nuc + IP (Intonation Pattern)

2. IP   → C (Contour) + JP (Juncture Point)

3. C   → $\begin{Bmatrix} \text{Disc(ontinuity)} \\ \text{Cont(inuity)} \end{Bmatrix}$

4. Disc → 001↓ (=any fall to 1 + terminal fade; 0=any pitch phoneme)

5. Cont → $\begin{bmatrix} \begin{bmatrix} 002↓ \\ 003↓ \\ 004↓ \end{bmatrix} \\ \begin{bmatrix} 021↑ \\ 032{-}↑ \\ 043{-}↑ \end{bmatrix} \end{bmatrix}$

It will be clear that this attempt merely expresses the descriptive categories of

Trager and Smith (1951) in another form, and therefore does not make any real contribution to the phonology of intonation itself. It assumes that there is one intonation pattern for every sentence, and, by separating syntax and intonation with an early rule, completely divorces the intonation pattern from the rest of the sentence. Subsequent work, summarized by Stockwell (1972), is rather more sophisticated, focusing less on the phonological form of intonation and more on the way in which intonation units may be derived from syntactic structure (cf. for example Bierwisch, 1966; Downing, 1970), thus integrating the rules for intonation with those of syntactic structure. An intensive debate in the early 1970s tried to determine how the location of the 'sentence stress' might be derived via syntactic rules, though it failed to resolve the issues adequately (Bresnan, 1971, 1972; Lakoff, 1972; Berman and Szamosi, 1972; Bolinger, 1972). As for the patterns themselves, Yorio (1973) suggests that these could be derived from rather abstract underlying structures involving performative verbs (cf. Austin, 1962; Ross, 1970). Thus, an utterance such as *This is a chair*, with a falling intonation, could be derived from something like *I declare that this is a chair*, while with a rising intonation it could be derived from *I ask if this is a chair*. Most linguists have found such proposals to be completely inadequate and unproductive.

5.3.5 THE LUND SCHOOL

Whatever the fate of these attempts to incorporate intonation into generative grammar, the principle that intonation patterns can be generated by the use of an appropriate algorithm has been widely adopted. One application of this is in the synthesis of artificial intonation contours, which has been undertaken by a number of scholars. Among these are Fujisaki and his colleagues, working on Japanese (e.g. Fujisaki and Nagashima, 1969), and especially Gårding and her associates at Lund (Bruce, 1977; Bruce and Gårding, 1978; Gårding, 1981, 1983), working primarily on Swedish and other Scandinavian languages.

Since Gårding's model was initially applied to Swedish, it has to deal not only with intonation but also the tonal accents of that language. It is 'based on an analysis which separates lexical prosody from phrase and sentence prosody' (Gårding, 1983), Thus, 'the input to the model is a sentence, equipped with markings for lexical accents or tones, accents (tones) at phrase and sentence level, morphological and phrase boundaries, and the mode of sentence intonation'. The principle is that 'all these factors combine and interact to produce the final temporal and tonal pattern of the actual speech signal'. In order to effect this interaction, Gårding assumes a top-down model of pitch assignment, in which the pitch features (high and low pitches) of the tonal accents are super-imposed on those of the phrase–accents, and the latter are superimposed on the overall sentence intonation. This is reduced to the informal algorithm given in Fig. 5.9.

Fig. 5.9   Rule 1.   *Sentence and phrase intonation*
Draw the tonal grid using sentence and major phrase boundaries

Rule 2.   *Sentence and phrase boundaries*
Insert highs and lows on the grid according to language and dialect

Rule 3.   *Sentence and phrase accent*
Insert highs and lows on the grid according to language and dialect

Rule 4.   *Word accent*
Insert highs and lows on the grid according to language and dialect

Rule 5.   *Contrastive word accent*
Adjust highs and lows according to language and dialect

Rule 6.   *Context rules*
Adjust highs and lows according to context

Rule 7.   *Concatenation*
Connect neighbouring generated highs and lows

In Fig. 5.9, Rule 1 creates a 'tonal grid', which is described as 'the global frame for the sentence intonation within which the local pitch movements can develop,' while Rules 2, 3, and 4 insert the pitch peaks and troughs on this grid corresponding to the sentence and phrase boundaries, the sentence and phrase accents, and the word accents, respectively. A grid of this kind is depicted in Fig. 5.10, where the broken lines represent the top and bottom of the normal pitch range, and the solid lines indicate the top and bottom values for normal accents within the phrase, the shape produced by the latter depending on the intonation pattern used. The dots indicate the highs and lows of the accents (cf. Gårding, 1983).

Fig. 5.10

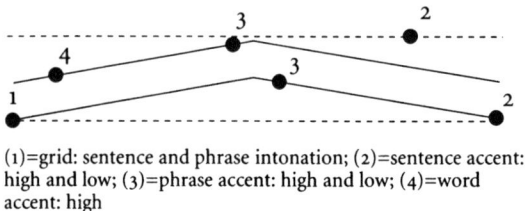

(1)=grid: sentence and phrase intonation; (2)=sentence accent: high and low; (3)=phrase accent: high and low; (4)=word accent: high

A characteristic of this model is that it separates accentual from intonational features in the input to the algorithm, but it explicitly allows for the integration of intonation with other pitch features and with the accentual features of the utterance as the algorithm is applied. A drawback is that it does not specifically identify the phonologically relevant characteristics of the intonation pattern, thus limiting its applicability as a phonological model of intonation The focus is on the process whereby an intonation pattern is generated on the basis of accentual and tonal features; the phonological features of the intonation pattern itself are less central, and in fact the model does not distinguish consistently between significant and insignificant pitch features.

The model has been applied to other languages besides Swedish, including Greek, French, and Chinese (Gårding, 1983; 1984). The algorithm is applied in a comparable fashion in each case, with a similar grid onto which accentual and tonal features are superimposed, though the details differ according to the specific pitch features of the different languages.

5.3.6 THE DUTCH SCHOOL

Among other proposed models, that adopted by researchers at the Institute for Perception Research at Eindhoven (IPO) is worthy of mention (Cohen and 't Hart, 1967; 't Hart and Cohen, 1973; 't Hart and Collier, 1975; 't Hart, Collier, and Cohen, 1990). This approach has a different starting point from that of most other schools, since it begins not with assumed phonologically distinct categories but rather with *perceptually* relevant features. Thus, the question asked here is 'Which properties of the acoustic signal are relevant for our perception of speech melody?' ('t Hart, Collier, and Cohen, 1990: 5).

In order to determine what the perceptually relevant properties of intonation are, the IPO approach adopts a methodology which involves the resynthesis of analysed intonation patterns using stylized pitch patterns. The principle here is to create stylized patterns which are simpler than, but perceptually equivalent to, the original, thus identifying the perceptually relevant features and eliminating imperceptible 'microintonation phenomena' (the minor rises and falls associated with individual segments and syllables). The assumption is not merely that such pitch fluctuations are not perceived, but also that their production is involuntary and not deliberate; thus, 'the F_0 curves that do contribute essentially to the perception of the speech melody are just those changes that are programmed and voluntarily executed by the speaker' ('t Hart, Collier, and Cohen, 1990: 40).

It may be questioned, however, whether the elaborate justification of intonational features on the basis of perceptual categories is really necessary. Though the analysis is claimed to be perceptually based, perception is inevitably largely determined by the phonologically relevant categories of the language in question, which are logically prior. Furthermore, it is acknowledged that not all pitch movements that are perceived are necessarily phonologically significant; the pitch movement must 'not only be above some psychophysical threshold, but at the same time be recognized as the result of some purposeful action on the speaker's side' ('t Hart, Collier, and Cohen, 1990: 70). Thus, in practice the IPO analysis is not really very different from other analyses which seek to establish phonologically relevant categories for intonation.

As far as the phonological analysis of the patterns themselves is concerned, the basic unit of intonation within this framework is the pitch *movement*, since this is claimed to be 'the smallest unit of perceptual analysis' ('t Hart, Collier, and Cohen, 1990: 72). The IPO approach thus rejects pitch 'levels' as the basic elements of intonation: 'we reject the alternative view that the speaker primarily intends to hit a particular pitch level' ('t Hart, Collier, and Cohen, 1990: 74). The pitch movement can, however, be decomposed into perceptual features, along a number of dimensions: direction, timing, rate of change, and size, along each of which the movement can be resolved into a number of discrete values, with precise phonetic definitions. For Dutch, for example, 't Hart, Collier, and Cohen (1990: 73) identify five different rising movements (labelled with Arabic numerals) and five falling movements (labelled with capital letters), which differ among themselves along the other dimensions. Movement 1 is an early, fast, full rise; movement 3 a late, fast, full rise; movement E an early, fast, half fall, and so on. Where there is more than one movement on a single syllable, the symbols can be linked, giving A&2, 5&A, B&1, and so on. Similar sets of movements can be established for other languages (on English see Pijper, 1983).

Pitch movements combine into *configurations*, though not all combinations of movements are found. According to 't Hart, Collier, and Cohen (1990: 78), 'rise "1" can be followed by fall "A" or "B", but never by fall "C". Fall "C" has to be preceded by rise "3", but the inverse is not true: rise "3" can also be followed by fall "B" ', and so on. A configuration belongs to one of three classes: *prefix*, *root*, or *suffix*, which combine into a *contour*. Prefix and suffix are optional, and the prefix may be recursive. Thus, the contour is constructed according to the formula (Prefix)^n Root (Suffix). This scheme invites comparison with the structures described in other frameworks, in particular the British nuclear tone approach, though it is evident that the pattern is here built up from its component parts in a manner which is not found in British analyses. The limited number of actually occurring contours can be generated by means of a complex transition network which specifies the permitted combinations of these

Fig. 5.11

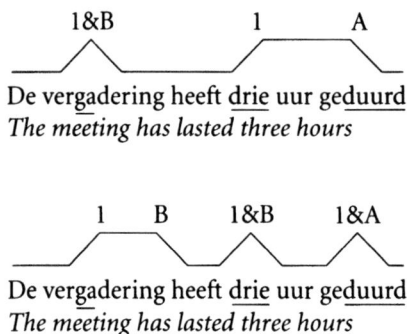

1&B   1 A

De vergadering heeft <u>drie</u> uur ge<u>duurd</u>
The meeting has lasted three hours

1 B 1&B 1&A

De vergadering heeft <u>drie</u> uur ge<u>duurd</u>
The meeting has lasted three hours

parts ('t Hart, Collier, and Cohen, 1990: 81). Examples of the analysis of actual patterns in these terms are given in Fig. 5.11.

5.3.7 INTONATION IN NON-LINEAR PHONOLOGY

More recently, intonation, like other prosodic features, has been interpreted in non-linear terms. Early work on intonation in this framework (Liberman, 1975; Goldsmith, 1976, 1978) recognizes 'tone melodies' which, like tone patterns in tone-languages (see 4.4.3), can be represented as a sequence of pitch levels— usually limited to High, Mid, and Low—on a separate autosegmental tier and linked to the string of syllables by rules of association. In order to align the pattern appropriately, Goldsmith adopts the 'star' convention used in the description of certain African languages (see 4.7.5), where tone is interpreted accentually. This enables him to capture the fact that the central part of the intonation pattern is associated with the main accent. Thus, assuming a basic melody Mid-High-Low, where the High pitch coincides with the nuclear accent, this is represented as M H* L. The nuclear accent of the utterance is similarly represented with a star, and the two marked elements are associated, as in Fig. 5.12.

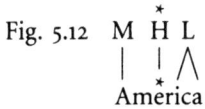

Fig. 5.12
$$
\begin{array}{ccc}
 & \overset{*}{\text{H}} & \\
\text{M} & \text{H} & \text{L} \\
| & | & \wedge \\
 & \overset{*}{\text{America}} &
\end{array}
$$

Longer utterances can be represented with a succession of such accents. An alternative question, such as the utterance 'Do you want coffee, tea, or milk?', with rising movements on the first two items and a fall on the last, is represented by Goldsmith as in Fig. 5.13 ($ represents a boundary).

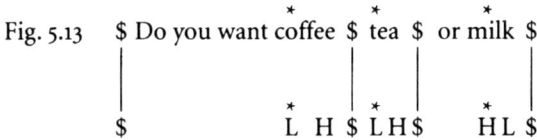

Fig. 5.13
$$
\begin{array}{c}
\overset{*}{}\quad\overset{*}{}\quad\overset{*}{} \\
\$ \text{ Do you want coffee } \$ \text{ tea } \$ \text{ or milk } \$ \\
| \qquad\qquad\qquad | \quad | \qquad | \\
| \qquad\qquad\;\; \overset{*}{}\; | \overset{*}{} | \;\; \overset{*}{} | \\
\$ \qquad\qquad\quad \text{L H } \$ \text{ LH} \$ \quad \text{HL } \$
\end{array}
$$

The most influential of recent non-linear contributions to intonation, however, has been the work of Pierrehumbert (1980). She adopts Goldsmith's star marking (each pattern with a star now being called a 'pitch–accent'), and adds a feature derived from the analysis of Swedish by Bruce (1977). Bruce seeks to reconcile the tonal accents of that language with the existence of intonational features by incorporating an intonational element (a 'phrase tone') *after* the tonal accents. Pierrehumbert applies this principle to English (where the pitch– accents do not, of course, have the tonal properties that the Swedish accents have), adding such a phrase tone after the last pitch–accent. Another principle which, according to Goldsmith (1978), derives from an idea by Sag, is to associate the final pitch feature with the boundary itself (a 'boundary tone'). All these various elements are combined, and English intonation patterns are represented as a sequence of pitch–accents, followed by a phrase tone and a boundary tone. The location of the pitch–accents is determined by the metrical structure of the utterance, a principle taken from Liberman and Prince (1977). Thus, a simple phrase such as *an orange ballgown*, pronounced with a neutral declarative intonation, can be assigned the pattern H* H* L L%, with two H* pitch–accents (on *o* and *ball*), a L phrase tone and a final L boundary tone (L%).

Pierrehumbert's model has been widely applied and developed (e.g. in Beckman and Pierrehumbert, 1986, Pierrehumbert and Beckman, 1988, and Ladd, 1996), and its transcriptional conventions, as applied to English, have been coded as the 'ToBI' (Tone and Break Index) system (Silverman et al., 1992; Pitrelli, Beckman, and Hirschberg, 1994).[13] Again, though the framework is rather different from others, there are parallels with other analytical frameworks, allowing conversion between them (cf. Roach, 1994). We shall consider aspects of this model further in the discussion in the remainder of this chapter.

5.4 The Analysis of Intonation

5.4.1 THE INTONATION UNIT

Having surveyed briefly some of the major approaches to the description of intonational phonology, we may now proceed to a more detailed examination of the specific proposals made. The starting point for the analysis of intonation is the concept of an *intonation unit*. All scholars who are concerned with intonation have identified—either overtly or tacitly— such a unit, variously called the 'sprechtakt' (Klinghardt), 'breath-group' (Jones), 'tone-group' (Palmer, Armstrong, and Ward, O'Connor and Arnold, Halliday), 'rhythm unit' (Pike), 'phonemic clause' (Trager and Smith), 'tone-unit' (Crystal), 'intonation-group' (Cruttenden), 'intonation phrase' (Pierrehumbert), among other terms. The neutral term *intonation unit* will be used here, though, as we shall see, this term may become ambiguous if more than one such unit is recognized. The intonation pattern associated with such a unit has been called a 'melody' (Klinghardt), a 'tune' (Armstrong and Ward), a 'tone-pattern' (Palmer), a 'contour' (Pike), among other terms.

Exactly which part of the sentence or utterance this unit corresponds to has been variously interpreted. The major question here is whether the unit is established on the basis of grammatical structure, or is essentially independent of this structure. There is certainly some correlation with grammatical units, especially

---

[13] This system is intended primarily for the annotation of prosodic features in computer corpora rather than as a phonological transcription system. It will therefore not be considered further here.

the clause,[14] and this leads some scholars to regard this as the norm.[15] However, because this correlation is frequently absent, many scholars regard the intonation unit as corresponding not to a grammatical unit, but to a 'sense-group' (Armstrong and Ward, O'Connor and Arnold) or 'information unit' (Halliday), which may have a variable relationship to syntactic units. Attempts have been made (e.g. by Lieberman, 1965, and Bierwisch, 1966) to derive intonation units by rule from syntactic structure, but these can only deal with arbitrarily-defined 'default' cases.

For our present purposes we are concerned not with any possible syntactic or discourse relevance of the intonation unit, but rather with its phonological characteristics. One of its properties, which we considered in Chapter 3, is that it is also a unit of accentuation, an 'accent phrase'. This means that it has a single 'sentence accent' (this term is, of course, inappropriate) or, in the terms used in Chapter 3, a Level 2 accent. The fact that the same unit is both accentual and intonational is, of course, significant for the relationship between accent and intonation. As far as the intonational characteristics of the unit are concerned, it has been said that there is a unity of pattern within it; what this means is that the intonation unit has a single intonation pattern, though this is, of course, circular, since a pattern may be defined as the pitch associated with the unit postulated. Nevertheless, the point is a valid one, if we interpret it as implying that the pitch pattern of the intonation unit has a certain internal structure, as will become clearer below. Another characteristic claimed for the unit, in those theoretical frameworks which include such a notion, is that it is bounded by a 'terminal juncture', or a 'phrase boundary'.

The term 'intonation-unit' implies that there is only one such unit, but this is not necessarily the case, and a number of scholars have suggested that there may be other units, which are hierarchically ordered. Trim (1959, 1964), for example, distinguishes 'major' and 'minor' tone-groups, the former consisting of combinations of the latter. A larger unit than the tone-group is suggested in Fox (1973, 1984b) on the basis of sequences of patterns; Beckman and Pierrehumbert (1986) introduce, in addition to their 'intonational phrase', a smaller 'intermediate phrase', initially for Japanese, but also for English. The equivalence between the different units established by different scholars is not always easy to establish, but there is at least some evidence for more complex intonation structures, which will be discussed below. This question has also been broached above in connection with accentual structure (3.4.2.2), where the possibility of higher

---

[14] Crystal (1969: 257–63) provides some statistics regarding the correlation between clauses and intonation units. In a comparison of English and German intonation (Fox, 1978: 519), a correspondence was found between clause and intonation unit in a quarter to a third of cases. In German data, the correspondence was found in about half of cases.

[15] Halliday (1967: 18–19) considers the correspondence of tone-group and clause to be the 'neutral term' in his 'tonality system'; non-correspondence is 'marked tonality'. Since, however, in some constructions non-correspondence is the norm, 'neutral tonality' may be functionally marked.

'degrees' of accentuation, resulting from subordination of intonation units to one another, was considered.

5.4.2 INTONATION AND ACCENTUATION

In 3.4 the accentual structure of utterances was discussed, and a distinction was made between Level 1 accentuation, involving rhythmical prominence in languages such as English, and Level 2 accentuation, found in many more languages, which characterizes a whole phrase. As we have observed, Level 2 accentuation has implications for intonation, since this 'tonic accent' (Arnold, 1957a, 1957b; Garde, 1968) corresponds to the nucleus of the British descriptive tradition, and thus constitutes the pivotal point of the intonation pattern. This applies not only in English but also in many other languages which do not have the accentual structure of English.

But there are also implications for intonation in Level 1 prominence, which, as we have noted, is a matter of rhythmical prominence at a lower level than the nucleus. Though this kind of accentuation has, of course, received ample discussion in works on stress, its significance for intonation has been somewhat neglected. One point that is seldom made, for example, is that there is a relationship between the intonation unit and the principle of isochrony, which defines the foot (see 2.9.3). It appears that the intonation unit is the unit over which isochrony is maintained. A new foot-length can therefore be established for each new intonation unit (Rees, 1975).

As far as the relevance of Level 1 accentuation for intonation is concerned, we have already observed that early writers on English intonation, such as Klinghardt, Armstrong and Ward, and others, do not subdivide the intonation group, but they nevertheless indicate the pitch of stressed syllables differently from that of unstressed syllables. It is clear, in fact, that the main burden of the intonation pattern, in a language such as English, is carried by the accented syllables. This is manifested phonetically in a number of ways. First, in an intonation unit with a number of pre-nuclear stresses, there tends to be a falling trend, with each stressed syllable pronounced at a slightly lower pitch. Kingdon (1958b: 63), for example, gives such a stepping sequence—given as Fig. 5.4—as 'the basic intonation of English', and a similar effect is noticeable in the example from Armstrong and Ward given as Fig. 5.5. The stressed syllables thus have a key role in the phonetic structure of the pattern. Second, and more significantly, in cases where there is no such simple falling (or rising) trend, and the pitch is more varied within the foot, successive feet tend to show a similar pattern. Again, some of the early auditory analyses demonstrate this principle; Palmer's 'broken scandent head' for example, consists of a series of rises. A similar phenomenon is recognized by Halliday (1967), several of whose 'pretonics' have a repeated foot-shape, for example, his 'bouncing' and 'listing' pretonics to his falling tone, Tone 1, both of which have a repeated rising foot movement. The same is found in other languages, though the typical foot pattern may be different. Such a situation naturally only occurs in languages which have this form of Level 1 accentuation; in French, there is, of course, no such accent, and no such recurrent pattern. Pierrehumbert's 'pitch–accents' also demonstrate the role of accentuation in the intonation patterns of English, with each such accent being associated with a metrically strong syllable.

Level 1 accentuation, and hence the foot, can thus be shown to have a significant role in the phonetic structure of the intonation unit. It is this that allows the use of such devices as 'tonetic stress marks' (Kingdon, 1939; Trim, 1964), where the stress mark is simultaneously an indication of the pitch pattern of the foot. It is therefore also possible to see each foot as a kind of intonation unit. This is the principle underlying the recognition of the 'minor tone-groups' of Trim (1959, 1964), mentioned above.[16]

5.4.3 THE ELEMENTS OF INTONATION

5.4.3.1 Introduction: Tunes

For some scholars, especially early writers on the subject, the pattern *as a whole* is the basic unit of intonation. In this approach, which we find in the works of Klinghardt and others (Klinghardt and Klemm, 1920; Barker, 1925; Armstrong and Ward, 1926), internal features may be recognized within the pattern, such as different pitch levels for stressed and unstressed syllables, and different pitches for syllables before the first stress and after the last stress, but these are seen as matters of phonetic detail. As we have noted, a number of different 'tunes' are recognized in this framework, each of which can be assigned a meaning; this view is also taken in some of the work of Bolinger, where specific discourse functions, for example 'accosting questions' (Bolinger, 1948) are assigned a range of patterns, with no attempt made to divide up the pattern into significant parts. Similarly, Liberman and Sag (1974) identify a 'contradiction contour' as a whole pattern with a specific contradictory meaning.

Those scholars who describe intonation in this way do allow for variant structures, where one or other part of the tune is absent. Armstrong and Ward (1926), for example, treat all of the illustrations of Fig. 5.14 as instances of 'Tune I'. These all have in common the falling pitch on the last accented syllable, but, since the parts are not considered to be independent, there is no grouping of *different* patterns together on the basis of some common feature.

---

[16] Bolinger (1955); suggests a different kind of interdependence between intonation and accentuation. According to him, the alternative pronunciation of words such as *'absolutely* as *abso'lutely* constitutes a case of intonation determining stress rather than the reverse; the former replaces the latter, and 'pitch allophones' are 'in complementary distribution with intensity allophones'. However, Bolinger's interpretation of this phenomenon is not the only one; a more plausible analysis is that the emphatic version involves a shift of accent rather than primarily of intonation, and the pitch features move with the accent.

Fig. 5.14 'Yes.

I can 'see it.

Quite 'right.

'Here's a pretty kettle of fish!

They 'came a to 'call 'yesteray 'after 'noon.

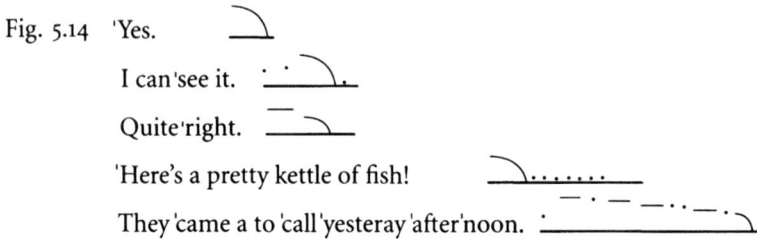

A related characteristic of intonation patterns is that they may expand or contract according to the amount of segmental material within the intonation unit. Thus, not only are patterns with different parts regarded as the same (as in Fig. 5.14), but also patterns which have exactly the same parts but differ in length. A characteristic example is the English 'rise–fall–rise' pattern, illustrated in Fig. 5.15, which can occur on a single syllable or upon a whole utterance. This expandability/compressibility of patterns[17] means that the pattern is in principle independent of the segmental or syllabic structure of the unit.

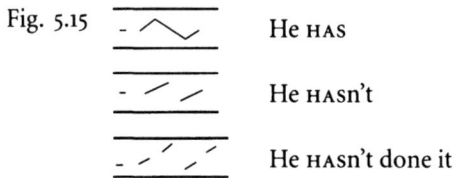

Fig. 5.15

He HAS

He HASn't

He HASn't done it

However, despite the flexibility demonstrated here, an approach which sees the pattern of the intonation unit as an indivisible whole does not seem to be very satisfactory. In the first place, there are many different patterns, with both similarities and differences between them, and these differences and similarities are localizable in specific parts of the pattern. Standard principles of linguistic analysis demand that we establish a structure with substitutable parts. Second, there must also at least be points in the pattern which must be aligned with appropriate parts of the utterance, and with other prosodic features. All of this suggests that the intonation pattern has a structure, and that it can be broken down into parts which have some degree of independence. This is, in fact, the assumption made by the majority of scholars, though they do not necessarily agree on the nature or scope of the parts, as we shall see in the course of this discussion.

In order to establish the structure of intonation patterns, we must first determine the nature of the elements in terms of which this structure is to be described. It is here, however, that some of the major differences arise between the various descriptive frameworks, with some scholars favouring elements of mini-

---

[17] Ladd (1996: 133–6) proposes the possibility of compression (vs. truncation) of patterns as a typological criterion for intonation systems. Cf. 5.8.1, below.

mal scope and others recognizing larger entities. There is, of course, a reciprocal relationship between the elements postulated and the structures which they are assumed to constitute: the simpler and more basic the elements, the more complex the structures that must be recognized to accommodate them. Hence, recognition of minimal elements does not necessarily achieve a more economical analysis, since it is balanced by the need to establish more complex combinations. Given this relationship between elements and structures, it is impractical to consider them separately, and we shall therefore consider the issues surrounding both of these under the same headings in what follows.

5.4.3.2 Pitch Phonemes and Pitch Levels

For Pike and the American structuralist tradition the basic elements of the intonation contour are specific points in the pattern, and, since these are just points, with no extent in time, the contrastive possibilities here differ only in their pitch level. Four levels are recognized by the majority of scholars in this framework. These 'pitch phonemes' are not in themselves meaningful; as Pike (1945: 26) puts it, 'it is the intonation contour as a whole which carries the meaning while the pitch levels contribute end points, beginning points or direction-change points to the contours—and as such are basic building blocks which contribute to the contours and hence contribute to the meaning'. Although contours containing certain pitch levels (e.g. level 1, the highest) may have some aspect of meaning in common (in the case of level 1, 'some element of surprise or unexpectedness'), Pike notes that more satisfactory generalizations can be made by grouping whole contours together which have a similar form. However, the basic elements of intonation are for Pike the pitch phonemes ('contour points') themselves.

For Wells (1945), and for other American structuralists such as Trager and Smith (1951) and Hockett (1955), the contour as a whole is an intonation *morpheme*, with no phonological status. However, the contour also includes terminal junctures, which constitute another kind of phonemic element. Trager and Smith (1951: 50) transcribe the utterance *How do they study?*, spoken with a rising intonation, as in Fig. 5.7, repeated here as Fig. 5.16, with the pitch phonemes /2 3 1/ followed by the 'double-cross' juncture /#/ indicating a terminal fall (note that Trager and Smith reverse Pike's numbers for pitch levels, so that 1 = low). For Trager and Smith, the pitch of the first three syllables, though rising slightly and therefore different in each case, can be regarded as phonemically the same, and, furthermore, there is only *one* occurrence of this phoneme, which consequently has 'scope'. Again, therefore, the basic element of intonation is the pitch phoneme, though with the addition of the terminal juncture phoneme. The whole contour is not a phonological element, since 'on the level of phonemics there are no such things as "intonations"' (p. 52).

Fig. 5.16 /²hǽw+də+ðèy+³stɑ́diy¹#/

Similarly, Hockett (1955: 45–51) describes English intonation in terms of three pitch phonemes (the fourth level of Pike and others is catered for by a phoneme of 'extra height') and three 'terminal contours', one of which is neutral (|) and has no effect on the pitch, while the other two provide for a final fall (↓) and a final rise (↑), respectively. Thus, an English utterance such as *It's three o'clock*, with a falling intonation, can be analysed as in Fig. 5.17(a), while *Is it three o'clock?*, with a rising intonation, is analysed as in Fig. 5.17(b).

Fig. 5.17   (a)   *²It's three o'³¹clock* ↓
            (b)   *²Is it three o'³³clock* ↑

The motivation for this approach is that pitch phonemes are *minimal*: the elements of the pattern are reduced to their minimal extent, and there are minimal contrasts between them. Analyses in these terms can thus claim to identify the basic, irreducible components of the pattern, and to be highly economical. This doubtless explains the continued use of levels in more recent theories, such as non-linear phonology. Liberman describes English intonation in terms of three contrasting levels (H, M, L) occurring at specific points, and Pierrehumbert specifies her pitch–accents and other pitch features in terms of an even more reduced set of contrasting levels, with a binary distinction between H(igh) and L(ow), though in the latter analysis larger units—the pitch–accents themselves—are also recognized. In order to accommodate the wide range of phonetically occurring pitch levels under the two levels, H and L, Pierrehumbert uses a number of other principles, such as *downstep*, whereby the level of a H tone is reduced following a L (see below).

Although the claims of such analyses to present a highly economical phonological description are considerable, other approaches have rejected them either as psychologically implausible, or as failing to allow the necessary generalizations across different patterns. These points will be taken up below.

5.4.3.3 Pitch Movements, 'Configurations', and Nuclear Tones

The 'nuclear tone' approach to intonational description has been widely adopted, and not merely in the British tradition, where it originated. Like the pitch phoneme approach, it recognizes that the most significant intonational feature is associated with the main accent of the phrase, but there the similarity ends, since it takes the whole shape, from the position of this accent onwards, as the distinctive element of the pattern. A division is often made between the nucleus proper (the pitch movement on the accented syllable) and the *tail*, but the latter is not regarded as phonologically distinctive; it is simply a means of specifying the phonetic shape of the pattern. The different pitch patterns associated with the nucleus are the 'nuclear tones' and a limited set of such tones is recognized for specific languages. They take the form of pitch *movements*, with labels indicating shapes, such as 'rise', 'fall', 'rise–fall', 'fall–rise', 'rise–fall–rise', etc., and also, where necessary, the height or range of the movement: 'high fall', 'narrow rise', etc. No two of the major analyses of English intonation within this framework have exactly the same set of tones; the differences derive largely from the different ways in which the phonetic pitch patterns are grouped together, for example, whether a high and a low fall are treated as two separate tones or as variant forms of the same tone.

Since the nuclear tone covers only the pitch pattern from the nuclear accent onwards, the part of the pattern preceding the nucleus is dealt with separately, as the *head*, though this is regarded as of secondary importance, since the main character of the pattern is determined by the nuclear tone, and the head is in any case optional. Again, a variety of different head-patterns are recognized by different scholars, differing in a number of ways, for example 'high', 'low', 'falling', 'rising', etc. Some of these heads may be phonetically quite complex, with various rises and falls coinciding, in languages with accents, with each accented syllable. In these cases it is not strictly true to say, therefore, that the head is a pitch *movement* in the sense that the nuclear tone is; it is rather a *sequence* of movements, which may be repeated as many times as there are accented syllables.

One further part of the whole pattern is also noted in this analysis: the *pre-head*, which consists of the unstressed syllables preceding the first accent of the head (or the nucleus itself, if there is no head).[18] Its distinctive status is marginal, and the possibilities are very limited. O'Connor and Arnold (1961) distinguish a 'high' and a 'low' prehead, but an inspection of the possible patterns given by them (p. vi) shows that these two are in complementary distribution.

Other approaches, which do not necessarily recognize nuclear tones, nevertheless regard the intonation pattern as consisting of movements rather than points. Delattre, Poenack, and Olsen (1965), for example, divide up the German pattern for 'continuation' into a number of essential sections (together forming the outline of a bird), but these sections are clearly phonetic elements and their phonological status is doubtful. Similarly, scholars working in the tradition of the Dutch school of analysis recognize movements as the basic elements. The work of 't Hart, Collier, and Cohen (1990) operates with pitch movements as 'the smallest unit of perceptual analysis' (p. 72). These movements—different kinds of rising and falling pitches—form 'configurations' (Prefix, Root, and Suffix) which are in turn concatenated into 'contours'. Another approach may also be mentioned which recognizes pitch movements, but reduces them to minimal terms: that of Isačenko and Schädlich (1966). They describe German intonation in terms of binary switches between high and low pitch (or the reverse), together with a timing distinction (the switch may be pre-ictic—before the accent—or post-ictic—after the accent). Whether this rather basic system can do justice to all the pitch patterns found in languages is doubtful, however.

---

[18] The prehead is not always considered to be completely unaccented; O'Connor and Arnold (1961: 22–3) allow the low prehead to contain stressed syllables in some cases, though they do not receive pitch prominence and are therefore not, in their terms, 'accented'.

5.4.3.4 Pitch–Accents, Phrase Tones, and Boundary Tones

The approach represented by the non-linear framework of Pierrehumbert (1980) and related works is in some ways intermediate between the pitch phoneme approach on the one hand and the nuclear tone approach on the other. Here, the intonation pattern is analysed in terms of *pitch–accents*; each pattern thus consists of one or more such accents, which may in turn consist of either one or two *tones*. The tones are restricted to a binary H vs. L. In the case of bi-tonal accents, one of the tones is starred so as to coincide with a metrically strong syllable. We thus may have H*, L*, H*+L, H+L*, L*+H, L+H* as possible pitch–accent types.[19] However, although these accents form the basis of the pattern, no specific category of nucleus or nuclear tone is recognized. Hence the nucleus is no different from any other pitch–accent within the phrase. In frameworks which recognize a nucleus, nuclear tones have a special status, not merely accentually but also in terms of their pitch pattern. In Pierrehumbert's model, this is not the case. The special pitch features associated with the nucleus in these other frameworks are accommodated in Pierrehumbert's model by associating pitch features with either a *phrase accent* or a *boundary tone*. Thus, pitch features of the nuclear tones of the British tradition may correspond to features which are distributed over several different entities in Pierrehumbert's approach.

A number of alternative proposals have been made within this framework, though none of them radically alter the approach (for discussion, see Ladd, 1996: 89–98). The most significant for the present discussion of the elements of intonation patterns is the recognition, by Beckman and Pierrehumbert (1986), of a further intonation unit, the *intermediate phrase*. Beckman and Pierrehumbert introduce this unit as a result of work on Japanese, which, as we saw in 3.3.4, has no (Level 1) accentuation, but has a single (Level 2) accent for each accentual phrase. In their analysis, such accentual phrases are grouped together into intermediate phrases, and the latter into intonation phrases.

The idea of a hierarchy of phrases in Japanese is not new, since groups of units have been discussed by other scholars (e.g. Jorden and Chaplin, 1963—see the discussion in 3.3.4). However, the status of the various intonation elements recognized by Pierrehumbert—the phrase accent and the boundary tone—is also affected here, since the hierarchy of units implies a hierarchy of boundaries. The original phrase accent of Pierrehumbert (1980) can then be reanalysed as the boundary tone of a lower-ranking prosodic unit, the intermediate phrase. This analysis can also be applied to English; Beckman and Pierrehumbert claim that 'the phrase–accent plus boundary–tone configuration of Pierrehumbert (1980) should be reanalysed as involving correlates of two levels of phrasing. The phrase accent would then be a terminal tone for the intermediate phrase, while only the boundary tone is terminal to the intonation phrase.' The original analysis of a

---

[19] A further pitch–accent, H*+H, was postulated by Pierrehumbert (1980), but later eliminated.

falling intonation given in Fig. 5.18(a), with a pitch–accent (H*), a phrase accent (L), and a boundary tone (L%), is thus replaced by that of Fig. 5.18(b), with a pitch–accent (H*), an intermediate phrase boundary tone (L%), and an intonation phrase boundary (L%).

Fig. 5.18 (a) [H* L   L%]
         (b) [[H* L%] L%]

A further characteristic of Pierrehumbert's analysis is the treatment of *declination*, the gradual fall in pitch which is characteristic of most (though not all) utterances. This is equivalent to *downdrift* in tone-languages (see 4.2.2.3; 4.3.4.5; 4.5.3). In British pedagogical works it is often accommodated by incorporating such a fall into the head (see the examples given in Figs. 5.4 and 5.5, above). Pierrehumbert accounts for the phenomenon in English by allowing it to be the result of the lowering of a High tone after a Low tone, in the manner of downdrift and downstep in African languages.[20] Thus, the pitch–accent H*+L is used exclusively for the purpose of inducing pitch lowering in a following H tone. Use of this pitch–accent not only caters for declination; it also enables Pierrehumbert to reduce drastically the range of levels necessary to the minimum contrast H vs. L.

5.5 Issues in the Analysis of Intonation

5.5.1 INTRODUCTION

Each of the major approaches to the analysis of intonation patterns that we have considered has its own strengths and weaknesses, and it is therefore not possible to determine in a simple manner which of them is to be preferred. On the one hand, they are not entirely incompatible with one another; the same patterns can be described as an undivided whole, as a series of pitch movements, or as a succession of points, and indeed all these three analyses could be equally correct, in the sense of providing an unambiguous characterization of the pattern. On the other hand, the different analyses are clearly not entirely equivalent, since each framework provides a different range of possibilities and allows different generalizations to be made. It is largely in terms of the efficiency and significance of these generalizations that a comparative evaluation of the different models can be undertaken.

The major issues in the phonological analysis of intonation can be conveniently grouped under a small number of headings, reflecting disputes as to the

---

[20] Pierrehumbert (1980) uses the term *downstep* for this phenomenon, though whether it is really analogous to this concept in African languages (see 4.2.2.3, 4.3.3, 4.3.4.5, 4.5.3) is, as Beckman and Pierrehumbert (1986) acknowledge, at best doubtful. The latter suggest *catathesis* as an alternative term, 'out of deference to the Africanist usage'.

kinds of units to be recognized, the structural parts of the intonation patterns, and the appropriate analysis of the major pitch features of the pattern. These headings do not cover all the possible questions that could be discussed here, but they allow us to focus on the most significant issues. No attempt can be made, of course, to include discussion of all the various theoretical positions taken in the extensive literature on these issues; again, it is primarily the most influential theories that will be considered, with only occasional mention of alternative points of view.

5.5.2 LEVELS VS. CONFIGURATIONS

As we have seen, a fundamental issue here is whether the distinctive elements of intonation are *points* in the pattern or whether they are pitch *movements*. In the former case the movements can be treated as automatic transitions from one point to the next; in the latter case the points are incidental consequences of the movements. At a purely descriptive level either analysis can be regarded as adequate, since the same overall pattern is produced; however, the question is which of these two approaches achieves the better result in theoretical terms. The issues raised here are parallel to those considered in relation to 'levels' and 'contours' with tones (see 4.3.2). The alternatives are illustrated in Fig. 5.19. Example (a) assumes that the pattern is specified in terms of the three points A, B, and C; example (b) assumes a Rise and a Fall, or a single complex movement, Rise–Fall.

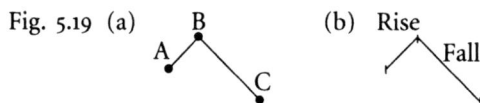

Fig. 5.19 (a)   B   (b) Rise
              A /•\   /\ Fall
              •/   \C   /   \
                    •   ↓

These different analyses lead to different types of structures and different systems of contrasts. In analysis (a) it will be necessary to determine (i) how many points are required to form the pattern, and (ii) how many distinct levels of these points should be recognized. The answer to question (i) is in principle given by the shape of the pattern itself. A single movement such as a rise or a fall requires two points, while a more complex movement such as a rising–falling or a falling–rising shape requires three points. A still more complex shape, such as a rising–falling–rising movement, will need four points. However, it is also possible to have more points than the minimum, for example if a simple fall is analysed in terms of a high point, a mid point, and a low point, or even a high point followed by two low points. Question (ii) cannot be answered by inspection of the pattern itself, but requires reference to the whole system of patterns, and to evidence of their distinctiveness, since phonetically distinct levels may be grouped together under a single phonological level where they are not distinctive. In analysis (b) there are analogous questions. We must again determine (i) how many pitch movements are involved, and (ii) which movements should be recognized. In this case, however, the answer to question (i) is not determined by the shape alone, since the shape of Fig. 5.19(b) could be analysed as a single rising–falling movement or as a rise followed by a fall. Again the answer to question (ii) depends on the system as a whole and the contrasts available within it.

The analysis of Fig. 5.19(a) is, of course, characteristic of Pike and the Bloomfieldian tradition, though in fact Pike also recognizes contours as well as pitch phonemes, and the latter can therefore be seen as features of the former. He is thus able, in a sense, to straddle the division between pitch movements, or 'configurations' on the one hand, and pitch 'levels' on the other, since he makes use of both, using levels to specify the shape of configurations. Nevertheless, the analysis of contours into phonemes is for Pike an essential step; though expressing admiration for Palmer's analysis, he laments (Pike, 1945: 6) the latter's 'oversight' in failing to analyse the patterns into distinctive levels, and offers similar criticisms of the work of Armstrong and Ward, Schubiger, and Kingdon. Trager and Smith (1951) recognize no contours at all, and abandon the structural parts recognized by Pike. For them, only the pitch phonemes exist as phonological entities.

The issue of the adequacy of these two approaches is raised by Bolinger (1951), who defends the configuration approach. He claims that experiments show that 'the basic entity of intonation is a pattern . . . in the fundamental down-to-earth sense of a continuous line that can be traced on a piece of paper'. The basis of Bolinger's argument can be sketched out as follows, with reference to the alternative representations given in Fig. 5.19. If we have a number of similar contours, for example those with a rising–falling shape, the relationships between them will of necessity be expressed somewhat differently in terms of the different conventions. The contours given in Fig. 5.19 could be described as 231 in a pitch-phoneme analysis (where 1 is low) and as a mid (or narrow) rise–fall in a configuration analysis; a contour that rises higher before falling would be 241 in the former representation and high (or wide) rise–fall in the latter. Given that these two contours are related phonetically and semantically, the issue is whether this relationship is best expressed in terms of levels or configurations. A configuration analysis is able to relate them quite easily, as they both have the same shape: rise–fall, which can be given whatever meaning this shape is deemed to have. The difference between the forms is one of range, which can again be correlated with a semantic parameter. By contrast, the levels analysis cannot relate the contours in terms of a common shape, since such shapes do not exist phonologically in this analysis. The relationship thus becomes an arbitrary one. As Bolinger (1951) puts it, ' "231 and 241" (plus a note on synonymy) is less efficient than "rise–fall" (plus a note on pitch range)'. A further criticism of the levels approach is that any such levels are inevitably arbitrary, since the distinction between a narrow rise–fall and a wide rise–fall, for example, is not a discrete one, but a matter of gradience.

Scholars in the tradition of the Dutch school ('t Hart, Collier, and Cohen,

1990) strongly advocate a configuration approach, arguing that it is pitch movements, rather than levels, that are perceptually significant. Thus, their 'Proposition 2' (p. 72) claims that 'At the first level of description, the smallest unit of perceptual analysis is the pitch movement', while 'Proposition 3' (p. 75) states unequivocally that 'There are no pitch levels'. 't Hart, Collier, and Cohen explicitly reject the view 'that the speaker primarily intends to hit a particular pitch level and that the resulting movements are only the physiologically unavoidable transitions between any two basic levels'. Like Bolinger, they claim that the range of the movement (which might require specification in terms of differences of pitch levels) is of only secondary importance in the definition of the different forms.

There would therefore seem to be good reason to adopt a 'configurations' rather than a 'levels' analysis of intonation patterns; the arguments in favour of the former presented above do indeed seem compelling; the recognition of contour *shapes* allows the sort of generalizations that are required, by excluding the range or extent of the pitch movement. Thus, for example, falling patterns can be grouped together phonologically on the basis of their shape without reference to the height of the start or the extent of the fall. This is not possible if the pitch level of specific points is the only phonological parameter at our disposal for distinguishing different contours.

Nevertheless, American scholars have largely continued to use pitch levels in the specification of intonation patterns. Thus, Leben (1976), Goldsmith (1978), Liberman (1975), and others, specify the patterns in terms of the occurrence of the pitch levels Low, Mid and High. Their systems would thus be unable to achieve the kinds of generalization to which Bolinger refers. The situation is somewhat different with the work of Pierrehumbert (1980), however, since, though adopting levels, she reduces these to a simple binary opposition of High and Low, and any intermediate levels are introduced as non-phonological consequences of downstep or of phonetic rules. This means that at least some of the desired generalizations are achieved automatically, since pitch range is eliminated from the primary specification of the pattern. In her approach, therefore, falls from high to mid, high to low, or mid to low, which would require separate specifications in a levels approach, will all receive the description H–L.

This approach can be said to adopt a similar compromise to that of Pike, since *both* levels *and* configurations are employed (the latter in the form of bi-tonal pitch–accents), with the shape of the accent being specified in terms of levels. Ladd (1996: 59), for one, considers that this theory 'successfully resolves this debate'. According to Ladd, this is not merely because the model has both levels and pitch–accents, but also because, as we have seen, the number of levels is reduced to two: High and Low, thus countering one of the further defects claimed for the levels approach, the arbitrariness of the number of levels distinguished.

Nevertheless, some desirable generalizations are still elusive in this framework, for example those that can be made across different contour shapes, such as the pairs fall–rise and rise–fall–rise, or fall and rise–fall. Each of these pairs of contours can be said to be related, both phonetically and semantically, but these relationships cannot be captured satisfactorily in either the configurational nuclear tone approach or the levels approach, including the binary framework of Pierrehumbert. It is therefore necessary to develop a means of achieving such generalizations. As we shall see below, this requires a cross-classification of patterns which can best be achieved by features rather than levels. There is no evidence that levels as such, whether multivalued or binary, can fulfil this role.

5.5.3 THE STRUCTURE OF INTONATION PATTERNS

In spite of different modes of analysis and representation, many scholars agree in dividing intonation patterns into two parts, which we may informally call a pre-nuclear part and a nuclear part. Opinions differ on the relationship between these two parts. In some works in the British tradition, such as Palmer (1922), O'Connor and Arnold (1961), and Halliday (1967), these parts are given some degree of independence: each of Palmer's four nucleus tones can combine with his three heads; O'Connor and Arnold's six nuclear tones can be combined with their four different heads. For both Palmer and Halliday, the nucleus or tonic is the determining element of the tone-group, the versions with different heads/pretonics providing variant forms. Halliday treats pretonic choices as 'secondary systems', with the choice being different for each nuclear tone. O'Connor and Arnold do not give such priority to the nucleus; the ten combinations recognized differ in *either* the nuclear tone *or* the head/prehead. Thus, for example, the first two tone-groups have a low falling nucleus, the second differing from the first in having either a stepping head with a low prehead or a high prehead and no head, as opposed to the low head and/or prehead of the first tone-group.

In Pike's analysis of English intonation, two structural parts of the pattern are also recognized, the precontour and the primary contour. These cannot be equated with the (prehead +) head and the nucleus (+ tail) of the British scholars, since for Pike each accented syllable is associated with a primary contour, and the precontour consists of the preceding unaccented syllables. There are no theoretical restrictions on combinations of the two; Pike (1945: 67) suggests that 'under the requisite contextual conditions, presumably any precontour could be combined with any primary contour', though not all combinations would be equally plausible. The precontours are regarded as subordinate to the primary contours in meaning ('the different precontours have meanings, but in general their implication of the speaker's attitudes is not so strong as that of the primary contours'—p. 30), but they are phonologically subordinate only in the sense that not all total contours contain precontours.

The Dutch school of intonation ('t Hart, Collier, and Cohen, 1990), which claims to identify perceptually relevant features, also establishes a number of structural parts of the intonation pattern. This approach groups pitch movements into 'configurations' which may be 'prefixes', 'roots', or 'suffixes', and these are in turn concatenated into 'contours', which are the largest units. The obligatory core of the contour is the root, which appears to correspond to the nucleus of British analyses; it may be optionally preceded by any number of prefixes, and optionally followed by a suffix. The prefixes thus appear to correspond to the British head, and the suffix to the tail. As far as possible combinations of these are concerned, 't Hart, Collier, and Cohen state that 'many sequences of Prefix, Root and Suffix are unlawful' (p. 80), and they therefore devise a complex set of constraints, in the form of a transition network, limiting their co-occurrence.

More controversial is the analysis of the prenuclear portion of the pattern itself. As we have seen (5.4.2), in a language such as English (and this applies to other Germanic languages, such as German and Dutch) the pre-nuclear pattern is built on the (non-nuclear) accented syllables, so that each such accent is the pivotal point of a pitch movement. Since these languages are 'stress-timed' languages (see 3.9.2.1) this is equivalent to associating these pitch movements with the foot. Thus, the 'head' (this term henceforth refers to the pre-nuclear portion of the intonation unit) may consist of a sequence of such 'tonal feet'.

In the British tradition, this structure is recognized phonetically, but no phonological subdivisions of the head are made. In some other analytical frameworks, however, each such tonal foot is accorded some independence. In the model of the Dutch School, for example, the 'Prefix' configuration may consist of, among other things, a rise and a fall, as in Fig. 5.11 (where it is 1&B), and this may be recursive. The basic unit here is thus not the head as a whole but merely the single tonal foot, and the head pattern arises through the concatenation of such feet. In Pierrehumbert's model, the head is again built up from pitch–accents. In both cases the concatenation of units is captured by the use of a finite-state grammar, which allows indefinite recursion of foot patterns.

The question that arises here is whether the distinctive phonological unit is the head as a whole or the individual foot/pitch–accent. If the former, then we would expect there to be recursion not merely of the foot/pitch–accent as a unit, but also of the pitch pattern associated with it; in other words, we should have a succession of tonally identical feet. We would also expect there to be pitch features which characterize the head as a whole, such as an overall upward or downward pitch tendency. In the case of the British descriptive tradition, both expectations are largely borne out. If we take the 'scandent head' of Palmer (1924: 16), for example, this takes the form of Fig. 5.20, with a series of rises, each beginning with an accented syllable. It will also be noted that there is a consistent downward trend (declination) characterizing the whole head.

Fig. 5.20 ╱ ╱ ╱ ╱

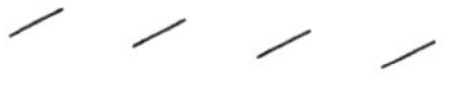

Similarly, Halliday (1970: 16) gives the example of Fig. 5.21(a) to illustrate his 'uneven pretonic' to the falling tone, and that of Fig. 5.21(b) to illustrate the pretonic to his low falling–rising tone (Halliday, 1970: 18; the nucleus begins with the upright line).

Fig. 5.21

(a)

why don't you / ask him to / give you your / money back

(b)

but it / certainly / couldn't be / animal

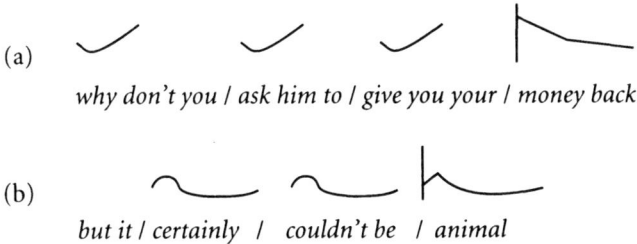

However, in other models this recursion of the pitch pattern does not seem to be insisted on. Both the Dutch and Pierrehumbert's model allow a free choice of prefix/pitch–accent within the head. Indeed, Halliday himself provides examples in which the different feet of his pretonic appear to have different shapes. One such is the 'listing pretonic', illustrated in Fig. 5.22. Halliday (1970: 16) explains that the basic pattern is mid rising, but that 'when an item in the list contains more than one foot, every foot in it except the last is at high level; only the last foot in each item displays the characteristic mid rising pattern.' Thus, the two feet of *a pound of apples* are different; the first is high level and the second mid rising.

Fig. 5.22

a / pound of / apples / ˏ a grapefruit / ˏ and / half a dozen / oranges

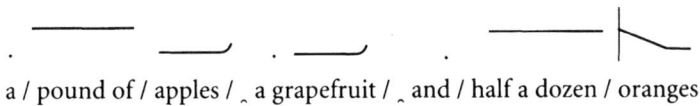

Many cases of this kind can, however, be accounted for in terms of the division into intonation units; there is often some indeterminacy with regard to whether such examples constitute a single unit or more than one, and most can be convincingly analysed as more than one, in which case the difficulty disappears. However, it is conceivable that, although it seems to be usual for each foot in the head to have a similar pattern, this is not always the case, and it would be unwise to elevate this to a principle. Nevertheless, Ladd (1996: 208, 211) is prepared to modify Pierrehumbert's model in such a way that the accents in the head 'represent a *single linguistic choice*' (the emphasis is Ladd's). The unity of the head is also reinforced, as we have seen, by its overall pitch tendency, which may be falling, rising, or level, and high, mid, or low. In Pierrehumbert's model, this trend is determined by the choice of pitch–accent; particular accents (in English specifically H*+L) may induce 'downstep', and since the choice of accents is free, the trend is not necessarily uniform throughout the contour. However, the majority of contours given by Pierrehumbert in fact show a sequence of downsteps, rather than isolated instances within the head, and thus confirm that the overall falling trend is a property of the head as a whole, rather than of individual pitch–accents.

5.5.4 NUCLEAR TONES VS. PHRASE TONES AND BOUNDARY TONES

With Pierrehumbert's model further questions arise as to the appropriate structure of the intonation contour. In this model the contour consists of a series of pitch–accents, followed by a phrase tone and a boundary tone. No specific 'nuclear tone' is recognized, so that the nuclear tone of the British tradition corresponds to the last pitch–accent together with the phrase and boundary tones (or, in the later version of Beckman and Pierrehumbert, 1986, the last pitch–accent together with two kinds of boundary tones). It is possible, in fact, to relate Pierrehumbert's combinations to typical British tones, though it should be borne in mind that no one definitive set of the latter exists. A table of such correspondences is given by Ladd (1996: 82). Though Ladd rightly points out that Pierrehumbert's aim is not to provide a new notation for existing categories, and her analysis should not, therefore, be judged by its ability to do this, a comparison is nevertheless of interest, as it throws light on the different categories involved.

The allocation of pitch features to nuclear tones or to boundaries could, in a sense, be seen as rather arbitrary, a matter of mere notation; since the nuclear tone is the last pitch movement of the intonation unit, the effect is the same whether we treat the end of this movement as a property of the nucleus or of the boundary. In the case of, say, a falling–rising pitch movement we could postulate either a falling–rising nuclear tone, or a H pitch–accent followed by a L phrase accent (or intermediate phrase boundary tone) and a H boundary tone. In either case, rules of realization can be devised which produce the same phonetic result. On this basis, therefore, it is not possible to determine which analysis is to be preferred.

We must therefore look to other criteria of evaluation, and to other kinds of evidence. One argument could relate to the location of the phonetic features; in the case of a rising pattern the rise does not, in fact, take place at the nucleus itself, but frequently tends to occur at the end of the unit. In an utterance such as *Are you sure he's coming?*, for example, with the nucleus on *sure* and a rising intonation, the pitch is generally low during *sure he's com-* and only rises on *-ing*. This might suggest, therefore, that it is appropriate to regard the final high pitch as a property of the utterance-final boundary. Unfortunately, the argument is nullified by the behaviour of the falling intonation pattern. In *I'm sure he's coming*, again with the nucleus on *sure* but with a falling pattern, the entire fall takes place at the nucleus, either on the nuclear syllable itself or on the immediately following syllable, so that the final low pitch would here seem to be more appropriately assigned to the nucleus than to the boundary. This makes it clear that the precise location of the high and low pitches simply reflects the nature of the pitch movement involved, and cannot be used as evidence for the structure of the pattern itself, unless we wish to argue—which would not seem plausible—that the structure of these pitch movements is actually different.

One criticism that could be made of Pierrehumbert's model, from the perspective of British analyses, is that there is a certain amount of indeterminacy regarding the analysis of contours, since it is not always clear to which of the latter's elements—pitch–accent, phrase accent, boundary tone—each part of the contour is to be assigned. Take, for example, the simple falling nuclear tone of the British analyses, which, as we have just noted, typically falls in the nuclear syllable and remains low thereafter. There would in principle be four different ways of representing this in Pierrehumbert's original model, given in Fig. 5.23.

Fig. 5.23

	Pitch–accent	Phrase accent	Boundary tone
(i)	H*	L	L%
(ii)	L*	L	L%
(iii)	H*+L	L	L%
(iv)	H+L*	L	L%

The British tradition usually recognizes two varieties of fall, high and low (though Halliday has a third, mid variety), and these may correspond to (i) and (ii) of Fig. 5.23, respectively, especially since the 'low' variety is frequently characterized by a drop on the nuclear syllable from a preceding higher pitch (indeed, it is so defined by Halliday). But a further possibility is (iii), which, as Ladd points out, would be the expected representation of a falling pitch–accent. However, Pierrehumbert does not, in fact, use (iii) in this way at all, but rather as a means of triggering a following 'downstep', as discussed above. In all of these cases there appears to be a considerable amount of redundancy in the specification of the pattern. A similar situation is found with rising patterns. Again, a variety of possibilities exists for the representation of such patterns (see Fig. 5.24), and again there appears to be some indeterminacy and redundancy, with either the phrase tone or the boundary tone being surplus to requirements.[21]

Fig. 5.24

	Pitch–accent	Phrase tone	Boundary tone
(i)	H*	H	H%
(ii)	L*	L	H%
(iii)	L*	H	H%
(iv)	L*+H	H	H%
(v)	L+H*	H	H%
(vi)	H+L*	H	H%

The only English contour where the whole of this structure appears to be needed is the 'rise–fall–rise' (and the rarer fall–rise–fall). Since this pattern has

---

[21] Omitted from Fig. 5.24 are a number of so-called 'stylized' patterns (cf. Ladd, 1978). These are specified by means of a low boundary tone following a high phrase tone. However, these are a special and rather exceptional category, which can probably be dealt with separately in a different manner.

three pitch movements it requires four reference points, and must therefore be specified with a bitonal pitch–accent, a phrase tone, and a boundary tone. Ladd (1996: 82) gives two possible representations of this pattern, L+H* L H% and L*+H L H%, though only the latter is the rise–fall–rise proper. Paradoxically, however, this pattern provides arguments *against* Pierrehumbert's analysis. Apart from the fact that this pattern is quite rare and very emphatic, and it would seem undesirable to complicate the analysis of all other forms in order to accommodate it, it also pinpoints a difficulty with the analysis as a whole. The evidence comes from cases where this nuclear pattern is preceded by a head.

A characteristic of the head before this nuclear tone (and, indeed, the other complex nuclear tone, the fall–rise–fall) is that each of its feet has a similar movement to the nucleus itself. This has already been illustrated in Fig. 5.21(b). The difficulty that this poses for an analysis of the nuclear tone as pitch–accent + phrase tone + boundary tone is that the prenuclear pitch–accents are not followed by the last two elements, and cannot, therefore, be analysed in this way. Unless, therefore, we are prepared to analyse prenuclear and nuclear versions of the same pitch–accent differently, we must conclude that the nuclear version, too, must be analysed without recourse to phrase tone and boundary tone. In fact, given Pierrehumbert's proposed set of pitch–accent types for English, it is not possible to analyse this pitch movement at all without recourse to phrase tone and boundary tone. This does not demonstrate the need for such elements, however; the point being made here is that we would need such elements for prenuclear pitch–accents, too.

Item (iv) of Fig. 5.23, and items (v) and (vi) of Fig. 5.24, raise a further question. Pierrehumbert allows for the alignment of either of the two tones of a two-tone pitch–accent with the metrically strong (accented) syllable, giving the four possibilities H*+L, L*+H, H+L*, and L+H*. But indeterminacy again arises here, since a sequence 'H L 'H could be analysed as H* L+H* or as H*+L H*,[22] while 'L H 'L could be L* H+L* or L*+H L*. Item (iv) of Fig. 5.23 represents (in terms of a British analysis) a low falling nucleus preceded by a high head or prehead, and, if the former, it is not clear why the high pitch should be part of the final pitch–accent (the nucleus) and not part of the preceding (non-nuclear) pitch–accent. The same question arises with items (v) and (vi) of Fig. 5.24.

A further controversial issue in Pierrehumbert's model is its rejection of a separate category of nuclear accent. The nuclear accent is not distinguished from the prenuclear accents, except in so far as it is followed by the phrase and boundary tones. Not all of Pierrehumbert's followers have endorsed this; Féry (1993), for example, distinguishes prenuclear and nuclear accents in her description of German, while Ladd (1996: 211) similarly reintroduces the distinction, and modifies Pierrehumbert's finite-state grammar to accommodate it. It could be argued

---

[22] The analysis H*+L H* for this pattern would not be possible under Pierrehumbert's assumptions, however, since this pattern is reserved for cases of downstep.

that the elimination of the distinction is desirable, inasmuch as it separates the intonation system proper from the accentual system. This issue has, as we saw in Chapter 3, a long history. Silverman and Pierrehumbert (1990) also justify the non-recognition of a distinction with instrumental evidence demonstrating that prenuclear and nuclear accents are subject to similar phonetic constraints. However, this clearly does not resolve the matter, since the issue is not that the two kinds of accent are phonetically different, but that they have a different phonological role. There is overwhelming evidence, accumulated in the literature on intonation over several decades, that the nucleus does have a distinctive phonological role, and is not merely the last pitch–accent within the pattern.

Though this discussion of Pierrehumbert's model has been brief, and undertaken largely from the perspective of the nuclear tone theory, it does seem clear that there are a number of grounds for questioning some of the details of the model. Whether these weaknesses are matters of detail only, or whether they fundamentally undermine the framework as a whole, is difficult to assess. Ladd, while voicing serious concerns about a number of issues such as those raised here, and advocating important modifications to Pierrehumbert's model, does not discard the model itself, but seeks 'to distinguish . . . the essential ideas of the autosegmental-metrical approach from the specific details of Pierrehumbert's analysis of English' (Ladd, 1996: 4); he wishes, therefore, to revise the latter without abandoning the former. Furthermore, there are certain aspects of Pierrehumbert's model which are certainly of interest and importance in the wider context of prosodic structure. This model sets intonational distinctions in a hierarchical prosodic framework, recognizing pitch features of various prosodic domains. Even though some of the claims made may be open to objection, this general principle is compatible with the approach advocated in the present book.

5.5.5 DECLINATION, HEIGHT, AND RANGE

As we have seen, one of the features of Pierrehumbert's analysis is its use of *downstep*. This concept is employed to account for declination,[23] the overall tendency for the pitch to fall throughout the utterance. Though described phonetically by many scholars, from Klinghardt onwards, declination has usually been considered to be an automatic feature, with no phonological implications. Discussions over the years include especially those of Pike (1945: 77), Cohen, Collier, and 't Hart (1982), and Ladd (1984).

Though apparently a straightforward matter, declination has proved to be controversial, as it raises a variety of both practical and theoretical questions. Among the practical questions is the manner in which declination is manifested phonetically, and hence how it should be measured. The downward trend may affect both the 'baseline' and the 'topline'—the lower and higher limits of pitch

---

[23] This term was first used by Cohen and 't Hart (1967: 184).

excursion, respectively—though it may be difficult to know exactly what to measure in the case of the latter, since, in a language with Level 1 accentuation, there are superimposed peaks corresponding to the accented syllables.

The major issue that is raised by declination is the extent to which it is an automatic feature or a deliberate, controllable parameter of intonation. Lieberman (1967) regards the falling pitch as a physiologically determined feature of the 'archetypal normal breath group' (p. 27); he does acknowledge, however, that speakers may override this fall in 'marked' cases by deliberately increasing the tension of the laryngeal muscles, resulting in a rising pitch. This would make declination controllable, but only for special effects. According to 't Hart, Collier, and Cohen (1990: 134–9), experiments suggest a compromise here, that speakers are able to control whether declination is applied or not, but that this is a once-for-all decision. 'Once it has been "switched on", declination follows automatically. In other words, it is not necessary to assume that the speaker controls the declining pitch syllable by syllable.'

Pierrehumbert does not regard declination as an independent parameter; rather it is the result of selecting the pitch–accent H*+L, whose automatic consequence is a lowering of a following H tone. It thus would correspond exactly to the mechanism generally assumed to account for downdrift in African tone-languages. However, this does not seem to be a particularly satisfactory approach, in part because this pitch–accent is used *only* to produce downstep, and hence it hardly makes sense to consider downstep to be an incidental effect of pitch–accent choice. Experimental evidence also undermines the approach, since, according to 't Hart, Collier, and Cohen (1990: 127), attempts to synthesize declination by producing smaller rises than falls—the mechanism implied by 'downstep'—produce unnatural-sounding utterances; declination requires a continuously sloping fall.

Ladd (1984) objects to Pierrehumbert's downstep analysis on a number of grounds. He argues that the use of the H*+L pitch–accent in this way is improper, since this would be the appropriate representation for a normal falling contour. He also considers downstep to be an independent choice, and represents it with a special downstep marker (¹) before the affected syllable, in the manner of Africanist analyses. This does not, however, answer the point that declination is a once-for-all choice in the utterance, and should therefore be considered to be a property of the pattern as a whole, rather than of individual accents. It also does not allow for the opposite phenomenon to declination: the raising of the pitch throughout the utterance. Though not as common as declination, it is not infrequent, and several scholars note the existence of rising heads. In Pierrehumbert's model this would require a further pitch–accent which is the converse of H*+L , such as L*+H, and which would induce pitch raising; Ladd's framework would need an upstep before each accent. Neither of these solutions has been proposed, however.

These various complications suggest that the issue is somewhat wider than merely a technical device for reducing the pitch level. There are, in fact, a number of different parameters here which affect the pitch level of the utterance at specific points, of which declination is only one. Utterances as a whole may differ from one another in pitch *height*, pitch *range*, and pitch *slope*. Pitch height refers to the average pitch level in relation to the speaker's normal pitch level. This has sometimes been considered under the heading of 'key', discussed by Sweet (1906: 70–1) and by Brazil (Brazil, Coulthard, and Johns, 1980: 23–37; Brazil, 1997: 40–66), and 'register' (Ladd, 1990; Clements, 1990). Pitch range refers to the difference between the top and bottom limits of the pitch pattern, while pitch slope is the overall downward or upward trend (which includes declination). These clearly overlap to some extent; declination (= downward slope) may involve a downward shift of pitch height and also a reduction of pitch range as the top limit is lowered. Nevertheless, these can also be implemented independently, with, for example, a downward shift of pitch height without a reduction in range, or a narrow pitch range at a high level, and so on. But the significant point to be made here is that these are parameters of the intonation unit *as a whole*, or indeed of larger intonation units.

With regard to declination, a further question here relates to the ability of speakers to 'look ahead' when planning their utterances. Since declination progressively lowers the pitch, the speaker must start the utterance high enough to prevent the pitch becoming too low too soon. This demands that speakers have some idea of the length of their utterance before they begin speaking, a requirement that not all scholars are prepared to accept. However, there is evidence that speakers do tend to reach approximately the same pitch level at the end of all their utterances, whatever their length ('t Hart, Collier, and Cohen, 1990: 134). There are also mechanisms available to speakers to revise their plans as the utterance proceeds: 'declination reset'. This phenomenon, whereby the downward trend is interrupted and begins again from a higher level, has long been observed; it is noted, for example, in Armstrong and Ward (1926: 18), and in many other works. It is also considered to give some sort of prominence to the point at which the pitch is reset, and therefore to have a communicative function ('t Hart, Collier, and Cohen, 1990: 148).

One final point may be noted. Although declination is a virtually universal phenomenon in languages, it is also constrained by the prosodic structure of the language in question, and is therefore implemented in different ways. We have already observed its operation in tone-languages, in the form of downdrift and downstep (see Chapter 4). Typically, downdrift can only be implemented when a High tone follows a Low tone; in other cases the identity of the tones is endangered. But there are also differences in non-tone languages. In French, the falling tendency is manifested as a gradual fall from syllable to syllable within each accentual phrase; an analogous process—though with the mora rather than the syllable as the unit—is involved in Japanese (Pierrehumbert and Beckman, 1988: 11–13). In English and German, on the other hand, declination is heavily dependent on the foot, defined by the occurrence of accented syllables, with the pitch falling from foot to foot, rather than syllable to syllable. Thus, though the principle is the same in all these languages, the details, and the mechanisms involved, are different. This issue will be considered further in 5.8, below.

5.6 Intonation Features

5.6.1 INTRODUCTION

We have so far considered primarily questions relating to the structure of into-nation patterns; we must now turn our attention to the analysis of systems of intonational contrasts. As we have noted, the paradigmatic dimension is directly dependent on the syntagmatic dimension, since the domain of contrast deter-mines which contrasts are operative. The 'pitch phoneme' approach essentially reduces the contrasts to a matter of different pitch levels, while in the 'nuclear tone' approach, and other approaches which recognize pitch movements rather than points, the contrasts are between different shapes, and therefore somewhat more complex.

As noted above, the number of levels recognized in the pitch phoneme frame-work is generally four, this being deemed the minimum number which allows specification of all the distinct contours of a language such as English. We have also noted, however, that a major criticism of the 'levels' approach is that it does not permit appropriate generalizations, since related patterns, differing in range of movement, cannot be treated together. This is possible in a 'configuration' approach, since different patterns may have the same shape, while differing in other respects, and they can therefore be assigned the same basic meaning. Since differences of pitch range are gradual rather than discrete, a further criticism of the 'pitch phoneme' approach is that the number of levels is inevitably arbitrary.

One feature of Pierrehumbert's approach, as discussed above, is that it recog-nizes *both* pitch–accents *and* 'tones', the former being complex elements which may have an internal structure, the latter being minimal segments and therefore specifiable only in terms of levels. However, the fact that these levels are reduced to a binary H vs. L means that the second criticism, the arbitrary number of levels, is effectively nullified, since pitch range cannot be accommodated in an analysis with only two levels, and must be referred to some other parameter. In this framework there are thus two kinds of paradigmatic contrast: the binary contrast between the two tones, H and L, and the contrasts between the different pitch–accents themselves. These contrasts are not simple, since there is not only a potential difference of *shape* (e.g. H+L vs. L+H), but also a structural differ-ence according to which of the tones is starred (e.g. H*+L vs. H+L*). Given a maximum of two tones for each pitch–accent, with either tone starred, the num-ber of pitch–accents is actually quite limited, with only ten possibilities. Pierrehumbert (1980) recognizes only seven of these: H*, L*, H*+L, L*+H,

H+L*, L+H*, H*+H. The missing patterns are H+H*, L*+L, and L+L*. However, H*+H has subsequently been eliminated, and a similar fate would have befallen the other combinations of like tones, in part because they violate the Obligatory Contour Principle (see 4.4.3.3). Further, the pattern H*+L is not really recognized in its own right, since it is simply used to initiate downstep. In any case, however, it is not possible to make further generalizations in this model.

A more fruitful enquiry into the nature of intonational contrasts is possible with the 'configuration' approaches, especially the nuclear tone framework of the British analyses. Although, as Bolinger (1951) demonstrates, this approach is better able to achieve generalizations of the sort discussed above, it is nevertheless open to the objection that it fails to break down the patterns phonologically into their minimal components, and hence is unable to make other kinds of generalizations across the different patterns. Thus, for example, we can easily group together different patterns with the same shape under a single heading such as 'fall–rise', but we are not able to state that a fall–rise has more affinity with a rise than with a fall. Pike (1945: ch. 4) attempts to make precisely this kind of generalization with his contours, but is hampered by his pitch–phoneme analysis, and can only group related contours together informally, 'according to the level from which they begin or end, and the direction of pitch change' (p. 44). He can therefore only list the related contours. In the following subsections we shall explore a possible way in which such generalizations can be made.

5.6.2 DIMENSIONS OF TONAL CONTRASTS

In order to determine how a set of nuclear tones might best be analysed in these terms, we shall examine a selection of the analyses of English intonation patterns made by British scholars. Our interest here is not in the features of English as such, but with the nature of the analysis, and these different descriptions of a single language within a single tradition provide a convenient source of homogeneous data and illustrations of the principles involved.

The earliest systematic analysis is provided by Palmer (1922). His system, presented in Fig. 5.25, is relatively small, with only four tones (fall, high rise, rise–fall–rise, and low rise), though he gives a rise–fall as an intensified variant of the fall, and a fall–rise as a less intense variant of the rise–fall–rise.

Fig. 5.25 *Palmer (1922)*

1. Falling   ⟍   or ⟍ (↷)

2. High rising   ⟋

3. Falling–rising   ⤳   (⌣)

4. Low rising   ⤳

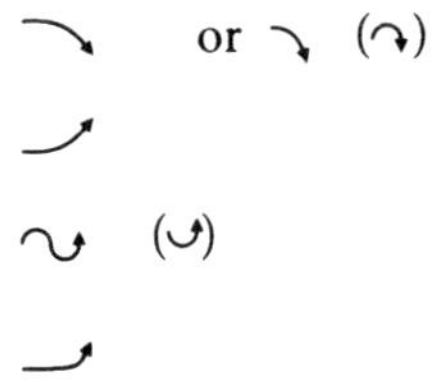

By contrast, Jassem[24] (1952) has a very large number of nuclear tones, recognizing similar varieties of pitch movement as distinct tones. He thus has three varieties of fall and rise, as well as different forms of level, falling–rising, and rising–falling tones. His system is given in Fig. 5.26.

Fig. 5.26 *Jassem (1952)*

1.	Full falling	↘
2.	Low falling	↘
3.	High falling	↘
4.	Full rising	↗
5.	Low rising	↗
6.	High rising	↗
7.	High level	→
8.	Low level	→
9.	Low falling–rising	∪
10.	High falling–rising	∪
11.	Low rising–falling	∩
12.	High rising–falling	∩

Fig. 5.27 gives the system of Kingdon (1958b), which has five nuclear tones, rising, falling, falling–rising, rising–falling, and rising–falling–rising. Two of these have variant forms. The fall–rise is given in two versions: undivided and divided, where the latter involves the separation of the fall, occurring on the nucleus, from the rise, which occurs at the end. More will be said about this variant below.

Fig. 5.27 *Kingdon (1958b)*

    I. Rising: (a) high ╱
                 (b) low ╱
   II. Falling: ╲ or ╲
  III. Falling–rising: (a) undivided ∨
                      (b) divided ╲..╱
  IV. Rising–falling: ∧
   V. Rising–falling–rising: ∿

Schubiger (1958) has a similar analysis, but does not recognize variant forms. She thus gives independent status to Kingdon's high and low forms (Fig. 5.28).

---

[24] Though Jassem is Polish, his analysis is in the same spirit as the British analyses, and can thus be included in the British School.

Fall–rise $\vee$
Rise–fall $\wedge$
Rise–fall–rise $\wedge\!\!\vee$

The system of nuclear tones given by O'Connor and Arnold (1961) is almost identical, the only difference being that it does not include the rise–fall–rise (Fig. 5.29).

Fig. 5.29 *O'Connor and Arnold (1961)*

1. Low Fall   ⌐
2. High Fall ⌐
3. Rise–fall ⌐
4. Low Rise   ⌐
5. High Rise ⌐
6. Fall–rise ⌣

Finally, we may give Halliday's system (Halliday, 1967; 1970), which includes variant forms of most of his five tones (Fig. 5.30). Not included here are his 'double tonics', which consist of the combinations 1+3 and 5+3.

Fig. 5.30 *Halliday (1967)*

1. Falling: wide (1+)   \
        medium (1)   \
        narrow (1–)   —
2. High Rising: straight (2)   /
        broken (2)   ∨
3. Low Rising: ⌿
4. (Rising–)falling–rising: high (4) ∿
        low (4)   ∿
5. (Falling–)rising–falling: high (5) ⌄⌃
        low (5)   ⌄⌃

As immediate observations on these systems of tones, we may note first that all are different in one respect or another, either in the number of tones recognized or in the particular patterns included. However, there are clearly similarities, too, and the differences are not primarily in the kinds of pitch movement identified (there are, of course, relatively few possibilities, with rise, fall, rise–fall, and fall–rise being predictable) but rather in how the various movements are grouped into classes or types. Many more variants are also included by the scholars concerned in their detailed discussions of the patterns. Especially significant, too, is that fact that several of these systems include more than one level of differentiation, with 'primary tones' and 'secondary tones'.

What is of interest to us here are first the criteria used by the different scholars, and second the ranking of the various criteria. Tones are not simply distinguished according to their shape; shape is clearly a relevant factor, but some of the systems group together tones with different shapes (such as fall and rise–fall). The main criteria appear to be:

(1) final pitch direction (falling, rising—occasionally level)
(2) complexity of the movement (1-directional, 2-directional, etc.)
(3) range of the movement (wide, narrow)
(4) height of the movement (high, low—occasionally mid).

There could theoretically be others, such as the speed of movement (fast, slow), the manner of movement (sliding, stepping, etc.), but these are not taken into account in distinguishing different tones.

Apart from the parameters themselves, there are also differences in how they are used in distinguishing different tones. Parameters may be ranked, some being used for primary and others for secondary distinctions; some are used consistently throughout the system, and others for some parts of the system but not for others, for example where 'high' and 'low' rises are distinguished but not 'high' and 'low' falls. Primary distinctions have to be categorical, and continuously variable phonetic parameters must be reduced to binary terms if they are to function in such distinctions; secondary distinctions may be matters of gradience.

In spite of such variation, it is clear that there is a *hierarchical* relationship among the different parameters, so that the above list also reflects their relative significance. Final pitch direction is used as a primary criterion in all the systems, and there is no instance of patterns differing in this respect being grouped together as a single tone. Complexity is used only slightly more sparingly; all except Palmer and Halliday distinguish all pitch movements which differ in these terms, e.g. rise–fall and fall. Range is used mostly as a secondary criterion, except in the case of simple rising tones, though Jassem, Schubiger, and O'Connor and Arnold use it to distinguish primary tones. Only Jassem uses height to distinguish primary tones. In no case is a parameter used for primary distinctions if a higher-ranking parameter is not so used. It is thus possible to consider that the different systems in fact use the same scale, and the differences between them are essentially a matter of where on this scale the divisions are made. This hierarchy also reflects differences of meaning, the major distinction being signalled by the final pitch direction, followed by complexity, and then range and height.

The only formal means of cross-classifying a group of items such as these nuclear tones is through a set of distinctive features. Features have been used for intonation by several scholars; we have seen, for example, their use in specifying accentual features, including intonation, by Vanderslice and Ladefoged (1972), who also propose the features [±cadence] and [±endglide] (see 3.5.2). Features have also been used by Hirst (1976; 1983; 1988). However, these features are largely ways of specifying levels, such as [±High], [±Low]; features of this kind are also implicit in Pierrehumbert's analysis, since H and L tones are merely abbreviations for [+High] and [−High], respectively.[25] If, however, we wish to devise a set of distinctive features for the nuclear tones, the evidence from this survey of some major analyses of English would suggest features which correspond not to levels but to the parameters just identified. A suggested set is presented in Fig. 5.31. The hierarchical relationship between these features can be captured by a set of implicational statements, such that, for example [±complex] implies [±high-ending]. However, no claim is being advanced here for the universality of these features or these statements, since they are based entirely on analyses of English. It is possible that other dimensions may be exploited in other languages, or that the same dimensions could be ranked differently. For example, there is some evidence that 'complexity' may be seen as a matter of timing, and that the feature [+delayed peak] proposed by Ladd (1983) might be employed here.

Fig. 5.31   [±high-ending]
      [±complex]
      [±wide]
      [±high]

The aim of this discussion has been to consider how we may achieve the necessary generalizations across the different types of nuclear tones on a different basis from those approaches which divide these tones into points or levels. What is important here is that the features recognized are regarded as properties of the nuclear part of the intonation unit as a whole, and thus avoid the arbitrariness of attempting to assign specific points of the pattern to 'pitch–accents', 'phrase tones', and 'boundary tones'. The generalizations cannot be made by the use of levels, even if these levels are reduced to a binary [±High].

5.7 Intonation and the Structure of Utterances

Most of the analyses presented and discussed so far are concerned with single intonation patterns applying to a basic intonation unit, called the 'tone-group' by scholars in the British tradition. The implication is that the intonation of utterances or conversations as a whole can be described in terms of a succession of such units, each of which has a structure and a pattern which are independent of the other units in the utterance.

A number of suggestions have been made at various points in the present book which indicate that there may be more to the intonation of such larger stretches of speech than merely the concatenation of these basic intonation units.

---

[25] In Pierrehumbert's case, this is a binary distinction, so that only a single feature is required. [+High, −Low] and [+Low, −High] would imply at least a ternary distinction, with a Mid [−High, −Low] tone, [+High, +Low] being unusable.

First, in our discussion of accentuation in Chapter 3, it was noted (3.4) that the hierarchical organization of utterances may extend beyond the Level 1 and Level 2 recognized there to include still higher 'levels', but that these levels are essentially a matter of intonation rather than accent. In other words, if Level 2 accentuation can be interpreted as nuclear prominence within the intonation unit, then it may be possible to recognize larger, more inclusive intonation units, whose most prominent points can be seen as higher-level accents. This argument is supported by Jorden and Chaplin's analysis of Japanese (1963), discussed in 3.3.4, where two levels of pitch–accent marking are employed (see Fig. 3.9).

A second observation relates to Beckman and Pierrehumbert's analysis of Japanese and English (1986) which, as we have seen, involves recognition of an 'intermediate phrase' as well as an 'intonation phrase', where the former is a constituent of the latter, and—in terms of their model—the final pitch–accent may contain an additional boundary tone which is attributable to the larger unit. Even without this latter point, it is still possible to recognize a hierarchical arrangement of units of this kind. As a number of scholars have pointed out, this hierarchy of units may be identified with that which has been postulated elsewhere, for example by Selkirk (1984), and by Nespor and Vogel (1986).[26]

The intonational evidence for such larger units is of several kinds. In the first place, certain overall pitch features of the utterance, including those identified above as properties of the intonation unit as a whole, such as the pitch height, range, and slope, are not confined to individual intonation units but may have larger domains. Lehiste (1982) notes that there are several such features, including non-intonational features such as length, which typically apply to stretches of speech longer than simple sentences, and 'speakers use phonological means to signal the beginning and end of such units'. Though each individual unit may have its own values for these parameters, there is nevertheless often an overall value for them which extends over larger stretches of speech. Take, for example, the height parameter. Certainly, the pitch pattern of each unit may be assigned a particular height, and this may differ from unit to unit. But the utterance as a whole, however many intonation units it contains, may also be characterized by a pitch level. This phenomenon is described by Sweet (1906: 70) under the heading of *key*; he notes that 'each sentence, or sentence-group, has a general pitch or key of its own'. Thus, 'the high key is the natural expression of energetic and joyful emotions, the low of sadness and solemnity' (p. 71). In addition to the overall key of the utterance, there are, according to Sweet, differences of key *within* utterances, with constant shifts up or down. Thus, 'questions are naturally uttered in a higher key than answers, and parenthetic clauses in a lower key than those which state the main facts. In all natural speech there is an incessant change of key' (ibid.). A similar point is made by Brazil (Brazil, 1975,

---

[26] The general characteristics of hierarchical structures for prosody will be considered in more detail in Ch. 6. The current discussion is restricted to the evidence from intonation.

1997; Brazil, Coulthard, and Johns, 1980), who adopts Sweet's concept of key and shows how it reflects the organization of utterances in discourse. Speakers may begin their utterances in a high key, and progress through a mid key to a low key, so that key becomes a marker of utterance structure. An example is given in Fig. 5.32. Brazil, like Sweet, recognizes three keys, but in fact this number is rather arbitrary, as there may be more than three height levels in the course of an utterance.

Fig. 5.32 *high*   WHY do you
          mid   // now TELL me //   // EAT // all that
          low   FOOD //

It will be observed that what is here seen as a system of different heights for individual intonation units, with a progressive lower overall pitch for each successive unit, can also be seen as a matter of downward slope (or declination) for the utterance *as a whole*. Though declination is usually seen as a feature of individual intonation units, it is here also a feature of the whole utterance. Similar remarks may be made about features such as pitch range; each individual intonation unit may have its range, but this is also true of whole utterances. What emerges here, therefore, is a framework in which there are (at least) two levels at which these overall pitch features may be said to operate.

Further evidence for different levels of structure in intonation, and in particular for a larger domain than the simple intonation unit, is provided by sequences of intonation patterns, specifically nuclear tones. It has long been reported that certain patterns are 'final' and others 'non-final'; Klinghardt (Klinghardt and Klemm, 1920; Klinghardt, 1927), for example, recognizes a difference between patterns which are *abschließend* ('conclusive') and those which are *weiterweisend* ('forward pointing'). However, this has generally been interpreted in purely linear terms. Another approach, adopted by Palmer (1922, 1924), is to recognize a *ranking* of tone-groups, such that some are *subordinate* to others. According to Palmer, there are two kinds of tone-sequences: co-ordinating (in which the tones of the sequence are identical), and subordinating (in which the tones are different. In the latter case the unit with the falling nucleus is 'the one expressing the more important and the other expressing the less important fact'. The sequences he identifies are given in Fig. 5.33. It can be seen that this creates a larger intonation unit, with a hierarchical structure, in much the same way that sentences may consist of clauses, some of which are co-ordinate and others subordinate.

Fig. 5.33 *Co-ordinating*
          1. [↘‖↘]   2. [↗‖↗]   3. [↜‖↜]

          Subordinating
          1. [↘‖↗]   2. [↗‖↘]   3. [↘‖↜]   4. [↜‖↘]

Crystal and Quirk (1964) and Crystal (1969) also put forward a 'theory of subordination' for intonation patterns, but on a rather different basis, indeed the reverse of Palmer's, since they regard as subordinate those cases where the tone is *identical* in successive units, and where the second tone has a narrower range than the first. Crystal and Quirk's approach is therefore purely phonetic, and it is not clear what phonological implications it may have, if any. Palmer's approach could be seen as more phonological, with the recognition of subordinating and co-ordinating relationships, expressed by different tones.

This principle is elaborated, along the lines suggested by Palmer rather than Crystal, in work by the present writer (Fox, 1973, 1978, 1982, 1984a, 1984b). Here, a larger intonation unit, the *paratone* or *paratone-group*[27] is explicitly established in which one or more *major* tone-groups are optionally preceded and/or followed by *minor* tone-groups.[28] Thus, an utterance such as *Whenever I see him, I get angry* is likely to be pronounced with two intonation units, with a rising or falling–rising pattern in the first unit and a falling pattern in the second, i.e. *Whenever I ʹsee him / I get ˋangry*. The first unit could be considered subordinate to the second, since it is dependent on it, so that the structure is minor + major. Other cases involve co-ordinate structures. For example an utterance such as *I missed the lecture, which was a pity*, pronounced with two intonation units and with a falling pattern in each, would constitute two co-ordinate units (the nuclear tone is indicated on the nuclear syllable): *I missed the ˋlecture / which was a ˋpity*.

Both types of structure are recursive; we might expand our subordinating example by the addition of further minor units, as in *Whenever I ʹsee him / and he talks about his new ʹcar / I get ˋangry*, while the co-ordinating example could be expanded to *I missed the ˋlecture / which was a ˋpity / as I really wanted to ˋhear it*. Both subordination and co-ordination can occur simultaneously, as in *Because the ʹtrain was late / I missed the ˋlecture / which was a ˋpity*. This has the structure minor + major + major. It is clear that the nature of the nuclear tone is an indicator of its function within the utterance; tones which end low are major, while those which end high are minor. However, high-ending tones may also be major where they are independent, for example in utterances such as *When you've finished ʹthat / are you coming to ʹlunch?*, where the structure could be seen as minor + major, in spite of the final high-ending tone.

It is important, of course, to note that we are here considering intonation structures, and not syntactic structures. Hence, although the structure minor +

---

[27] The term 'paratone' has been employed by several scholars, for example Brown, Currie, and Kenworthy (1980); Yule (1980); Couper-Kuhlen (1986), though the present writer may claim to have been the first to use it, in an unpublished paper given in Edinburgh in 1968. The term 'paratone' was used in early published work (Fox, 1973) as a designation for a larger unit; it was later replaced by 'paratone-group' (Fox, 1978), in order to make it parallel to 'tone-group', and as part of a systematic extension of Halliday's framework—then widely adopted—to larger intonation structures.

[28] This usage of 'major' and 'minor' differs from that of Trim (1959, 1964).

major is typical for an utterance such as *Whenever I ´see him / I get `angry* , and this is parallel to the subordinate + main clause structure of the sentence, the same pattern is typical even when the order of the clauses is reversed, as in *I get ´angry / whenever I `see him*. As with other aspects of intonation, there appears to be a relationship to syntactic structure, such that some types of syntactic construction are likely to occur with certain intonation structures, but the intonational choices are in principle independent.[29]

One characteristic of English intonation structure which does not appear to be common in other languages is the occurrence of minor intonation units following major ones, giving the structure major + minor. This has been described—though not in these terms—by a number of scholars, for example Kingdon (1958b) and Halliday (1967, 1970). Kingdon describes this pattern as a 'divided' fall rise (see Fig. 5.27); Halliday describes it as a single tone-group with a 'double tonic'. The first unit has a fall or rise–fall, and the second a low rise. It should be noted that this fall + rise pattern of English is quite distinct from the fall–rise nuclear pattern.[30] Halliday (1970: 12) gives the examples *Arthur's been here `twice in the last ,year or so* , and *He's never taken ^Jane on any of his ,visits though*. These patterns are rather anomalous in Halliday's framework, since they are single patterns with two nuclei, and the second nucleus—the low rise— cannot have a head. But these can simply be regarded as cases of the structure major + minor; indeed Halliday (1967: 42) gives it precisely this analysis in terms of its functional role, where it is said to indicate major + minor 'information point'. This relationship is clear from the fact that it is often possible to maintain the 'information structure' of an utterance when the order of clauses is reversed by changing the intonation structure. In Fig. 5.34, the version in column 1 is much closer in meaning to that of column 2 than that of column 3, despite the reversal of the order, because the patterns of column 2 have the structure major + minor, while those of column 3 have minor + major. There is thus an equivalence between a preceding minor intonation unit and a following one.[31] However, the intonation structures involved here are not necessarily found in other languages; German, for example, does not permit following minor intonation units (Fox, 1982).

[29] Some details of the types of construction which prefer co-ordinate structures are given in Fox (1984b).
[30] See Halliday (1970: 20) for a detailed description. Gussenhoven (1983: 321) commits the common error of confusing the two when he criticizes the analysis of the utterance *they're all the `same these poli ,ticians* in Fox (1982), which he wrongly takes to be a fall–rise, as major + minor, thus 'missing the generalization that postposed non-focus elements like *these politicians* are appended as tails'. The rise of a fall–rise is certainly a tail to the fall, but the rise of the fall + rise pattern is not. His analysis of comparable utterances in Coleman (1914) and elsewhere, which again he treats as cases of the fall–rise, is similarly flawed, thus vitiating much of his argument (1983: 314–21) that there are no 'double-focus' contours in English.
[31] For further discussion of this approach see especially Fox (1973, 1984b).

Fig. 5.34

1	2	3
minor + major	*major + minor*	*minor + major*
If it ´rains /	We can't `go /	We can't ´go /
we can't `go	if it ,rains	if it `rains
On ´Wednesday /	I'll be in `London /	I'll be in ´London /
I'll be in `London	on ,Wednesday	on `Wednesday

Sequences of patterns, especially nuclear tones, thus constitute further evidence for larger units of intonation, in addition to the overall pitch features of height, range, and slope. According to the proposals put forward here, such a larger unit would contain one or more major intonation units, with optional accompanying minor intonation units which may precede or follow them.[32] A question that arises here is whether there is just one level of subordination of intonation units, or whether subordination is a recursive process. In syntactic structures, the latter is the case, with, for example relative clauses inside relative clauses (*this is the cat that caught the rat that ate the cheese* . . ., etc.), but the evidence for such recursive subordination in intonation is by no means certain, since potential cases are open to an alternative interpretation. Consider, for example, the recorded utterance:

because I feel sure if they `did this / the students would ,work / for everything that really `mattered

It would be possible to consider that there are two levels of subordination here, with the second unit subordinated to the third and the first to the second, giving the structure ((1 2) 3), where the underlining reflects the subordination. However, it is equally plausible that the first two units are subordinated to the third, giving only one level of subordination. The subordination of the first unit to the second is probably purely syntactic rather than intonational. There is no convincing evidence for more than one level of subordination in intonation.

We may also note that there are implications here for accentual structure. It was argued in Chapter 4 that any 'degrees' of accentuation above Level 1 can be seen as matters of intonation rather than of accent proper, with Level 2 accentuation being the nuclear accent of the intonation unit. It was also noted that degrees above Level 2 would require larger intonation structures. The implication of the proposal made here is that, if we choose to regard intonational prominence as accentual, then we could postulate a further level of accentuation (Level 3) corresponding to the larger intonation unit. The lack of further hierarchical structure for intonation would mean that there could be no 'Level 4' accentuation.[33]

---

[32] A formula to generate the possible structures here is $(minor_0 \ major \ minor_0)_1$, where subscript numbers give minimal values.

[33] Ladd (1996: 241–4) argues, however, that the hierarchy of units is in principle indeterminate. For further discussion see Ch. 6.

5.8 The Typology of Intonation

5.8.1 INTRODUCTION: UNIVERSALS AND TYPOLOGY IN INTONATION

There is a fundamental flaw in the discussion of intonation in this chapter so far: it has been too restricted in scope, dealing primarily with English, and with some languages of similar structure, and only occasionally taking account of other languages and other language types. This narrow range is largely inevitable, because most descriptive and theoretical frameworks for intonation have been based on the characteristics of English, and it has therefore been necessary, in evaluating these frameworks, to place the phenomena with which they are concerned in the forefront of the discussion. But this restriction is clearly undesirable, since there is no guarantee that English intonation is representative of other languages, and indeed it is a priori unlikely, since intonation is known to interact with other prosodic features, such as tone, tonal accent, and pitch–accent, which English does not have. We therefore need to broaden the perspective to include languages of other prosodic types.

It is possible, nevertheless, that English, as a non-tone language, represents one end of a spectrum of intonational complexity, and that languages of other types will have simpler systems. This is effectively the claim made by Pike, who summarily dismisses the view that tone-languages can have more than a limited kind of intonation. He observes (1948: 16–17) that 'all tone languages have intonation of the emotional type, with the general height of voice affected, and so on, but I have not seen reported for them a highly organized contrastive system with a limited number of relative levels controlling the formation of intonations that carry shades of meaning'. Thus, according to Pike, intonation can have only a limited place in tone-languages; it may 'modify the phonetic character of the tonemes or temporarily obliterate their contrasts, or even constitute narrative versus interrogative contours, and the like, which are superimposed on the lexical pitches' (p. 17). This would contrast with the role of intonation in non-tone languages, such as English, where more complex, and more meaningful, contrasts are in evidence.

Pike's claim cannot necessarily be wholly endorsed, however. One would certainly expect intonation to be different in languages with and without tone, and tone is likely to limit the role of intonation, since pitch is already pre-empted for lexical contrasts. But additional complications may also ensue, since there will be potential interaction, even conflict, between the two uses of pitch. An instance of this is the case of downdrift and downstep in African tone-languages, which arises as a result of the interplay between the maintenance of tonal contrasts and the tendency towards intonational declination. Comparable, though different, interactions may be expected in a pitch–accent language such as Japanese, or a tonal accent language such as Swedish.

The starting point here is the *universality* of intonation. That intonation is universal in languages is not really in doubt, in spite of Pike's reservations; what is at issue is the nature of the parallels in its form and use. Several scholars, such as Abe (1955), Bolinger (1964, 1978), Cruttenden (1981), and Ohala (1983), attempt to identify such similar properties of intonation in a range of different languages. Typical universal findings include the occurrence of high or rising pitch in questions and in non-final parts of utterances, and low or falling pitch in statements and utterance finally, as well as the role of intonation in breaking up the utterance into communicative chunks. Significant though these features are, they are at too general a level to be particularly useful, and they are to some extent outweighed by the many obvious differences that we find between the intonation systems of specific languages, for example in the types of pattern allowed, in the presence or absence of an intonational nucleus, and so on. Ladd (1981) therefore argues against this kind of universalist approach (which he calls the Strong Universalist Hypothesis), favouring the more discriminating model of the Nuclear Tone Hypothesis, which, he argues, is better able to identify the differences between languages.

A less ambitious approach is to establish a typology of intonation. This allows differences between languages, but keeps them within definable limits. It is not clear, however, what the parameters of such a typology should be. As with all typologies, it is not necessarily sufficient to identify features which occur in some languages but not in others; in order to qualify for the status of typological parameters, any differences need to have wider significance, with a range of other differences being dependent upon them. Few, if any, of the suggested parameters seem to have such status.

Ladd (1996: 119) enumerates four different ways in which languages may differ intonationally:

1 Semantic—'differences in the meaning or use of phonologically identical tunes'
2 Systemic—'differences in the inventory of phonologically distinct tune types'
3 Realisational—'differences of detail in the phonetic realisation of what may be regarded phonologically as the same tune'
4 Phonotactic—'differences in tune-text association and in the permitted structure of tunes'.

Ladd gives illustrations of differences falling under these various headings, but none of them seem to be sufficiently important to justify typological status. One interesting illustration given of a typological parameter (pp. 132–6) is the 'compression' vs. 'truncation' dichotomy (the terms are from Grønnum, 1991). According to Ladd, English is 'a compressing language *par excellence*'; a complex pattern, such as a rise–fall–rise, associated with a polysyllabic utterance, may be compressed onto a single syllable (an illustration is given in Fig. 5.15). Other languages may not allow such compression, and may prefer to simplify or truncate the pattern. As an example of a language which avoids compression, Ladd suggests German. Thus, in the examples of Fig. 5.35, sentence (a) is a typical high fall–rise question, with a high-pitched nucleus (here capitalized), and a following fall and rise on the remaining syllables. Sentence (b) has the same pattern, but compressed onto two syllables. In sentence (c), however, the nucleus contains only a single syllable; here, according to Ladd, the compression 'sounds odd phonetically', and a simple high rise would be preferred. German, according to this view, prefers to truncate rather than to compress.

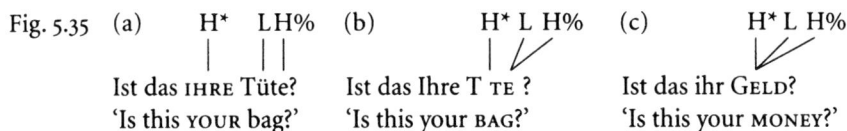

Fig. 5.35 (a)   H* LH%   (b)   H* L H%   (c)   H* L H%

Ist das IHRE Tüte?   Ist das Ihre T TE ?   Ist das ihr GELD?
'Is this YOUR bag?'   'Is this your BAG?'   'Is this your MONEY?'

However, this is not the only interpretation of these data. First, the pattern here should not be equated with the English (rise–)fall–rise, which is used to demonstrate the compressibility of English contours. The latter does not occur in German (see Fox, 1981; 1984a), and the question of its compressibility does not arise. The German fall–rise is a variant of the rise, which is also found in English—Halliday (1967, 1970) describes it as the 'broken' or 'pointed' rise. It differs from the (rise–)fall–rise in having a higher overall pitch level, and in consisting of two separate movements with a sharp change of direction in the middle (Halliday, 1970: 20). Second, English is also somewhat reluctant—if perhaps a little less so than German—to compress this form. An utterance such as 'Is this your HAT?' would be less likely to have this fall–rise than 'Is this your um-BRELla?'. In any event, the situation here is exactly the same in the two languages. If German has a greater tendency to avoid the fall–rise on a single syllable (and this is by no means certain), it is more likely to be due to the fact that German, on the whole, prefers jumps to glides and cannot accommodate the necessary glides on a single syllable, than to the setting of any 'truncation' parameter.

This example has been discussed in detail because it demonstrates the difficulty of establishing typological parameters for intonation. The differences between the two languages at this point are (i) the absence of a pattern corresponding to the English rise–fall–rise, and (ii) the preference of German for jumps rather than glides. Neither of these seems to be of sufficient significance to justify being regarded as a major typological parameter. The presence or absence of individual patterns in the inventory is relatively superficial, and the preference for jumps or glides is a matter of phonetic realization rather than phonology. The latter is, furthermore, not absolute, as English, too, may use jumps in certain speech-styles. There does not seem, therefore, to be the basis for a typology here. English and German are in any case so close in their prosodic characteristics that we would not expect them to be typologically different.

There are other problems here. Given the absence of a uniform descriptive approach, differences are often as much to do with the model or framework adopted as with the facts of the language in question. Widely different descriptions have been given, for example, of languages with very similar prosodic systems, such as English, German, and Dutch, and even of different varieties of

Prosodic Features and Prosodic Structure

English. The 'nucleus', which is fundamental to the description of intonation in the British tradition, is not recognized in most American models, including that of Pierrehumbert (1980); it is called into question by Brown, Currie, and Kenworthy (1980) for Scottish English, and its existence is explicitly denied for Danish by Thorsen (1983). But it is difficult to assess to what extent these different claims relate to the languages or varieties themselves and to what extent they are merely differences in the theoretical framework adopted.

We are more likely to identify typological differences when we look at intonation from the wider perspective of languages of different prosodic types—tone vs. non-tone languages, languages with different kinds of accentual structure, and so on. In what follows, we shall examine some of the properties of intonation in such languages.

5.8.2 A FRAMEWORK FOR INTONATIONAL TYPOLOGY

5.8.2.1 Introduction

If we are to establish a genuine typology for intonation, then we cannot necessarily use the sorts of descriptive categories that are found in some of the standard analyses, since these are generally restricted to a narrow range of languages of the European type, and primarily English. As a convenient framework for an overview of this kind we need to adopt rather more general categories which are not so restricted in their application. Somewhat impressionistically, we shall use three very general categories of intonational phenomena which are likely to be relevant for all languages (cf. Fox, 1995):[34]

  (i)   envelope features
  (ii) prominence features
  (iii) modality features.

By *envelope features* is meant the set of pitch features which are applicable to the utterance as a whole, and which form a setting for the other intonational features. Such envelope features include principally pitch *range*, pitch *height*, and pitch *slope* (which includes *declination*). *Prominence features* are those where pitch is used to pick out and give prominence to a part of the utterance. This would include the features associated with an intonational nucleus, but also other cases of pitch prominence where there are no accentual implications. *Modality features*—the name is perhaps not ideal—are those local pitch features which carry the typical intonation meanings, such as the rises and falls associated with nuclear tones or their equivalent in languages such as English or German.

---

[34] The discussion here is based on a study of the typology of intonation whose results are summarized in Fox (1995).

These categories are intended to be general in the sense that they take no account of *how* the particular features are realized in different language types. The features in each category may need to take on different forms of realization according to the nature of the prosodic structure of the language concerned, as discussed below.

5.8.2.2 Envelope Features

Envelope features are those pitch features which characterize the utterance as a whole, or major portions of it. They comprise mainly pitch range, height, and slope, as discussed in 5.5.5, above, and they include declination. Similar use is made of pitch range and height in languages of very different types, with the overall pitch level and range of movement affected in similar ways by various discourse factors. Of more interest is declination; an overall falling tendency is attested in very many languages, but its implementation is constrained in different ways in different cases. In French, for example, it takes the form of a gradual fall from syllable to syllable, as in Fig. 5.36 (Coustenoble and Armstrong, 1934; MacCarthy, 1975).

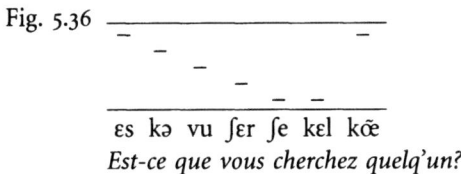

Fig. 5.36

ɛs kə vu ʃɛr ʃe kɛl kœ̃
Est-ce que vous cherchez quelq'un?

English, unlike French, has accented and unaccented syllables within the intonation unit, and it is the accented syllables which implement the downward trend, while the unaccented syllables may continue at the same level, or even rise. This was illustrated above in Fig. 5.5, taken from O'Connor and Arnold (1961), which is repeated here as Fig. 5.37. It can be seen that declination here proceeds in a stepwise fashion, with a lower pitch for each accented syllable, represented by the larger circles.

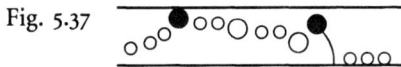

Fig. 5.37

In tone-languages the same declination effect has been widely observed. In languages of the South East Asian contour-type (see 4.3.2), the downward trend does not need to interfere with tonal contrasts, and each tone may simply be pronounced at a slightly lower level than its predecessor. For Mandarin Chinese, Chao (1968: 40) notes that 'in longer sentences, there is a slight tendency for the pitch to trail off to a lower key toward the end', though he suggests that the fall is slight and not necessary. Shen (1989) gives many examples where a sequence of identical tones is pronounced at a progressively lower pitch. A similar case is reported in Fox (1995), where each of the tones of an utterance such as *Zhōng cān, xī cān, tā dōu chī* ('He eats both Chinese and Western food'), which are all high level, is pronounced at a slightly lower pitch than its predecessor, producing an overall fall.

In African tone-languages of the 'register' type, the implementation of declination is less easy, as it endangers the distinctiveness of the tonal levels. Here, as we observed in Chapter 4, the downward trend is restricted to certain places where its effect on the tonal contrasts is minimal, namely where a High tone follows a Low tone, resulting in downdrift, and this has even been phonologized in the form of downstep. A typical instance from Igbo (Emenanjo, 1987) was given as Fig. 4.5, and is repeated here as Fig. 5.38.

Fig. 5.38   L H L H H H H L H

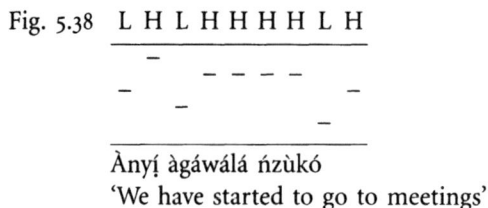

Ànyị̀ àgáwálá ńzùkó
'We have started to go to meetings'

In Japanese, a similar downward trend occurs, though here it is limited by the presence of the pitch–accent. Pierrehumbert and Beckman (1988: 57–91) distinguish three kinds of 'downtrend': *catathesis*, which is, in their analysis, the result of a downstep; *declination*, which is a purely phonetic matter; and *final lowering*, which occurs at the very end of a phrase. However, these are probably all instances of the same phenomenon. Here, the pitch lowering proceeds from mora to mora.

A number of general points can be made here. First, envelope features such as declination occur in languages of widely different prosodic types; second, that the actual implementation of these features may vary considerably; and third, that the particular implementation found is a direct reflection of the prosodic characteristics of the language concerned, for example, whether it is tonal or not, and what kind of accentual structure it has, if any.

5.8.2.3 Prominence Features

By prominence features is meant those pitch features which serve to single out a particular point, or points, in the utterance. In English two basic kinds of pitch prominence are generally recognized: that associated with the intonational nucleus, and that associated with non-nuclear accented syllables, which, as we saw in Chapter 3, are made prominent largely by pitch. But the situation is different in other languages. In French the latter form of prominence is absent, but there is occasional use of emphatic prominence, involving higher pitch, which is independent of the normal phrase–accent, for example the syllables in bold type in *c'est absolument impossible* or *c'est magnifique*. In Japanese, too, there are no non-nuclear accented syllables; as we have seen, the phrase–accent is a matter of pitch alone, and it is possible to achieve greater prominence by raising the pitch of the accented mora. As in French, pitch prominence can also be achieved elsewhere, in this case on the second mora of the phrase, which regularly has the first high pitch.

Tone-languages also have the possibility of pitch prominence. Fox (1995) gives evidence from Mende, Cantonese, and Mandarin Chinese of prominence obtained by raising (or, in the case of the low tones, lowering) the pitch of individual syllables. Another means of achieving pitch prominence is to defer declination. Different versions of the Mandarin sentence *Zhōngsan xīngqīsān tīng shōuyīnjī* ('Zhongsan listens to the radio on Wednesdays'), with high level tones throughout, were elicited in such a way as to vary the focus, which fell on *Zhōngsan, xīngqīsān* and *shōuyīnjī* in different utterances. In each case, declination was deferred until after the focal item, the pitch remaining at a more or less high level until after this item. In Zulu, which has a phrase–accent as well as tone, the accented (penultimate) syllable is distinguished by higher pitch.

As in the case of envelope features, therefore, we may conclude that pitch prominence can be achieved in all these different languages, but that the way it can be achieved depends on the prosodic structure of the language.

5.8.2.4 Modality Features

Modality features are the specific pitch patterns used to distinguish utterances, such as 'fall', 'rise', etc. Once more, languages of various prosodic types make use of pitch in this way, though again it is clear that their capacity for doing so, and the manner in which such pitch features can be realized, depends on the nature of the overall prosodic structure, and in particular on the extent to which pitch features are pre-empted for other purposes.

The starting point is the nuclear tone of the British tradition, which associates the major features of modality with the nuclear accent. The term 'associates' is used advisedly, since the pitch features of the nuclear tone are not necessarily located in the nuclear syllable itself. As we noted in 5.5.4, above, in English a falling nuclear tone will usually have the fall on the nuclear syllable, the following syllables being low, but in the case of the rising tone the nuclear syllable itself is usually low and level, and the rise does not take place until the end of the intonation unit.

In Japanese, however, although a nuclear accent (the pitch–accent of the phrase) can be recognized, it cannot in principle be the location of intonational modalities, since its pitch pattern is predetermined: the accented mora is high and it is followed by a low pitched mora. This does not prevent the use of modality features in Japanese, however, since these features are placed at the *end* of the unit, often supported by a particle such as *ka* or *ne*, which thus becomes the bearer of the pattern. This situation is also common in tone-languages, where modality features cannot occur in the body of the utterance as they would interfere directly with lexical tones. These features are therefore often appended to the final syllable, or an additional syllable is added with the sole function of carrying the intonation pattern. In both Mandarin Chinese and in Cantonese particles such as *a* may be pronounced with a range of pitch patterns.

We must again conclude, therefore, that there is evidence for modality features of intonation in languages with different prosodic characteristics, but again there are different ways in which they are implemented, according to the constraints imposed by the language type.

5.8.3 CONCLUSION

Several conclusions can be drawn from this discussion of typological features of intonation. We have seen that languages of various prosodic types, with different tonal and accentual features, can be said to have the same kinds of intonational features—envelope, prominence, and modality features—but that these features may be implemented and realized in different ways, and that these different realizations depend on non-intonational features of the prosodic structure of the language. It would appear, therefore, first that the presence or absence of such intonational features is unlikely to yield a satisfactory typology, and second that a typology based on differences of implementation or realization will be a typology not of intonation as such but of overall prosodic structure. The conclusions from this would be that a typology of intonation as such is therefore not really feasible.

It is still possible, of course, to recognize purely intonational differences between languages, but it seems that any such differences are relatively trivial, concerned with the inventory of patterns and their phonetic realization; such differences may be considered to lie below the typological 'threshold'. Any more significant intonational differences between languages are likely to be due to differences in the prosodic structures through which intonational features are realized.

5.9 Conclusion: Intonation and Prosodic Structure

This chapter has considered a number of frameworks for the description of intonation. We have seen that, despite the problems involved in analysing intonation phonologically and the lack of attention to the phonological basis of the analysis, and despite the very divergent views of the different schools as to the concepts and categories to be employed, we may nevertheless discern a number of significant characteristics of the phonology of intonation.

Crucial to the analysis of intonation is the question of prosodic *structure*. Given that the scope of intonation is so large, extending to utterances as a whole, there are many different ways in which its organization and structure can be described, and the particular intonational contrasts that are recognized inevitably depend on the nature of the units and structural categories that are established. As we have seen, some schools attempt to describe intonation in terms of minimal units, or points in the pitch pattern. However, this approach fails to provide for the necessary generalizations, which require reference to shapes rather than points. Similarly, it can be argued that we must recognize structural parts of intonation patterns, incuding 'heads' and 'nuclei', if we are to capture the appropriate generalizations.

An important characteristic of the overall structure of intonation is that it is hierarchical, in the sense that we can recognize a number of domains of intonation of different sizes, the larger including the smaller. Thus, in a language such as English, in which accentual features play a part in the structure of the intonation patterns, accentual units (feet) have their pitch patterns, as do larger entities (intonation-units, 'tone-groups') and larger units still, as discussed in 5.7. In this, of course, intonation resembles the other features that we have examined in previous chapters, but, unlike the situation with other features, the hierarchical arrangement extends to the utterance as a whole. The precise nature of the hierarchy may differ from language to language, since in languages without Level 1 accentuation the accentual foot is lacking and cannot constitute an intonation unit.

6

Prosodic Structure

6.1 Introduction: The Concept of Prosodic Structure

In the preceding chapters we have looked in some detail at individual prosodic features, principally length, accent, tone, and intonation, though others, such as rhythm, have also been considered, and we have examined the ways in which these features can be systematized phonologically. Each feature has been discussed largely in its own terms, as an independent prosodic system, taking account of its individual phonetic and phonological properties, and the means of specifying them.

Yet it is evident that these various prosodic features are not completely independent of one another. The discussion of each feature has involved frequent cross-references to other features which are relevant to its systematization. The discussion of length, for example, requires reference to accent as a determining factor in many languages; for its part, accent leads to a consideration of intonational prominence; the systematization of tone involves both length and accent, while intonation is also seen to be heavily dependent on accentual features. There are thus considerable mutual dependencies and interactions among the prosodic features.

In addition to these interactions, prosodic features have many things in common. Features often share their phonetic foundation; tone and intonation have a common basis in pitch, while accent, too, has been shown to be in part often a matter of pitch prominence. Length, along with accent, has by some been considered to be a manifestation of greater 'intensity'. More significantly, however, what unites these features more than any phonological interaction or common phonetic basis is *the way they fit together*; they share a common organization, a common structure which they collectively create and on which they all depend. This common prosodic structure is the focus of the present chapter, in which we shall examine the way in which these features are organized and the characteristics of the structures involved.

The notion of *structure* is a crucial one for the present discussion, but it is open to a variety of interpretations and is thus not unambiguous. In its most common linguistic usage, it refers to the organization of a sentence or other unit of language in terms of the relationships between its parts. It is thus an essentially syntagmatic concept, being concerned with the relationships between co-occurring elements. Crystal (1997: 367) notes that the term may be used in a narrow sense to mean 'a particular sequential pattern of linguistic elements', for example when we describe the structure of a sentence as a string of elements such as subject, verb, and object, or the structure of a syllable in terms of a particular sequence of consonants and vowels. However, the concept may be understood more broadly to cover not just the concatenation of elements which constitute a particular unit but other kinds of relationship, involving a variety of different dimensions. In this sense, the structure of a linguistic unit cannot be stated merely by listing its constituent parts but must also include a description of the relationships between these parts. The kinds of relationships that are assumed to be involved here vary from theory to theory; in syntactic theories a wide range of specific formal and functional relationships have been recognized; in phonology the range of relationships appears to be narrower. There are nevertheless a number of different dimensions here, which will be considered in the course of this chapter.

In this general sense, 'structure' is also not intended to be limited to the 'structuralist' frameworks which characterized the formative period of twentieth-century linguistics, still less to the particular methodological approach of 'American structuralism', which has generally been rejected since Chomsky's criticisms (Chomsky, 1964, 1965). The concept of structure as *organization* is as valid for generative as for pre-generative frameworks, though the place of such a structure in individual models may need to be reinterpreted. Structuralist scholars considered the identification of the network of relations to be the goal of linguistic investigation, invoking the Saussurean concept of a *system*; classical generative grammarians, however, subordinated structure to the *grammar*, seen as a set of ordered rules. Whatever the merits of rule-based approaches to phonology, their weakness—seen especially in Chomsky and Halle (1968) and related works—is that the form of the actually occurring utterances becomes the arbitrary result of the application of the rules, and hence has no inherent structure of its own.

More attention has been paid to phonological structures in more recent theories, especially in non-linear models, with a concern for the nature of *phonological representations*. In these models, a more elaborate, multi-dimensional form is assumed for utterances, manifested either as a hierarchical organization, as in metrical phonology and a number of other models, or as a set of parallel and interacting tiers, as in autosegmental theory. Though such models remain generative in the broad sense, they presuppose the existence of a number of constructional principles on which the output of the grammar is based, and by which the rules are constrained. Given such a view, it is evident that utterances can no longer be seen merely as the product of the rules; they must be regarded as having an independently motivated structure which constrains the operation of the rules.

The assumption underlying the discussion in the present chapter is therefore that such an independently motivated structure exists in the area of prosodic features; the task is therefore to determine its nature and examine the place and role of the prosodic features within it. Such a structure must be recognized whatever form the specification of prosodic features may take, including rule-based generative models. How the constraints imposed by this structure are to be captured in a linguistic description depends on the theoretical assumptions underlying the description itself. In a structuralist framework the structure is seen as the framework for the operation of linguistic contrasts, and is not explicitly generated. Within a generative framework several different possibilities are available. The structure may be construed as the result of an elaborate *conspiracy* between phonological rules (Kisseberth, 1970), in which different formal processes lead to the same result; we could see prosodic structure as a complex set of *output conditions* or *surface phonetic constraints* on the rules of the grammar, constraining the rules to produce the desired outcome (Shibatani, 1973); or we could interpret this structure as a set of *filters*, allowing well-formed structures to pass but blocking ill-formed ones, in the spirit of Chomsky (1981).

A more recent trend, *Optimality Theory* (Prince and Smolensky, 1993; McCarthy and Prince, 1993; Archangeli and Langendoen (eds.), 1997), is based on similar principles, but it takes them further. Like the Principles and Parameters approach of Chomsky (1981), Optimality Theory assumes a set of constraints which take the place of rules; unlike other approaches, however, which attempt to establish exceptionless constraints, or regard the constraints as parameters applying in some languages but not in others, it regards these constraints as *violable*, and therefore not absolute. They are *ranked* in such a way that some may take precedence over others. The constraints are universal, but the ranking is language-specific. As in other constraint-based approaches, only forms which comply with the constraints can be sanctioned—or 'licensed'—by the grammar.[1]

This model has been applied to the specification of prosodic features by a number of scholars; an outline is provided by Hammond (1997). He suggests that the fact that segments are grouped into syllables in English can be stipulated by the constraint of SYLLABLE LICENSING, while the existence of a peak in each syllable is covered by the PEAK constraint. It is claimed that not all languages comply with these constraints; in some there may be segments which do not belong to syllables. English, with its consonant clusters, must violate a further constraint, *COMPLEX, which stipulates that there should be only one consonant in the syllable margin.[2] In order to deal with stress and feet, several further constraints can be invoked (Hammond, 1997): ROOTING ('words must be stressed'), TROCHAIC ('feet are trochaic'), and PARSE-SYLLABLE ('two

---

[1] Considerable claims have been made for this theory by its proponents; for Archangeli (1997) it is 'THE linguistic theory of the 1990s', and 'the dominant paradigm in formal phonology'. On the other hand, she concedes that 'there is very little published work available on Optimality Theory'. Some (published and unpublished) work in this framework is available at the Rutgers Optimality Archive (http://ruccs.rutgers.edu/roa.html).

[2] The asterisk here indicates a negative constraint, in this case that complex syllable onsets do not occur.

unfooted syllables cannot be adjacent'). In so far as they are valid, the same principles could presumably be extended to other parts of the prosodic hierarchy.

It is likely that, given a suitable set of constraints, much of prosodic structure
could be specified in these terms. That this approach—along with rule-based and
other constraint-based approaches—is not pursued here rests on a number of
considerations. In the first place, the focus in the present chapter is on *the
nature of the structure itself* rather than on the mechanisms whereby it might
be specified. Second, it is evident that any such constraint system is actually
derivative; it depends on a prior understanding of the structures which are to
be specified. The structures are therefore here taken to be primary, and the
means by which they are specified, whether through rule systems, constraints,
or any other formal devices, are from the perspective of this discussion regarded
as of secondary importance.

As a further justification for the primacy of structure, we may also claim that
this structure is not just an abstraction, present only in assumed mental representations of utterances, but has a physical basis. At various points in our discussion in the previous chapters we have seen that prosodic features rest on
fundamental aspects of the speech process itself; accentual features, for example,
have a rhythmical basis. This may be extended to units such as the syllable,
which, it has been claimed (Fry, 1964, 1968), is a basic unit of neurological pro-
gramming in speech. All of this entails recognition of prosodic structure not
as a mere formal device for the linguistic description of utterances but as the
fundamental basis for the production of speech.

Since the prosodic structure of different languages is not the same, it is clear,
nevertheless, that this structure is not wholly determined by physiological constraints. There are certainly some universal characteristics of prosodic structure
(such as the syllable) whose universality can legitimately be claimed, and which
in all probability are dependent on neurological or physiological principles.
There are also some differences between languages—for example, the different
bases of rhythm—where a similar principle (that of timing) is implemented in
a limited number of different phonetic ways; these differences might be accommodated by means of different 'parameter settings' in different languages. This
still leaves scope for many significant differences between the prosodic features
of different languages. Nevertheless, the fundamental *structure* of prosody in all
languages is heavily dependent on the requirements of the speaking process, and
it is this which will be considered in the remainder of this chapter.

6.2 The Nature of Prosodic Structure

6.2.1 PROSODIC DOMAINS

As we saw in Chapter 1, one possible definition of prosodic, as opposed to segmental, features is that they can be said to apply to, or be properties of, larger

stretches of speech than the individual segment. We must also note that different stretches of speech may be involved even for a single feature, so that the feature can be described as *stratified*; length, for example, may be a property not only of segments but, as we saw in Chapter 2, of syllables and feet; tone may apply to syllables, but again it may be associated with larger units, such as feet, as discussed in Chapter 4 (see 4.7.4); intonation patterns are parts of larger units, though here it is matter of some controversy what the basic units are (see Chapter 5).

We may call the stretch of speech to which we assign a particular feature its *domain*. The concept of a domain for a particular feature is a useful one, but it is not without its problems, since some features may be said to have two sorts of domains, which we may term the *domain of application* on the one hand and the *domain of relevance* on the other. A feature such as tone or accent may *apply to* a particular domain in the sense that it is a phonetic property of that domain, in this case generally the syllable. On the other hand we may say that the contrasts for which the feature *is relevant* can only be established over a larger domain—in the case of accent, for example, the foot.[3] This dual notion of domain is an inevitable consequence of the syntagmatic nature of prosodic features, which involve relationships between different points within a particular stretch of speech.[4]

Different features may share domains; both the syllable and the foot are domains for a number of prosodic features. The fact that such domains are shared means that we can establish a small set of prosodic *units* which can serve as prosodic domains. The basic units have been considered at various points in the preceding chapters, where we have recognized syllables, feet, and intonation units (other possible units have been discussed by different scholars, including especially the mora, the prosodic word, and the superfoot). Although the basic units are found in many languages, they are not universal: the foot is not a prosodic unit in languages which lack the Level 1 accentuation discussed in Chapter 3.

The existence of such prosodic units, and their importance as domains for more than one feature, suggests that the systematization of prosodic structure depends to a large extent on the systematization of these units and the relationships between them. This is not just a matter of relating the units to one another, however, but also of accommodating various other dimensions of

---

[3] As noted in Ch. 3, a distinction is made along these lines in the case of accent by Garde (1968: 12), who distinguishes between the *accentable* unit (the syllable) and the *accentual* unit (the foot).

[4] This is particularly true of accent, and of those cases where tone or quantity have an accentual role. For example, in two-tone systems with H and L tones, the H tone may be restricted in its occurrence so that its location takes on syntagmatic significance. It is in such cases that tone has been interpreted as accent by some scholars (see 4.7.5). The same might be true of quantity systems where 'long' vs. 'short' can be interpreted syntagmatically. Here, too, 'long' is likely to be interpreted as 'accented' and 'short' as 'unaccented'.

prosodic structure which depend in different ways on these units. This will be clarified and developed in the remainder of this chapter.

6.2.2 THE PROSODIC HIERARCHY

In our consideration of the individual prosodic features, one property of prosodic structure has repeatedly emerged: its hierarchical nature. In many cases where units such as the syllable, the foot, and the intonation unit, as well as less universally recognized units such as the mora, have appeared in the discussion, it has been in the context of an arrangement with smaller and larger units, where the larger can be said to contain the smaller. But though the existence of some sort of hierarchy in phonology is hardly controversial, the units involved, the precise nature of this hierarchy, and the strictness with which it is adhered to, are more contentious matters.

The concept of hierarchy in language is a very traditional one. Abercrombie (1949) draws attention to the hierarchical arrangement of units that was present—often implicitly rather than explicitly—in the descriptions of classical and traditional grammarians: 'human speech (*vox articulata et literata*)', he writes, 'the subject matter of grammar, may, according to this doctrine [viz. that of the Greeks and Romans], be split up into progressively smaller units: sentences, words, syllables and letters'. This hierarchy is depicted in Fig. 6.1.

Fig. 6.1   sentence
          word
          syllable
          letter

The hierarchy of Fig. 6.1 is, however, unsatisfactory because it is a conflation of different hierarchies, phonological, morpho-syntactic, and even orthographic.[5] If we invoke the 'double articulation' of language, we can split it into two parallel hierarchies, a grammatical and a phonological one (cf. Fudge, 1969). Fig 6.2 gives one version of a possible grammatical hierarchy.

Fig. 6.2   sentence
          clause
          phrase
          word
          morpheme

This hierarchy is inherent in many grammatical models, though it does not necessarily appear explicitly. Much grammatical analysis is based on the Immedi-

---

[5] It is, however, unjust, as Abercrombie (1949) makes clear, to see the incorporation of the 'letter' as a confusion of speech and writing; the term 'letter' was explicitly used to cover 'speech sound' until the invention of the latter technical term in the 19th century.

ate Constituent approach begun by Bloomfield (1935: 160-1) and developed by Wells (1947), which, though hierarchical, concentrates on the branching tree structure rather than on the units involved. Bloomfield describes the structure of the sentence *Poor John ran away* in terms of immediate constituents, but simply labels each constituent, apart from the individual morphemes, as a 'form'; Wells refers informally to 'sentences', 'words', and 'morphemes', but does not explicitly label constituents in terms of these units. Thus, no specific set of units is recognized here. Immediate constituents are also incorporated into the earlier versions of Generative Grammar, where structures are specified by Phrase–Structure rules. Chomsky (1957) describes the structure of the sentence *The man hit the ball* as in Fig. 6.3; it will be noted that he not only describes immediate constituents, but also gives them a category label—NP, VP, T, N, Verb—and the whole is labelled 'Sentence'. Since the labels NP and VP stand for phrase-types, and T, N, and Verb are word-types, the hierarchy of Fig. 6.2 is evidently implicit in the diagram, and in the rules which generate it.

Fig. 6.3

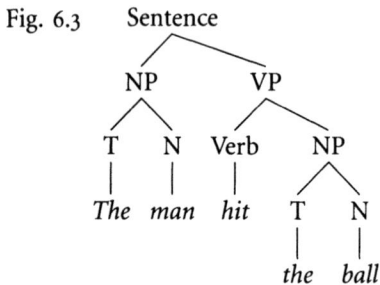

In more recent versions of phrase–structure grammars, too, such as X-bar syntax (Jackendoff, 1977), there is a similarly implicit hierarchy. In the diagram of Fig. 6.4 (Jackendoff, 1977: 17), X'' represents a phrasal category, and X a word type, with X' as an intermediate entity between the two, though no category labels as such are indicated.

Fig. 6.4

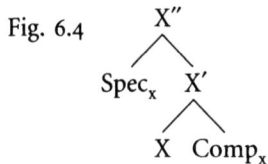

Such principles can also be applied to phonology. Although Wells (1947) considers phonological categories in his discussion of Immediate Constituents and there was an early analysis of the syllable in these terms by Pike and Pike (1947)—see Fig. 2.19—there were few attempts to incorporate a phonological hierarchy explicitly into the phonological theories of the 'classical' structuralist schools. Notable exceptions are the work of Hockett (1947, 1955), the 'scale and category' (later 'systemic') theory of Halliday (Halliday, 1961; Halliday, McIntosh, and Strevens, 1964: 51), the 'tagmemic' theory of Pike (1967: ch. 9), and a few others, all of which provide a hierarchy of phonological units. 'Classical' generative phonology (Chomsky and Halle, 1968) has no use for such structures, since on the one hand phonological structure is considered to be merely the concatenation of segment-sized feature-bundles, and on the other hand the domains of phonological processes affecting prosodic features are considered to be largely morpho-syntactic rather than phonological, and hence larger phonological domains are unnecessary or irrelevant.[6] This approach is still prevalent, as we have seen in several places in the preceding chapters, notably in the attempts to derive accentual and intonational structures from syntactic bracketing. Hence scholars in the generative tradition have felt the need to establish the credentials of a purely *phonological* structure. Inkelas and Zec (1990: xiii) support a proposal for the emancipation of phonology from syntax which 'consists of positing a new level of representation, prosodic structure, which serves as a mediator between the two components of phonology and syntax, and provides a locale for stating restrictions on their interaction'. This proposal, while not denying the relevance of syntax to prosodic structure, in effect restricts its influence to determining the boundaries of prosodic domains. More recent non-linear theories, especially Metrical Phonology (Liberman and Prince, 1977; Hogg and McCully, 1987; Goldsmith, 1990) have attempted to redress the balance, and have not only accepted the independent status of prosodic structure, but have also frequently employed hierarchical tree-structures. One approach which has explicitly recognized and advocated the use of such a hierarchy is Prosodic Phonology (Nespor and Vogel, 1982, 1983, 1986).

The simplest conception of a hierarchical phonological structure is as a set of units of different sizes or scopes, with the smaller progressively nested within the larger. The utterance *Every student must attend the lecture*, for example, would, in a typical pronunciation, contain ten syllables, with each odd-numbered syllable accented, and the last such accented syllable bearing the intonational nucleus. With the accented syllables marked with ' and the nucleus printed in capitals, this utterance could be transcribed as in Fig. 6.5(a). Expressing this in terms of a hierarchy of units, we would obtain the representation Fig. 6.5(b). Three units are needed, *intonation unit, foot,* and *syllable*, and their boundaries are represented by //, /, and ·, respectively. Since the boundaries of the units at different levels are assumed to coincide (an intonation unit boundary is also a foot boundary and a foot boundary is also a syllable boundary),[7]

---

[6] This view may in part be a reaction against the Bloomfieldian 'separation of levels' which generative phonologists were eager to abandon.

[7] Whether this is actually the case is a matter of some interest. On the whole this principle seems to apply fairly consistently, so that, for example, foot boundaries appear always to coincide with syllable boundaries. However, in sequences of intonation units, their boundaries do not necessarily coincide with those of feet, though the exact location of intonation unit boundaries is not always easy to determine.

these three levels can be combined in one representation, given in Fig. 6.5(c).

Fig. 6.5 (a) 'every 'student 'must at'tend the 'LECture

    (b) Intonation Unit: // ɛvriː stjuːdnt mʌst ətend ðə lɛktʃə //
           Feet: / ɛvriː / stjuːdnt / mʌst ə / tend ðə / lɛktʃə /
           Syllables: · ɛv · riː · stjuː · dnt · mʌst · ə · tend · ðə · lɛk · tʃə ·

    (c) // ɛv · riː / stjuː · dnt / mʌst · ə / tend · ðə / lɛk · tʃə //

Another way of representing this structure is in the form of a branching tree, as in Fig. 6.6(a), where I = 'Intonation Unit', F = 'Foot', and σ = 'Syllable'. It would also be possible to divide this utterance into two intonation units, as in Fig. 6.6(b), where U = 'Utterance'.

Fig. 6.6 (a)

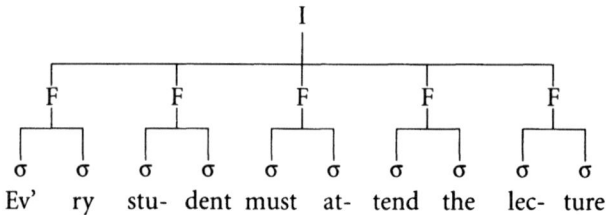

(b)

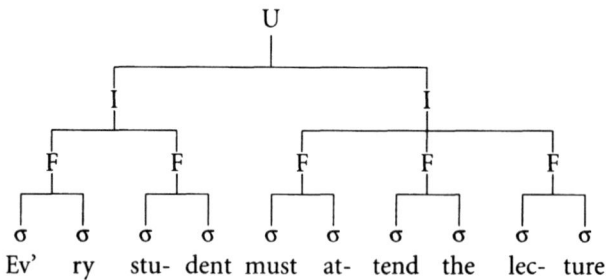

As can be seen from these figures, the fundamental principle assumed in this model is that there is a set of units of different sizes, with smaller units included within larger ones. At its strictest—the 'strict layer hypothesis' of Selkirk (1980)—the model claims that any utterance in the language can always be described without residue at any level; units at any one level will consist entirely of one or more instances of the unit below. The set of units themselves can be represented in a simple hierarchy, as in Fig. 6.7.

Fig. 6.7 utterance
       intonation unit
       foot
       syllable

The hierarchy of Fig. 6.7 is that used by Abercrombie (1964) and, following him, by Halliday (Halliday, McIntosh, and Strevens, 1964: 51; Halliday, 1967); similar sets of units are suggested by other scholars, though the number of units recognized, as well as the terms used, varies. Pike's 'Tagmemic' theory (see especially Pike, 1967, ch. 9; E. V. Pike, 1976) distinguishes between a 'phoneme' and a 'hyperphoneme', the latter being 'any phonological unit which is larger or higher ranking than a phoneme' (Pike, 1967: 364). Among these hyperphonemes are the 'emic syllable' (or 'syllabeme'), the 'emic stress group' (or 'abdomineme'),[8] and the 'emic pause group', together with an indeterminate number of larger units, beginning with the 'emic breath group', the 'emic rhetorical period', and the 'emic phonological section'. Pike's hierarchy of hyperphonemes is presented graphically in Fig. 6.8.

Fig. 6.8   emic phonological section
          emic rhetorical period
          emic breath group
          emic pause group
          emic stress group ('abdomineme')
          emic syllable ('syllabeme')

Such a hierarchy has also been adopted by a number of scholars working in current non-linear frameworks. Liberman and Prince (1977) discuss different phonological units, and Selkirk (1980) incorporates them more formally into the model. Her basic categories are given in Fig. 6.9.[9]

Fig. 6.9   prosodic word (ω)
          stress foot (Σ)
          syllable (σ)

Finally, we may note the hierarchy advocated by Nespor and Vogel (1982, 1983, 1986) in their 'Prosodic Phonology'; this is given as Fig. 6.10.

Fig. 6.10   phonological utterance
           intonational phrase
           phonological phrase
           clitic group
           phonological word
           foot
           syllable

Despite the differences between these hierarchies—they differ primarily, but not exclusively, in the number of units recognized at the top end of the

---

[8] This rather inelegant term reflects Pike's view of the nature of stress, which, as will be clear from Ch. 3, is not adopted in the present book.
[9] Selkirk also makes occasional use of a 'superfoot', intermediate between the stress-foot and prosodic word. Its status is, however, doubtful. See 6.5 below.

scale—they all agree in establishing a simple scale, with smaller units included in larger ones. As we shall see in what follows, this conception is of fundamental importance for prosodic structure, though it must be supplemented by a variety of other principles and categories.

6.2.3 DIMENSIONS OF PROSODIC STRUCTURE

Not all published prosodic hierarchies are of quite the form given in Fig. 6.7. In Hockett's description of Mandarin Chinese phonology (Hockett, 1947), for example, we find the arrangement depicted in Fig. 6.11. Here, the utterance is divided into two Immediate Constituents, *register contour* and one or more *macrosegments*; the latter is divided into *intonation* and one or more *mesosegments*; the latter is in turn divided into a *stress contour* and one or more *microsegments* and the last of these finally into *stress, tone,* and *residual structure* (the last of these corresponds to the segmental phonemes). This tree is clearly quite different from the simple, non-branching hierarchy presented in Figs. 6.7 to 6.10.

Fig. 6.11

```
                    (utterance)
         ┌──────────────┴──────────────┐
   register contour              macrosegment
                      ┌───────────────┴───────────────┐
                 intonation                      mesosegment
                            ┌──────────────┴──────────────┐
                      stress contour                 microsegment
                                           ┌──────────┼──────────┐
                                         stress     tone   residual structure
```

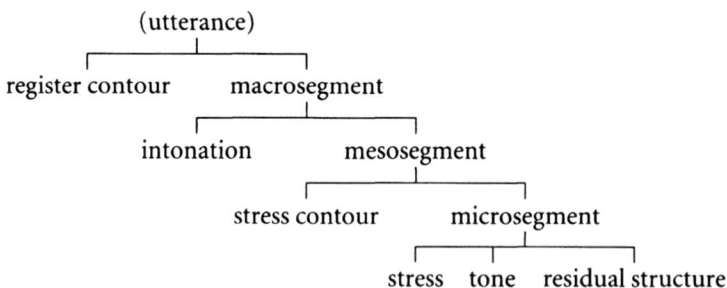

Some of the differences here are merely terminological; Hockett's microsegment is the syllable, his mesosegment is the foot, and his macrosegment is the intonation unit. But what differentiates his tree from those of Figs. 6.7 to 6.10 is that it has *branches*, but, unlike the branching tree of Fig. 6.6, there is more than one kind of element at each level. The mesosegment (foot), for example, does not only consist of microsegments (syllables), but in addition contains the stress contour; the macrosegment (intonation unit) does not just consist of mesosegments (feet) but also contains the intonation.

Hockett has clearly included in his tree not merely units as such, but also *features of units*: intonation, stress contour, stress, and tone. That such features are in some sense part of the units they characterize is not in doubt, but their status is evidently very different from units as such, which are the *domains* of features. The difficulty that arises in putting both units and features on the same basis can be seen in the different treatments given to features in different works by Hockett. In the analysis of Fig. 6.11, from his work of 1947, the macrosegment consists of intonation and mesosegment; in his *Manual* of 1955, a different view of this structure is presented. Here, the Immediate Constituents of the macrosegment are given as 'intonation' and 'remainder', and then, by a terminological sleight of hand, the latter is renamed 'macrosegment' (Hockett, 1955: 51) and divided into 'stress contour' and 'mesosegment'.[10] The two configurations are given in Fig. 6.12.

Fig. 6.12 (a) (1947)   (b) (1955)

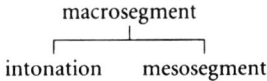

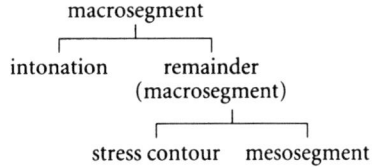

Hockett is evidently unsure whether features (intonation, stress contour) should be regarded as *daughters* of the units they apply to (here the macrosegment and mesosegment) or their *sisters*, that is, whether the configuration should be that of Fig. 6.13(a) or 6.13(b), where units and the features which apply to them are identified by identical subscripts. This uncertainty evidently arises from attempting to include features in the hierarchy alongside and equivalent to the units which they characterize, whereas they belong to a different dimension of prosodic structure, and do not sit comfortably on the tree at all.

Fig. 6.13 (a)   (b)

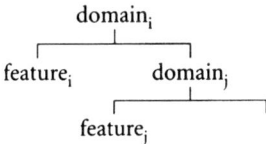

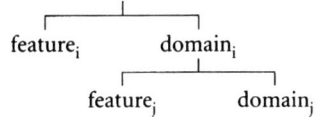

Similar difficulties arise with other discussions of hierarchical structures in phonology. A European structuralist attempt to provide a richer prosodic structure is found in Togeby's glossematic description of French—one of the few detailed applications of this theory to an actual language (Togeby, 1965). Like that of Hockett, his model is hierarchical, with the *phrase de modulation* as the highest unit: *la procédure prosodique consiste à diviser ces phrases de l'expression en leurs parties constituantes immédiates, par exemple en groupes de syllabes, ceux-ci à leur tour en syllabes, celles-ci en accent + thème syllabique, etc.* This hierarchy is represented in the form of a *table prosodique*, given here as Fig. 6.14, which lists *units*

---

[10] Hockett remarks (1955: 51) that 'the term "remainder" is so awkward that we shall now make a terminological shift, using henceforth the term "macrosegment" itself for what we have previously been calling a "macrosegment" *minus* its intonation'.

('unités') and their *parts* ('parties'). The items in brackets do not apply to French.

Fig. 6.14

Unités	*Parties*
texte	ligne de l'expression + ligne du contenu
ligne de l'expression	phrases de modulation
phrase de modulation	phrase + modulation
phrase	groupes de syllabes
(groupe syllabique)	(syllabe à accent faible + syllabe à accent fort)
syllabe	(accent + thème syllabique)
thème syllabique	centre vocalique + marge consonantique
groupe d'éléments	voyelles, consonnes

There are some difficulties of interpretation here which are not solved by Togeby's discussion (pp. 31-49), and these make it difficult to convert his table into a tree-diagram. Nevertheless, a corresponding tree is presented in Fig. 6.15, with the omission of the top two lines; Togeby's brackets are ignored; the square brackets are added for the reasons discussed below. Like Hockett, Togeby includes features as well as units in the tree; his *phrase de modulation* (intonation unit) and his syllable have the intonation pattern and the accent as constituents. But his table presents a number of further problems. The *groupe syllabique* is divided not simply into syllables but into *syllabe à accent faible* and *syllabe à accent fort*, while the syllable (or rather the *thème syllabique*—the syllable *minus* the accent) is divided not into phonemes (the term *phonème* does not appear in his table at all, though it occurs in his discussion) but into *centre vocalique* and *marge consonantique*. In order to proceed to the next lower level in the tree, it is necessary to group the two categories together again as *syllabe* and *groupe d'éléments* respectively—the square brackets are put in here to signal this. In the same way, the *groupe d'éléments* is further divided into *voyelles* and *consonnes*. There are thus a number of intermediate levels here whose status is not clear.

In order to explain these additional levels we must make a further category distinction: between a *unit* on the one hand and a *structural or functional constituent* of a unit on the other. This distinction is familiar from syntactic discussions as the difference between categories such as 'phrase' on the one hand, and functional labels such as 'subject' or 'object' on the other. Here, 'phrase' is a particular unit of the grammatical hierarchy; 'subject' is a functional category within the sentence. An analogous phonological distinction would be that between 'phoneme' on the one hand, and 'onset' or 'coda' on the other. A phrase may function as subject, and a phoneme may constitute the coda to a syllable, but these are different categories, established on a different basis, and they must be kept apart. Some of the problems with Togeby's framework can be attributed to a failure to do so. His *thème syllabique* is divided into peak (*centre vocalique*) and margin (*marge consonantique*); this is a perfectly legitimate analysis into functional constituents, but it should not be included in the same tree or table as units as such.

Fig. 6.15

```
                    phrase de modulation
            ┌────────────┴────────────┐
       modulation                   phrase
                                      │
                             groupe de syllabes
                              (groupe syllabique)
                        ┌────────────┴────────────┐
                   syllabe à                   syllabe à
                  accent faible              accent fort
                        └────────────┬────────────┘
                                 [syllabe]
                        ┌────────────┴────────────┐
                     accent              thème syllabique
                                  ┌───────────┴───────────┐
                               centre                   marge
                              vocalique              consonantique
                                  └───────────┬───────────┘
                                     [groupe d'éléments]
                                  ┌───────────┴───────────┐
                              voyelles                 consonnes
```

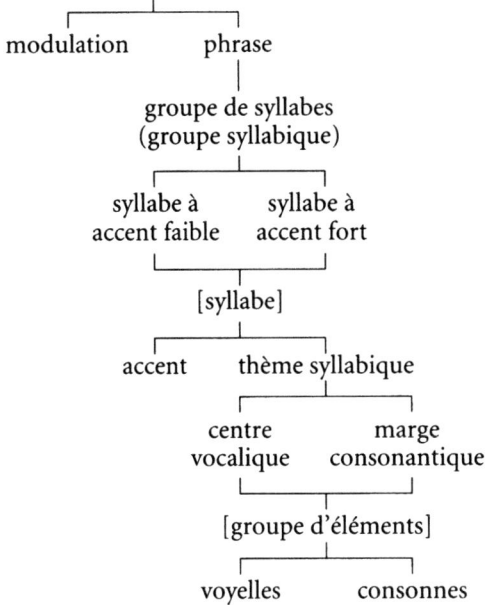

There remain further items in Togeby's framework which require explanation. He divides the *groupe syllabique* (equivalent to the foot) into *syllabe à accent faible* and *syllabe à accent fort*, and the *groupe d'éléments* (a cluster of phonemes forming a syllable peak or margin) into *voyelles* and *consonnes*. We thus have two different kinds of syllables and two different kinds of phonemes. The distinctions made here by Togeby involve different *types* or *classes* of units, and this again constitutes another dimension from the simple units themselves, and adds to the complexity of the tree.

Again a grammatical parallel may help to clarify the situation. A grammatical hierarchy might include such units as 'phrase', 'word', and 'morpheme', and these may be subclassified into types, such as 'noun phrase' and 'verb phrase', 'noun' and 'verb', and 'root' and 'affix'. Again this is a legitimate and necessary dimension of classification, but it is, of course, different from the identification of the units themselves. The relationship between 'word' and 'morpheme' is one of composition; that between 'word' and 'noun' is one of subclassification at the same level. Togeby's division of the *groupe syllabique* into two kinds of syllables (those with strong accent and those with weak accent) involves two dimensions of analysis simultaneously: the analysis of a group of syllables (presumably an accentual unit such as the foot) into its component syllables, and a simultaneous subclassification of the syllables into accented and unaccented. A similar analysis is involved in the case of the *groupe d'éléments*, which consists of vowels and consonants. The latter are two different classes of phonemes.

These various confusions and difficulties make it clear that there is a fundamental difference between a hierarchy of *units* on the one hand, and a hierarchy
of *attributes of units* on the other. The units themselves form a legitimate hierarchy, where the higher units include the lower. *Features* of units, their *functions*,
and the *classes* of units, on the other hand, are hierarchical only by virtue of
being properties of units which are arranged hierarchically. Their apparent hierarchical arrangement, with intonation higher up the tree than stress, and stress
higher up the tree than segmental features, and similarly with functions and
classes, is simply the result of the hierarchical arrangement of the units to which
they apply. We may therefore distinguish between the *primary hierarchy* of units
on the one hand and what may be called the *secondary hierarchies* of features,
functions, and classes on the other. The hierarchies in the latter case are not
autonomous; their hierarchical nature is parasitic upon the primary hierarchy
of the units themselves.

This distinction is important for the present discussion. A wide range of different and competing hierarchies have been proposed in the phonological literature, but the majority of them are found on closer inspection to be secondary,
since they presuppose and depend on a primary hierarchy. The conclusion that
we are forced to draw is that the only truly hierarchical structure that can be
recognized here is that of a set of units such as that of Fig. 6.7. The prosodic
hierarchy is thus basically one-dimensional in the sense that there is a simple set
of units, related by composition, and observing the 'Strict Layer Hypothesis' of
Selkirk (1980). The other 'hierarchies' are secondary, and, while clearly important, they must be referred to other dimensions of prosodic structure which
depend on the hierarchy, but are not in themselves hierarchical.

As an illustration consider the question of syllable structure. In terms of the
primary hierarchy of units this can be stated in terms of 'phonemes' or some
other such segmental unit. A syllable such as *ground* (/graund/), for example,
consists of 5 or 6 phonemes, according to how the diphthong is analysed.
An alternative analysis is available, however, in which these segments are classified as C (consonant) and V (vowel): CCVVCC. These two analyses, given as
Fig. 6.16 (σ = syllable; π = phoneme), appear to give hierarchies with different
sets of units, but that of Fig. 6.16(b) in fact includes two dimensions: the units
themselves, on different levels (syllable and phoneme—in the latter case implicit
in the symbols C and V), and the classification of units into types at a single
level (C and V). While the first of these dimensions is a primary hierarchy, the
second is not, so that Fig. 6.16(b) conflates two dimensions.

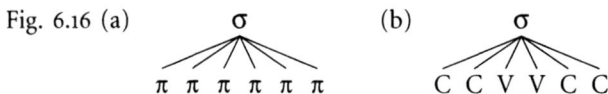

Fig. 6.16 (a) σ (b) σ

π π π π π π C C V V C C

More elaborate views of syllable structure are also found, as illustrated in
Fig. 6.17(a) (cf. Hockett, 1955: 52; Kahn, 1976) and in the 'syllable template'
(Selkirk, 1980) of Fig. 6.17(b). In the case of Fig. 6.17(a) the situation is analo-

Fig 6.17 (a)   (b)

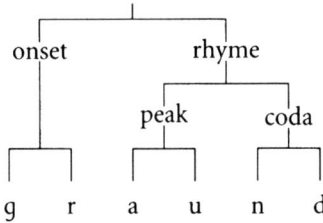 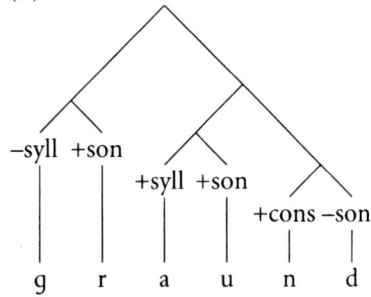

gous to that found in syntax, where alongside such categorial notions as NP, PP, etc. (themselves part of a secondary hierarchy as types or classes of units—cf. C and V in Figure 6.16(b)) we find functional categories such as 'subject', 'adjunct', etc. It is possible to draw syntactic trees to display the structure in terms of either, though following Chomsky (1965: 68) it has generally been assumed that the latter are relational labels which can be derived from the configuration of the tree itself. But in any case it is clear that the functional categories belong to a secondary hierarchy, since the functions are exercised by units of the primary hierarchy.[11] The functions are hierarchically ordered because the units themselves are. In Fig 6.17(b) the labels are those of *features* of the units in question, which again constitute a secondary hierarchy. In both (a) and (b) of Fig. 6.17 the primary units are implicit in the tree, even though there are no unit labels.

Applying these concepts to higher levels of prosodic structure using the sample sentence of Fig. 6.5a, we might designate the functional parts of the intonation unit (I) the 'head' and the 'nucleus', and, following Halliday (1967), the

Fig. 6.18

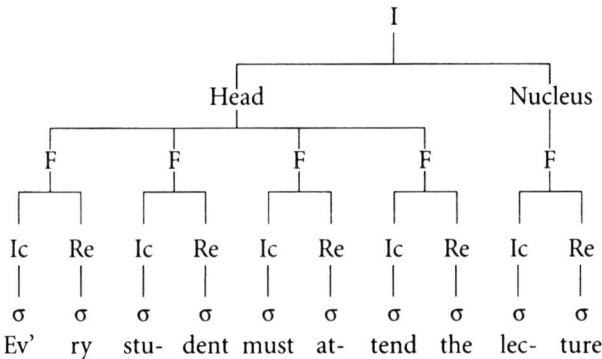

---

[11] This is only true in so far as functional roles are exercised by single occurrences of units. The categories of Fig. 6.17(a), for example—onset, rhyme, peak, and coda—evidently do not correspond to units of the primary hierarchy, since they consist of *groups* of units. This question will be considered further below.

functional parts of the foot (F) the 'ictus' (Ic) and the 'remiss' (Re). If we were to include these in our hierarchy we would obtain the tree of Fig. 6.18. The problem is immediately obvious: further 'secondary' units are introduced into the hierarchy in addition to the 'primary' ones, obscuring the nature of the prosodic hierarchy itself.

As we have noted in a number of places in this book, one form of representation in Metrical Phonology (Liberman and Prince, 1977; Hogg and McCully, 1987; Goldsmith, 1990; Hayes, 1995) takes the form of a branching tree, with nodes labelled s(trong) and w(eak), as in Fig. 6.19 (repeated from Fig. 3.14).

Fig. 6.19

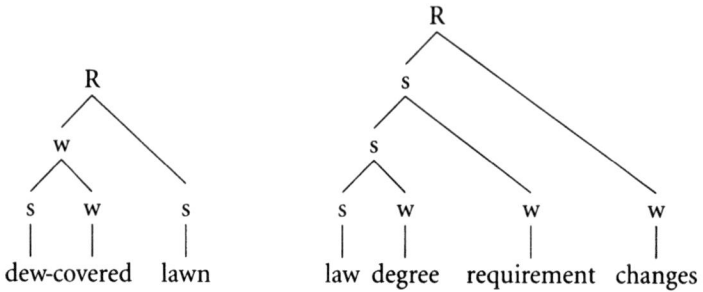

Here we apparently have a hierarchy not of units but of 'strong' and 'weak' nodes. It is clear, however, that such a hierarchy is not independent, but reflects an implicit hierarchy of unidentified units that are so labelled. The hierarchy of s and w nodes is therefore a secondary one. Indeed, we regularly find 's' and 'w' used as subscripts to unit labels such as 'syllable'. For example, Selkirk (1980) and Hayes (1981) give representations such as those of Fig. 6.20 (repeated from Fig. 3.20), with syllables, feet and 'phonological words' labelled 's' or 'w'.

Fig. 6.20

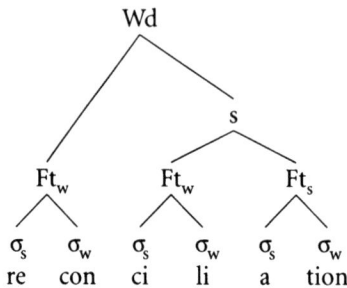

Giegerich (1984: 2) recognizes that there is, in effect, a double hierarchy in metrical trees such as that of Fig. 6.19, the 'hierarchy of phonological constituents', and the 'hierarchy of relative prominence', which correspond to what we have called 'primary' and 'secondary' hierarchies respectively. However, he rejects the former, arguing that it is derivable from the latter: 'I assume . . . that all such notions are relationally defined in metrical phonology and needn't therefore be stated in the tree' (1984: 13). Similar claims are made by Selkirk

(1984: 31). However, the apparent economy achieved by this is purely notational, since the primary hierarchy is in any case implicit in the representation, and there are further dangers in assuming the autonomy of the metrical 'hierarchy', since it can lead to the introduction of spurious units.

It is of interest, nevertheless, that the same categories, strong and weak, are used to label the whole tree, in spite of the fact that different units are involved at different levels; s(trong) and w(eak) are, of course, purely 'relational' labels, with no intrinsic content, and it is this which allows the use of these categories at different levels. They represent not phonetic features but *structural* categories. In fact, the s category represents nothing more than the *head* constituent at a particular level of structure. That the s vs. w categorization is particularly applicable to accentual features is also due to the assumed binary nature of accentual distinctions: the syllables of a foot may be accented or unaccented; the feet of an intonation unit may be nuclear or non-nuclear. By equating the more prominent and less prominent elements at each level we obtain a single dichotomy: strong vs. weak. It is probable, therefore, that these labels are in fact cover terms for different distinctions at different levels.

From this discussion we may draw some conclusions about the nature of prosodic structure. At the heart of this structure is a set of units, hierarchically ordered, serving as the domains of the prosodic features. In addition, there are a number of other dimensions which depend on these domains: functional categories in terms of which the structure of the units can be described, classes of units determined by their role in this structure, and features themselves. The set of units forms a primary hierarchy, while the dependent categories can be called secondary hierarchies, as their hierarchical arrangement is due to the hierarchical arrangements of the units of the primary hierarchy.

6.2.4 PROSODIC MODELS

Given the approach outlined above, we need to consider how the various categories discussed can be integrated into an overall framework. A number of structuralist models have been developed which attempt to accommodate multi-dimensional frameworks of this kind, notably the 'tagmemic' framework of Pike (1967) and the 'systemic' framework of Halliday (1961), the latter at least in its early version of 'scale and category' grammar. It is worth considering some of the principles adopted in these models in order to clarify the issues and identify the problems here, though not with a view to adopting either of these as a definitive model.

As we have seen, Pike's 'tagmemic' theory establishes a hierarchy of units (Fig. 6.8); it accommodates other dimensions by applying the concept of a 'tagmeme', which is a 'slot' + 'filler' relationship, the slot being, in effect, a structural element of a unit, and the filler being the class of the lower unit which occupies the slot. At the grammatical level, this would involve, for example, a combination such as 'Subject: Noun Phrase'; at the phonological level we could have 'Syllable Margin: Consonant' (Pike restricts the term 'tagmeme' to the grammatical level; the parallel phonological notion is the 'phonemic slot–class correlative' (1967: 340)).

A similar framework is provided by Halliday (1961), again not specifically phonological. The units of his hierarchy (the 'rank scale') are each described in terms of their 'elements of structure', each such element defining a 'class' of the unit below, which occurs as (part of) the element in question. Thus the element of structure 'S' (Subject) of the sentence defines a particular class of phrases (viz. Noun Phrases) which can function as the subject. Applied to prosodic structure, this theory would recognize, for example, 'ictus' and 'remiss' as elements of structure of the foot, defining two classes of syllable: 'salient' and 'weak', equivalent to accented and unaccented, respectively (Halliday, 1967: 12).

In both these phonological frameworks we therefore find analogous concepts: not only is phonological structure seen as a hierarchical arrangement of units, each unit forming part of the unit above, but the structure of any unit can be described in terms of certain parts ('slots', 'elements of structure') and hence the lower units of which a unit is composed can be subcategorized into types ('fillers', 'classes') according to their position in this structure.

The aim here is not to give a detailed exposition of either tagmemic or systemic grammar, still less to adopt them as models, but rather to see how the various dimensions of prosodic structure identified above can be related to one another. We must also take account, therefore, of some of the limitations of this kind of description, and of the criticisms that have been made of these theories. Since most of the discussion has been concerned with the application of these models to grammatical structure, we shall initially consider the problems that arise in the syntactic area before examining their phonological analogues.

One complication with a fixed set of units is that the structure occurring at each level may be quite complex. Each 'slot' or 'element of structure' may contain more than one occurrence of the unit below. We could recognize, for example, 'subject' as a slot in the structure of a clause, but in a co-ordinate structure there will be more than one phrase occupying this slot. Similarly, a compound word will have more than one root and an inflected word may have more than one affix. This is not in itself a problem for the different theories; Pike accepts as the filler for a slot not just a single unit but also a 'syntagmeme', which is a concatenation of units. More problematic is the fact that the structure of a unit is not necessarily a simple linear one, but may itself be hierarchically organized. A noun phrase such as *the big red book*, for example, consists of words, but there may be intermediate nodes between the phrase and the word, labelled X and Y in Fig. 6.21. It is these nodes that are covered by the single-bar category (X') in Fig. 6.4, above; indeed this category is introduced precisely to deal with recursive structures of this sort. The same is true in phonological analysis. We may regard the syllable as consisting of phonemes or some other segmental unit, but the structure of the syllable is not necessarily linear, as the analysis of Pike and Pike (1947), Kahn (1976), and Selkirk (1978, 1980), show.

Fig. 6.21

```
         NP
      ┌───┴────┐
      │        X
      │     ┌──┴───┐
      │     │      Y
      │     │   ┌──┴──┐
     Det    A   A     N
      │     │   │     │
     the   big red   book
```

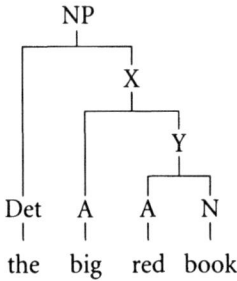

Another problem with a fixed hierarchy of units is the occurrence of units at a higher or lower level than normal. An instance of the former would be a conjunction (a word) linking two clauses, in which case it is immediately dominated by the sentence node, without intervening phrase and clause nodes. An instance of the latter would be the occurrence of a relative clause as part of a noun phrase. Such problems disturb the neatness of the hierarchy of units, and for many linguists they fatally undermine the concept of a hierarchy of units. Matthews (1966), for example, argues that as a result of such deviations from a strict hierarchy, 'the concept of rank is at once stripped of its theoretical significance'. Longacre (1970) concedes that 'attempts to define hierarchy overly rigidly in terms of exclusively descending exponence can only lead to complete jettisoning of the notion of hierarchy'.

Special provision has to be made for these complications in any theory. In tagmemic analysis notions such as 'nesting' and 'recursion' are invoked, as well as the concepts of 'level-skipping' and 'back-looping' to accommodate units occurring at a higher and a lower level than usual respectively (Longacre, 1970). Halliday (1961) calls the latter 'rank-shift'. Longacre sees 'descending exponence' (higher units consisting of lower ones) as a principle to which utterances must ultimately conform, but which may be temporarily interrupted by the complications just described. The analogy is with a river: 'often, the course of the river is smooth (descending hierarchy); there may be however, a cataract here and there (level-skipping), or eddies of various degrees of turbulence (back-looping) or lakes (recursions). The presence of cataracts, eddies and lakes in no way contradicts the fact that the river is progressing in a general downward direction.' Hence, 'both recursion and back-looping must, eventually, terminate and give way to the downward thrust' (Longacre, 1970: 186).

As for the intermediate structures that occur between units, Huddleston (1965) recognizes that the complexities may go beyond an arrangement of fixed units. He extends Halliday's scales to include not only 'rank' (the hierarchical arrangement of units) but 'depth', which is a measure of the extent to which an item is embedded within such a structure. For Huddleston, 'depth is helpful in describing the layering of structural constituents', but rank is 'deeper', and more important, since 'the rank scale enables us to assign features to the appropriate stretch of the text'. Halliday similarly defends the fixed rank scale, on the grounds that 'it facilitates generalization about syntagmatic and paradigmatic relations' (1966: 115).

So far, our discussion has been primarily in terms of syntax, and we would expect the same principles—and the same criticisms—to be carried over into the phonological domain. But this is not always the case. In the first place, there is no 'level-skipping' in phonology. We do not find, say, phonemes appearing directly as constituents of feet, or syllables as constituents of intonation units. It is always possible to assign such phonemes to syllables and such syllables to feet. Second, there is no equivalent of 'back-looping' or 'rank-shift' in phonology; we do not find feet appearing in the structure of syllables, or intonation units in the structure of feet. To this extent, then, a phonological hierarchy is less problematic than a grammatical one, and many of the criticisms that have been directed to the latter simply do not apply to the former. That the phonological hierarchy is more robust and less subject to disruption than the grammatical one is probably to be attributed to the fact that it is not just an arbitrary, formal, and abstract construct but is phonetically based. Units such as the syllable or the foot are not merely categories of phonological organization but have their roots in the neural and physiological constraints of the articulatory mechanism itself.

There remains, however, the problematic relationship between the hierarchy of units as such and the nodes of a constituent structure tree. On what grounds do we establish a fixed set of units, whatever the structural complexity involved? Given a structure such as that of Fig. 6.17(a), repeated here as Fig. 6.22, why is it that the top node is a syllable, and the terminal nodes are segments (phonemes), while the intermediate nodes have no status as units?

Fig. 6.22

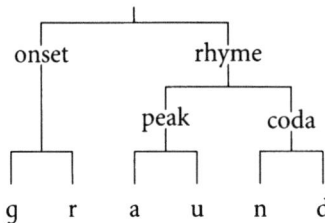

In order to answer these questions we must first recall that the structural parts (slots, elements of structure) may consist of more than one instance of the unit below; the 'onset' slot of Fig. 6.22 consists of two segments. A group of units of this sort has been called an 'expansion' of a single unit (Wells, 1947). Typically, the basic unit in such a construction is regarded as the *head*; the remaining units are subordinate to the head in the sense that they cannot occur without the head, though the head can occur independently. Pike (1974) refers to a 'paired hierarchy', in which each unit has a corresponding expansion, as in Fig. 6.23.

Fig. 6.23 | *Basic unit* | *Expansion* |
| --- | --- |
| dialogue | conversation |
| paragraph | monologue |
| clause | sentence |
| word | phrase |
| morpheme | stem |

Tench (1976) establishes a similar paired hierarchy (which he calls 'double ranks') for phonology, given in Fig. 6.24.

Fig. 6.24 | *Basic unit* | *Expansion* |
| --- | --- |
| phonological exchange | phonological conversation |
| phonological paragraph | phonological discourse |
| intonation unit | intonation group |
| syllable | rhythm group |
| phoneme | cluster |

The principle behind these paired hierarchies is clear enough: the expansion is a group of units whose role is the same as that of the basic unit which constitutes its head. Thus, a consonant cluster forming a syllable onset, or a vowel cluster forming a syllable nucleus, are both expansions of a single consonant or vowel. We may extend this to higher levels; a group of unaccented syllables in the 'remiss' part of a foot (e.g. -ical in 'phono'logical), or a group of non-nuclear feet forming the 'head'[12] of an intonation unit would also constitute an expansion of a single unit in these positions. Unfortunately, the distinction between expansion and higher unit is hard to draw, and neither Pike nor Tench is consistent. Pike regards the phrase as an expansion of the word, and a sentence as an expansion of the clause, but in neither case does the latter have the same function as the basic unit. Similarly, Tench treats the foot (rhythm group) as an expansion of the syllable, but again this is inappropriate, since the foot does not have the same role as a syllable in the structure of higher units. Though the principle of expansion is a valid one, therefore, these particular implementations of it are unsatisfactory.

Expansions account for the occurrence of more than one unit in a particular structural or functional position, but they do not account for the additional hierarchy of Fig. 6.22. The concept can, however, be extended to include such a hierarchy, since it is clear that the intermediate nodes are the result of recursive application of the same principle. Thus, if an expansion of X is $(X(\underline{X}))$, giving the tree of Fig. 6.25(a) (the head is underlined), then a further expansion of $(X(\underline{X}))$ will yield $(X(\underline{X(X)}))$, which gives the tree of Fig. 6.25(b). Applied to the

---

[12] 'Head' is here the conventional label for the prenuclear part of the intonation unit, and *not* the head constituent of a structure.

structure of a syllable or other prosodic unit, the principle of expansion is therefore able to account for the hierarchical intermediate structure.

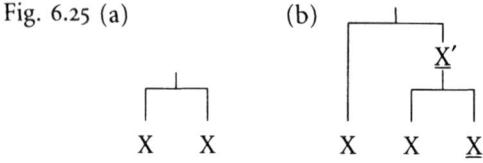

Fig. 6.25 (a)   (b)

$$X'$$

X   X   X   X   X

Again it is questionable, however, whether such a structure is really to be equated with the primary hierarchy of units. The hierarchy of expansion is not a matter of composition as such but of *dependency*: it indicates the recursive head-dependent relationship between parts of a structure.[13] In the trees of Fig. 6.25, the underlined X nodes are the heads of their expansions; in the tree of Fig. 6.25(b), the X' node (the original expansion) is also the head of the further expansion. But the whole structure does not *consist* of X and X' in the sense that it consists of Xs, since all these elements are at the same level.

The distinction between the primary hierarchy of units on the one hand, and the hierarchy obtained by progressive expansions, is also distinguished by Halliday in later work (Halliday, 1985: ch. 2). He distinguishes between *minimal* and *maximal* bracketing, where the former reflects 'ranked constituent analysis' (i.e. in terms of the primary hierarchy of units) and the latter 'immediate constituent analysis'. Taking the phrase *those two splendid old electric trains*, he gives the two different trees of Fig. 6.26, where (a) is based on minimal bracketing and (b) on maximal bracketing. With a ranked constituent analysis, each node

Fig. 6.26   (a) ranked constituents

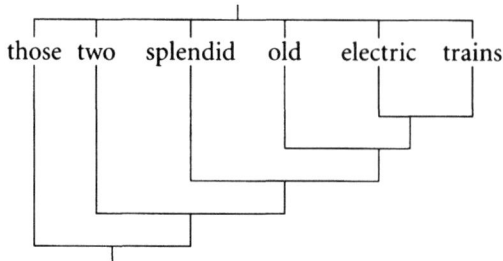

those two   splendid   old   electric   trains

(b) immediate constituents

[13] This claim runs counter to the established view that constituency and dependency are two quite different kinds of relationship. They are not, though dependency involves the additional concept of a *head*. Dependency trees can always be derived from constituency trees once the head constituent is known. The point being made here is that *both* dependency and constituency are concerned with relationships between parts of the structure at a single level, and thus differ from the relationship between units in the primary hierarchy.

corresponds to a basic unit of the primary hierarchy, which in this case gives only phrase and word, whereas immediate constituent analysis gives intermediate nodes. For Halliday, minimal bracketing 'means putting together as constituents only those sequences that actually function as structural units in the item in question' (1985: 26). Maximal bracketing, on the other hand, expresses 'the order of composition of the constituent parts' (ibid.).

Again, this discussion is based on syntactic relations, but it is equally applicable to phonology. The trees of Fig. 6.16(a) and Fig. 6.17(a), given above, are instances of minimal and maximal bracketing, respectively. They can be combined as in Fig. 6.27. Similarly, at a higher level, we might compare the representation of Fig. 6.6, which gives minimal bracketing, with that of Fig. 6.18, which gives maximal bracketing.

Fig. 6.27   (a)   ranked constituents

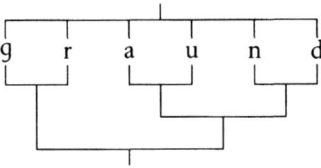

(b)   immediate constituents

We may note in passing that some of the differences in the representations of maximal bracketing result from the application of another, independent principle: that of binarity. For some scholars, binarity in the representation of immediate constituents is axiomatic, so that structures such as that of Fig. 6.18 are inadmissible. Minimal bracketing cannot be purely binary, of course, since units can consist of more than two of the unit below. That some structures are binary is hardly in doubt; binarity is, for example, a defining characteristic of the head/dependent dichotomy. But to elevate this to a universal principle seems unjustified. For example, in the description of foot-structure, all models would agree on the binary nature of the accented/unaccented (stressed/unstressed, strong/weak, etc.) distinction; this identifies the head of the foot. But there seems to be little justification for extending the binary principle to the unaccented syllables in trisyllabic feet such as *deepening* ('diːpənɪŋ) or *happily* ('hæpɪliː), which can be said to have the structure s w w. It is possible to build up the structure of these feet in a binary fashion, since the structure s w w can be regarded as a double expansion of the simple s, viz. (((s) w) w), with the structure Head + Dependent in each case, but, given the equal status of the unaccented syllables relative to the accented one, it is legitimate to ask whether the relations are not better captured by a single expansion ((s) w w).

In this connection we may also briefly consider another model: the *CV Phonology* of Clements and Keyser (1983). This framework is interesting in the present context because it attempts to deal with some of the dimensions of prosodic structure discussed above. It is largely restricted to the structure of the syllable, but the principles it embodies may be relevant for prosodic structure as a whole. Clements and Keyser adapt autosegmental tiers to the needs of phonological structure, placing different dimensions of this structure on different tiers. There is thus a 'syllable display' and a 'segmental display', representing two different levels of structure, but also a distinct 'CV tier' in which the different classes of segment are represented, and a separate 'nucleus tier', which indicates the nucleus of the syllable (see 2.7.4.2). Since all of these are placed on independent tiers, the problems arising from the inclusion of different dimensions in a single hierarchy do not arise. Nevertheless, it is possible—'for expository convenience'—to combine representations where tiers are shared, resulting in '*three-tiered* displays consisting of two-dimensional conflations of two-tiered displays sharing a tier in common' (Clements and Keyser, 1983: 17). The syllable *stout*, for example, is represented in Fig. 6.28(a) as a 'three-tiered syllable display' and in Fig. 6.28(b) as a 'three-tiered nucleus display', where σ = syllable and v = nucleus. It will be observed that the inclusion of the CV tier, categorizing the segments according to their role in the syllable, together with the nucleus tier, renders reference to a branching structure, including 'onset' and 'coda', unnecessary, and also results in the abandonment of the principle of binary-branching.

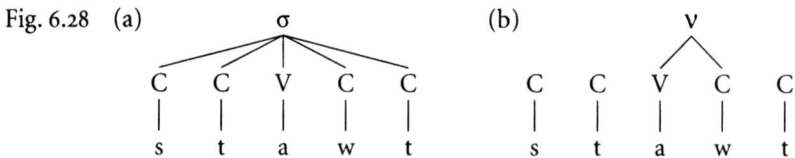

Fig. 6.28   (a) σ (b) v

```
         C   C   V   C   C          C   C   V   C   C
         |   |   |   |   |          |   |   |   |   |
         s   t   a   w   t          s   t   a   w   t
```

Though primarily concerned with the structure of the syllable, Clements and Keyser also extend these principles to include a 'foot-tier'. It would be possible, though they do not pursue this, to incorporate other tiers corresponding to the CV and nucleus tiers at higher levels. Since C and V are classes of segments, and the nucleus is the head constituent of the syllable, analogues at the foot level, using the terminology employed earlier for syllable categories and structural parts of the foot, would be a 'salience tier' (with the categories of syllable 'salient' and 'weak'), and the 'ictus tier', representing the accented portion of the foot. It is an open question whether there would be a role for such tiers in an expanded model along the lines proposed by Clements and Keyser.

Clements and Keyser also distinguish (p. 18) between *structural tiers* and *phonetic tiers*. The former include the σ tier, the CV tier, and the nucleus tier; the latter the segmental tier and the tonal tier, among others. The elements of the former are 'not defined in terms of phonetic features with specifiable physical correlates but are rather structural units, representing the higher-level serial organization of speech units that appears to be a general characteristic of linguistic structure at all levels'. This distinction would appear to correspond to that between the units, structural categories, and classes of unit on the one hand (structural tiers) and prosodic and segmental features on the other (phonetic tiers). Clements and Keyser's model is thus able to recognize, in a fairly explicit way, the different dimensions that we have discussed in this chapter, though these are largely limited to the structure of the syllable, and are not extended to higher levels. The issues raised by extending the model to other levels are thus not explored.

6.3 Prosodic Units

We have so far assumed a relatively small set of prosodic units comprising those illustrated in Fig. 6.7: syllable, foot, intonation unit, and utterance. Several scholars also include a number of others, at the bottom, in the middle, or at the top, though the status of these is not always clear. The difficulties here are in part terminological, since different labels are given to the same unit, particularly those at the top of the scale, and there are also typological differences between languages, so that the units required may differ.

The basic prosodic unit, probably recognizable in all languages, is the *syllable*.[14] The syllable is the domain of several different prosodic features, such as tone, and it is generally the unit which can be regarded as 'accented'. Length, too, may also be associated with the syllable, as discussed in 2.6. The *foot*, however, is not a universal, as it is restricted to languages with Level 1 accentuation, though some analyses give it a role in other languages, too. The *intonation unit* goes under a variety of names; since it is the domain of one kind of accent (Level 2 accent) it may be the same as the 'accentual phrase' of some analyses. Again, however, it is probably a universal, as all languages have intonation of some kind. Since all analyses recognize these three units (or two, in languages without the foot), we shall not need to justify them here.

We must consider, however, the possibility of other units in the hierarchy. As we saw in Chapter 2, many scholars recognize the *mora* as a legitimate unit (see 2.5.4; 2.8.3; 2.8.4; and elsewhere), though its relationship to the syllable is somewhat uncertain. The mora has often been included in the hierarchy as a unit below the syllable. The hierarchy of McCarthy and Prince (1995) is of this type; it was illustrated in Fig. 2.74(a), repeated here as Fig. 6.29(a). As noted in 2.10.1, however, it is more satisfactory, in the majority of cases at least, to regard the mora count as a property of the syllable, and therefore associated with it rather than a constituent of it. The mora thus becomes part of a secondary hierarchy rather than a primary unit. Since the foot, too, may have its quantity, we may

---

[14] The literature on the syllable is extensive, and no attempt will be made to review it here. For a recent discussion see Blevins (1995).

also postulate a parallel 'Quantity Tier' at the foot level, as in Fig, 6.29(b) (repeated from Fig. 2.74(b)).

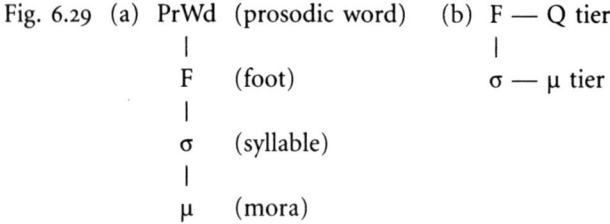

Fig. 6.29 (a) PrWd (prosodic word)   (b) F — Q tier
                | |
                F   (foot)   σ — μ tier
                |
                σ   (syllable)
                |
                μ   (mora)

There is nevertheless an argument for a typological distinction here. Trubetzkoy (1939) distinguishes syllable languages from mora languages, and syllable-counting languages from mora-counting languages, and later scholars, too, have identified languages in which the mora plays a more significant role than, say, in English. Japanese is clearly such a language, since here the mora can be regarded as the unit of timing (see 2.3.9.5), and the syllable has a subordinate role. Pierrehumbert and Beckman (1988: 21) therefore include the mora in their representations of Japanese prosodic structure, given here as Fig. 6.30, which describes the structure of the utterance *ane-no akai seetaa-wa doko desu ka?* ('Where is the big sister's red sweater?').[15] For Japanese, this representation is certainly more appropriate than for English, and it is therefore possible that a typological distinction can be made here between languages with the mora as a unit, and languages without.

Fig. 6.30

ane-no akai se'etaa-wa do'ko desu ka?
'Where is the big sister's red sweater?'

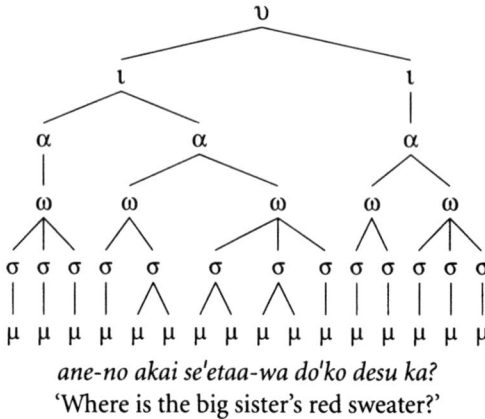

A number of scholars also introduce intermediate units between the syllable and the intonation unit. One such is Selkirk's 'stress superfoot' (Selkirk, 1980),

---

[15] Pierrehumbert and Beckman also include pitch features in their representation; these have been omitted here for clarity.

which was discussed in 3.5.3, and illustrated in Fig. 3.23, repeated here as Fig. 6.31. It is clear, however, that this is a spurious unit; it is an artefact of the insistence on binary-branching, which creates the foot (Σ) -*meri*- and then attaches the further syllable -*ca* requiring a higher node (Σ'). The foot here consists of the three syllables -*merica*, and no 'superfoot' is required.

Fig. 6.31

ω

Σ'

Σ_w Σ_s

σ σ_s σ_w σ_w

A   me   ri   ca

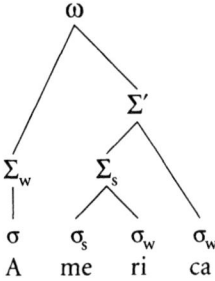

Several scholars (Liberman and Prince, 1977; Selkirk, 1980; Nespor and Vogel, 1986, among others) introduce the *phonological word* as a unit above the foot level. Since the word itself is a grammatical unit, its introduction into a phonological hierarchy requires justification, and Nespor and Vogel admit that it is not a purely phonological notion, but 'represents the interaction between the phonological and the morphological components of the grammar' (p. 109). Following the 'Strict Layer Hypothesis', they claim that 'each foot is . . . exhaustively included in a ω [= phonological word]; that is, it is never the case that the syllables of a single foot belong to different phonological words' (ibid.). It is clear from this claim that the phonological word cannot be co-extensive with the grammatical word, since otherwise the claim would be immediately disproved by any simple phrase such as *ripe bananas*, where the foot division does not correspond to the word-division: /raip bə/nɑːnəz/. According to Nespor and Vogel, there are some cases where the two do tend to coincide, for example in Modern Greek and Latin (1986: 110–17), but the phonological word may be smaller or larger than the grammatical word, as in Sanskrit, Turkish, or Hungarian (pp. 117–24). The criterion used for determining such a unit is the scope of phonological processes; in Turkish and Hungarian, for example, the phonological word is the domain of vowel harmony, so that non-harmonizing affixes are regarded as forming separate phonological words. Similarly, processes such as assimilation and elision may take place only *within* certain domains rather than across them, again justifying the recognition of the phonological word as their domain. For example, Nespor and Vogel show that in northern Italian intervocalic voicing of *s* takes place only within a domain which includes a simple morpheme (*a*[z]*ola*, 'button hole'), between a lexical morpheme and an inflectional morpheme (*ca*[z]*e*, 'houses'), between a lexical morpheme and a derivational suffix (*ca*[z]*ina*, 'little house'), and between a derivational prefix and a lexical morpheme (*re*[z]*istenza*, 'resistance'). But there are also instances where this voicing does not take place, for example, in *a[s]ociale*, 'asocial', which is also between a derivational prefix and a lexical morpheme, and between the two members of a compound, as in *tocca[s]ana*, 'cure-all'. The last two example are therefore regarded as consisting of two phonological words, while the remainder consist of only one.

There is, however, a difference between the domain of segmental phonological processes and units of the prosodic hierarchy. There is certainly a tendency for them to coincide, but, as the examples given by Nespor and Vogel show, the coincidence is not obligatory. There seems to be little justification for treating expressions such as *re[z]istenza* and *a[s]ociale* as *prosodically* different, merely because they behave differently with regard to segmental processes. Prosodic units proper have a more fundamental organizational role in prosodic structure than merely being the domain of such processes, which, as Nespor and Vogel acknowledge, may be subject to morpho-syntactic conditioning. This is not to dispute the existence of such domains, but merely to exclude them from the hierarchy of prosodic units.

Another unit recognized by Nespor and Vogel is the *clitic group*. Clitics are semi-independent elements which cannot stand alone but are attached to other words, examples being the Latin particle *-que* ('and') and the object pronouns in Spanish and Italian, and other Romance languages. The former becomes part of the word to which it is attached, for example with regard to stress rules, giving *'virum*, 'man' (accusative), but *vi'rumque*, 'and the man'; the latter do not: Spanish *'dando*, 'giving', but *'dandonoslos*, 'giving them to us' (Nespor and Vogel, 1986: 146). Nespor and Vogel claim that, in Italian and other languages, clitics have a special status, and that there are processes applying to groups containing them which do not apply elsewhere, justifying the recognition of the clitic group—consisting of a clitic and its host—as a prosodic unit. However, as far as the prosodic organization of utterances is concerned we must again conclude that this is unaffected by whether the expressions contain clitics or not, and the clitic group does not need to be recognized as a distinct unit in the hierarchy.

A final area of difficulty is with higher units than the intonation unit. We saw in 5.7 that it is possible to recognize higher intonation units, which might justify a 'Level 3 accentuation', and various scholars, such as Beckman and Pierrehumbert (1986), have proposed more than one unit to accommodate intonational phenomena. The difficulty here, however, is knowing when to stop. Nespor and Vogel (1986) recognize three higher units above the clitic group: phonological phrase, intonation phrase, and phonological utterance; Pike (1967: 364) has four such units above the foot: emic pause group, emic breath group, emic rhetorical period, and emic phonological section. Since the length of an utterance is theoretically indeterminate, it is always possible to recognize larger stretches of speech, but this does not necessarily justify the inclusion of further units in the prosodic hierarchy. At least two levels of intonation structure seem justifiable, as discussed in 5.7, but there is no real evidence for anything more; the higher intonation unit is probably to be identified with the utterance itself, and any larger stretches of speech can be regarded as sequences of discrete utterances. However, this is a matter on which it is not possible to reach a definitive conclusion.

6.4 Prosodic Features and Prosodic Structure

6.4.1 INTRODUCTION

In the light of this discussion of prosodic structure and prosodic units, we may now return to the prosodic features themselves, and consider how they relate to the various dimensions of prosodic structures that we have considered in this chapter. These features have often been seen as phonetic properties of units, and consequently have been specified in terms of phonetic features such as [±stress], [±tense], [±high], and so on. As we have seen in the preceding chapters, however, this approach is too simplistic; these features relate to prosodic structure in a variety of different ways, and cannot necessarily be specified in these terms.

In the first place, the majority of the features are *stratified*, in the sense that they apply at different levels of structure simultaneously, though they may have a particular domain where they are most relevant. Length, for example, is usually considered in relation to segments, but we have seen (2.6) that it is also relevant for the syllable; accent has been described in terms of Level 1 (the foot level), and Level 2 (the intonation-group level); tone is predominantly associated with the syllable, but it can in some cases be assigned to the foot (4.7.3). More important than this stratification, however, is the fact that the different features have a quite different status with respect to their place and role within prosodic structure. We have noted, for example, that accent has an organizational role; it forms a fundamental part of the structure. Tone, on the other hand, applies to and depends on this structure but does not play a part in its organization. In what follows we shall consider the place and role of each feature.

6.4.2 ACCENT

Several schools, including Bloomfieldian structuralism and classical generative phonology, treat accent paradigmatically, as a feature comparable to segmental features. For Trager and Smith (1951), for example, there are four 'stress phonemes' (3.3.2), while Jakobson, Fant, and Halle (1952) use a feature [±stress], and Chomsky and Halle (1968) have a multi-valued feature [1 stress], [2 stress], etc. (3.5.2). This position is modified in Metrical phonology, which reduces stress to a binary relational feature which is derived from metrical trees, or equivalent grids, with syllables designated as strong or weak (3.5.3). This in effect interprets accent as a class of syllable. However, this can in turn—in the case of Level 1 accent—be regarded as deriving from the role of the strong syllable in the structure of the foot: it forms the ictus, and is therefore the head of the foot. Thus, accent is ultimately not a phonetic property but a matter of *structure*, and this is reinforced by its role in the rhythmical organization of the utterance.

Level 2 accent is to be interpreted differently, but analogously. In a language which also has a Level 1 accent, such as English, Level 2 accent can also be interpreted structurally, as the head of the unit, in this case designating the nuclear foot of the intonation unit. In languages without a Level 1 accent, such as French or Japanese, Level 2 accent still has the same role, here characterizing one of the syllables or moras, respectively, of the intonation unit/accent phrase.

It is because of this structural role that the place of accent in prosodic structure is more basic than that of other features, justifying Beckman's claim (1986) that it is 'organizational', in the sense that it is not merely a property associated with specific prosodic units but is rather a defining characteristic of the structure itself.

6.4.3 LENGTH

Length is in some ways one of the most difficult prosodic feature to characterize, in spite of its apparent simplicity, as its status is ambivalent. As we saw in Chapter 2, it can be analysed in a variety of ways. At its simplest, it can be regarded as a phonetic feature which is a property of specific units. Vowel or consonant length can therefore be specified by a feature such as [±long] or [±tense], equivalent to other segmental features such as [±nasal] or [±round] (see 2.4.3).

As we have seen, however, such a paradigmatic analysis is too simplistic, firstly because it ignores the fact that length has syntagmatic implications. Various means have been devised to represent it syntagmatically, in particular by analysing long segments as sequences of short ones (2.5). Formally, this has been achieved by attributing the length of segments to different numbers of structural positions or timing slots. In this approach, length is no longer a phonetic feature of segments but again a matter of *structure*, in this case dependent on the number of occurrences of the relevant unit.

An alternative view of length is as a *prosodic* feature, a property of larger units. Apart from the rather inexplicit formulation of this approach in terms of 'chronemes' (2.8.2), the most clearly articulated version is found in Moraic Theory (2.8.4), which takes up the concept of the mora, used in Prague School theory (2.5.4). As we saw in 6.3, most formulations of this approach treat the mora as a constituent of the syllable, in which case length is specified in terms of the primary hierarchy of units, but it is possible to see the mora not as a unit but as a property of an existing unit, the syllable, as a feature representing a measure of syllable length, as illustrated in Fig. 6.29(b). As noted above, this difference of treatment may reflect a typological difference in the role of the mora in different languages. We have also seen that it is possible to represent syllable quantity in an analogous fashion, as a property of a higher unit (2.10.1).

6.4.4 TONE AND INTONATION

Tone is always treated as a feature of an existing unit, rather than as a unit or a structural property in itself. The majority of descriptions associate it with the syllable, though it has also been considered to be a property of the mora or the vowel (see 4.4). In tonal accent languages, such as Swedish or Serbo–Croat, it is more appropriately associated with the foot (4.7.3). In current theory, tone is usually represented autosegmentally, which allows features on the tonal tier to be associated with the appropriate tone-bearing units. In the case of tonal accent languages, a comparable tier at the foot level can be envisaged.

The place of intonation in prosodic structure is more difficult to establish. Traditional pedagogical analyses in the British tradition (cf. 5.3.2) in effect treat it as a property of the whole intonation unit (tone-group), but in other approaches parts of the intonation pattern are allocated to smaller units. The Bloomfieldian tradition regards the elements of the pattern as pitch phonemes, which are, like tone, assigned to individual syllables or vowels; more recent theory, especially the influential approach of Pierrehumbert (1980), analyses the pattern into foot-sized elements with each of which a 'pitch–accent' is associated, though here there are also boundary tones associated with the edges of the unit as a whole. Even in the British tradition, the phonetic specification of the pattern requires reference to smaller parts which are, in effect, co-extensive with feet, so that the pattern as a whole consists of a series of such foot-length patterns. Again, therefore, the stratification of this feature is evident.

6.4.5 CONCLUSION

This discussion shows that the relationship of the major prosodic features to prosodic structure differs from case to case, and that they cannot simply be regarded as a set of phonetic properties comparable to segmental features, such as voice, nasality, or lip rounding. This difference of status is clearest in the case of accent; in this case, as we saw in Chapter 3, it is difficult to associate any consistent phonetic property with accentual 'features', which is entirely consistent with its structural, rather than phonetic, role in prosodic structure. The interpretation of length is more variable, but here, too, a structural interpretation is justifiable, at least in some cases. On the other hand, tone and intonation are more clearly phonetic properties, though their interactions with accent means that they cannot be regarded as simple features. In all cases, too, the stratification of the features means that account must be taken of different levels of structure, and that a single specification ([±long], [±stress], etc.) is insufficient for this purpose.

6.5 The Specification of Prosody

The prosodic structure under discussion here, though clearly a theoretical construct, is not intended to be dependent on a particular theoretical model. It is assumed that such a structure underlies actual utterances, not merely in the sense of being, as a phonological framework, an abstract representation of utterances, but also ultimately in having a phonetic basis, and reflecting physical properties of the speech signal, as discussed in 6.1, above.

It is necessary, nevertheless, to consider how such a structure relates to widely accepted modes of linguistic description, and in particular to rule-based models such as those of classical generative phonology, more recent non-linear approaches, or constraint-based models. Since it is assumed that this prosodic structure characterizes actual utterances, in terms of rule-based grammars it must be seen as the output of the grammar. Since, further, this structure is by no means arbitrary, but is highly constrained, we must assume that the rules themselves are constrained by this output structure; the role of the grammar is therefore to specify utterances in terms of the kind of structure that we have identified in this chapter. In keeping with the principles outlined in 6.1, no attempt will be made here to formalize the rules of any such grammar; the focus is on the structure itself rather than the means by which it may be derived. Nevertheless, we can consider some of the general principles involved.[16]

Specification of prosodic structure may take several forms. One approach, adopted in classical generative phonology, is to assign appropriate feature values to the smallest units and to apply a series of recursive processes, which depend particularly on morpho-syntactic structure, and which combine and modify these feature values until the maximal domain is reached. This approach is used by Chomsky and Halle (1968) to assign stress patterns in English, and by McCawley (1968) to derive the pitch patterns of Japanese. It is also the means used to build metrical trees (Liberman and Prince, 1977). This may be termed the *bottom-up* approach. Its main claim is that it captures the principle that the whole is determined by its parts.[17] However, it suffers from the complementary

---

[16] This structure will not be treated here in terms of the principles of more recent Optimality Theory, in which rules are entirely replaced by ranked constraints (see 6.1, above). See Hammond (1997) for the beginnings of such an approach.

[17] One important theoretical model which also adopts a bottom-up approach is that of Lexical Phonology (Mohanan, 1982, 1986; Kiparsky, 1982). This theory has also been applied to prosodic features (e.g. Pulleyblank, 1986). The distinctive contribution of this theory is primarily to the mode of specification of phonological features rather than to the nature of prosodic structure itself, and for that reason it is not discussed in this book.

weakness that it does not allow the parts to be determined by the whole. In the case of prosodic features arranged in a hierarchical prosodic structure this is a serious disadvantage, since it seems clear that features of larger units provide the setting for those of smaller units. Intonational features, for example, determine the overall pitch level for the realization of tones. Features such as downdrift (see Chapter 4) can therefore not be ascribed to an overall tendency characterizing the whole unit, but must be derived by mutual interactions between the features of lower level units.[18] In the case of accentual features, the bottom-up approach is responsible for the mistaken claim (Liberman and Prince, 1977) that 'relative prominence tends to be preserved under embedding' (see 3.5.4), since it assumes the embedding of an already specified accentual structure into a larger unit. Whatever its merits in dealing with mutual interactions of low-level features, therefore, the bottom-up approach fails to accommodate satisfactorily the features of higher-level units.

An alternative view may be called the *top-down* approach. Here, it is assumed that the specification of prosodic structure and prosodic features begins with the highest levels and progressively superimposes the structure and features of lower units. This approach is adopted particularly, but not exclusively, by those concerned with the computer generation of synthetic prosodic patterns. Among them are Fujisaki and his associates (e.g. Fujisaki and Nagashima, 1969) and the Lund School of intonation studies (cf. 5.3.5, above). The latter produces a model of pitch assignment in which accentual and tonal features of lower units are progressively superimposed on the intonation features of higher units, according to the procedures specified in Fig. 5.9.

There is a further possibility for the specification of prosodic structures and features: the *left-to-right* model. If the bottom-up model reflects the principle that the parts determine the whole, and the top-down model reflects the fact that features of lower units are determined by the overall pattern of the higher units, then the left-to-right model embodies the basically linear nature of the speech-event itself. There are elements of this model in a number of theoretical frameworks. In the autosegmental specification of tone, for example, a common principle has been that, in default cases, tones and tone-bearing units are associated in a left-to-right sequence, this being the Universal Association Convention (Goldsmith, 1976: 117; cf. 4.4.3.2). Further, such phenomena as downstep, upstep, and downdrift (Chapter 4), and declination (Chapter 5) assume left-to-right recursive processes, while Pierrehumbert uses a left-to-right finite-state grammar for the generation of intonation contours.

This linear principle reflects the on-going, improvisatory aspect of utterance production. There is some evidence, however, for an element of forward planning which constrains this principle, since the speaker is able to look ahead.

---

[18] It will be recalled (5.5.5) that this is precisely the mechanism employed to achieve declination ('downstep') by Pierrehumbert, using the H*–L pitch–accent.

Thus, although declination results in a progressive lowering of pitch, 't Hart, Collier, and Cohen (1990: 134) claim that the end point reached in all utterances, regardless of their length, tends to be approximately the same. This implies that speakers have some idea of the length of their utterance when they begin it, and are therefore able to commence at a higher pitch to allow for the declination, or to adjust the rate of declination, in order not to reach too low a point too soon. This means that, although there is clearly a linear, left-to-right dimension to the specification of utterances, the process cannot necessarily be specified entirely from left to right. The element of forward planning here does not justify the recognition of an additional right-to-left dimension to the specification of prosody, however.

The fact that these three different modes of specification can all be applicable at different stages and for different phenomena suggests that there is an element of all three involved in the specification of prosodic structure. Accentual features have typically been derived by means of a bottom-up procedure, which may reflect the principle that accentual contrasts are built up in layers, as it were, with Level 2 accentuation superimposed on Level 1 accentuation. This is less satisfactory for features of tone and intonation, where it is more appropriate to see pitch features of smaller units as modifications of those of larger units; a top-down approach is more suitable here. The inclusion of left-to-right process- ing caters for the linearly recursive nature of many prosodic patterns, such as rhythm and intonation. Thus any grammar of prosody may need to incorporate a range of different mechanisms in the specification of prosodic structure and prosodic features. Since intonational features may require a top-down approach, while their realization also depends on accentual features which may need to be specified from the bottom up, and the recursive elements of the pitch pattern are most appropriately dealt with from left to right, it will be clear that consider- able demands will need to be made on any system of rules or constraints which aims to provide an explicit characterization of prosodic structure. Though cur- rent models may provide some of the necessary elements of these processes, it does not appear that they can provide them all.

The various dimensions of prosodic structure identified in 6.2.3 must also be expressed in the specification of prosodic structure. Current theories can accom- modate them, though they do not necessarily do so in an explicit fashion, nor necessarily in the most appropriate way. The primary hierarchy of units is speci- fied directly in most theories, though, as we saw in 6.2.3, the hierarchy is often made more complex by the inclusion of other dimensions which are more prop- erly assigned to secondary hierarchies. The structural or functional parts of units—ictus and remiss for the foot, head, and nucleus for the intonation unit, and comparable categories at a higher level—are usually specified by assigning 'word accents' and 'sentence accents', so that these categories are represented by features; classes of unit, on the other hand, are usually accommodated by the apportionment of 'strong' and 'weak' nodes in the metrical tree. Features themselves, especially those of tone and intonation but also potentially length, are properties of the units, and can be located on accompanying tiers.

As explained in 6.1, however, the formalization of an explicit system of rules goes beyond the brief of the present chapter and the present book, in which the major concern is to understand the nature of prosodic structure itself.

References

Note: in cases where a book appears in several editions, the earliest edition is usually cited.

ABE, Isamu (1955). 'Intonational patterns of English and Japanese.' *Word* 11: 386–98.

ABERCROMBIE, David (1949). 'What is a letter?' *Lingua* 2: 54–62.

—— (1964). 'Syllable quantity and enclitics in English.' In D. Abercrombie *et al.* (eds.), pp. 216–22.

—— (1965). 'Steele, Monboddo and Garrick.' In *Studies in Phonetics and Linguistics*, London: Oxford University Press, pp. 35–44.

—— (1967). *Elements of General Phonetics*. Edinburgh: Edinburgh University Press.

—— (1971). 'Some functions of silent stress.' In A. J. Aitken, A. McIntosh, and H. Pálsson (eds.), pp. 147–56.

—— (1976). '"Stress" and some other terms.' *Work in Progress*, Dept. of Linguistics, University of Edinburgh 9: 51–3.

—— and FRY, Dennis B., MACCARTHY, Peter A. D., SCOTT, Norman C. and TRIM, John L. M. (eds.) (1964). *In Honour of Daniel Jones*. London: Longman.

ABRAMSON, Arthur S. (1962). *The Vowels and Tones of Standard Thai: Acoustical Measurements and Experiments*. Bloomington: Indiana University Press.

AGARD, Frederick B. and DI PIETRO, Robert J. (1965). *The Sounds of English and Italian. A systematic analysis of the contrasts between the sound systems*. Chicago: University of Chicago Press.

AHOUA, Firmin (1986). 'The autosegmental representation of tones in Akan: more evidence for the tone mapping rule with reference to Baule.' In K. Bogers *et al.* (eds.), pp. 63–78.

AITKEN, A. J., McINTOSH, Angus and PÁLSSON, Hermann (eds.), (1971). *Edinburgh Studies in English and Scots*. London: Longman.

ALARCOS LLORACH, Emilio (1968). *Fonología Española*. 4th edn. Madrid: Editorial Gredos.

ALKON, Paul K. (1959). 'Joshua Steele and the melody of speech.' *Language and Speech* 2: 154–74.

ALLEN, G. D. (1975). 'Speech rhythm: its relation to performance universals and articulatory timing.' *Journal of Phonetics* 3: 75–86.

ALLEN, W. Sidney (1964). 'On quantity and quantitative verse.' In D. Abercrombie *et al.* (eds.), pp. 3–15.

—— (1965). *Vox Latina*. Cambridge: Cambridge University Press.

—— (1968). *Vox Graeca*. Cambridge: Cambridge University Press.

—— (1973). *Accent and Rhythm*. Cambridge: Cambridge University Press.

ALLEN, W. Stannard (1956). 'Stress marks.' *Le maître phonétique* 105: 15–16.

ANDERSON, Stephen R. (1974). *The Organization of Phonology*. New York: Academic Press.

—— (1978). 'Tone features.' In V. A. Fromkin (ed.), pp. 133–75.

—— (1984). 'A metrical interpretation of some traditional claims about quantity and stress.' In M. Aronoff and R. Oehrle (eds.), pp. 83–106.

—— and KIPARSKY, Paul (eds.) (1973). *A Festschrift for Morris Halle*. New York: Holt, Rinehart, & Winston.

ARCHANGELI, Diana (1997). 'Optimality theory. An introduction to linguistics in the 1990s.' In D. Archangeli and D. T. Langendoen (eds.), pp. 1–32.

—— and LANGENDOEN, D. Terence (eds.) (1997). *Optimality Theory. An overview.* Oxford: Blackwell.

—— and PULLEYBLANK, Douglas (1986). *The Content and Structure of Phonological Representations*. MS.

ARISTE, Paul (1939). 'A quantitative language.' In E. Blancquaert and W. Pée (eds.), pp. 276–80.

ARMSTRONG, Lilias E. (1934). 'The phonetic structure of Somali.' *Mitteilungen des Seminars für Orientalische Sprachen zu Berlin* 37.3: 116–61.

—— (1940). *The Phonetic and Tonal Structure of Kikuyu*. London: Oxford University Press.

—— and WARD, Ida C. (1926). *A Handbook of English Intonation*. Cambridge: Heffer.

ARMSTRONG, Robert G. (1968). 'Yala (Ikom): a terraced-level language with three tones.' *Journal of West African Languages* 5.1: 49–58.

ÁRNASON, Kristján (1980). *Quantity in Historical Phonology: Icelandic and Related Cases.* Cambridge: Cambridge University Press.

ARNOLD, Gordon F. (1957a). 'Stress in English words.' *Lingua* 6: 221–67.

—— (1957b). 'Stress in English words II.' *Lingua* 6: 397–441.

ARNOTT, D. W. (1964). 'Downstep in the Tiv verbal system.' *African Language Studies* 5: 34–51.

—— (1969). 'Tiv.' In E. Dunstan (ed.), pp. 143–51.

ARONOFF, Mark and OEHRLE, Richard (eds.) (1984). *Language Sound Structure. Studies in phonology presented to Morris Halle by his teacher and students.* Cambridge, MA: MIT Press.

ASONGWED, Tah and HYMAN, Larry M. (1976). 'Morphotonology of the Ngamambo noun.' In L. M. Hyman (ed.) (1976), pp. 23–56.

AUSTIN, John L. (1962). *How to Do Things With Words*. Oxford: Clarendon Press.

BABIĆ, Zrinka (1988). 'Accent systems in Croatian dialects.' In H. van der Hulst and N. Smith (eds.) (1988a), pp. 1–10.

BALASUMBRAMANIAN, T. (1980). 'Timing in Tamil.' *Journal of Phonetics* 8: 449–67.

BAO, Zhi-Ming (1990). *On the Nature of Tone*. Doctoral Dissertation, MIT.

BARKAÏ, M. (1974). 'On duration and spirantization in Biblical Hebrew.' *Linguistic Inquiry* 5: 456–9.

BARKER, Marie (1925). *A Handbook of German Intonation for University Students.* Cambridge: Heffer.

BEACH, Douglas M. (1924). 'The science of tonetics and its application to Bantu languages.' *Bantu Studies* 2: 75–106.

—— (1938). *The Phonetics of the Hottentot Language*. Cambridge: Heffer.

BECKMAN, Mary E. (1982). 'Segment duration and the "mora" in Japanese.' *Phonetica* 39: 113–35.

—— (1986). *Stress and Non-Stress Accent*. Dordrecht: Foris.

BECKMAN, Mary E. (cont.) (1992). 'Evidence for speech rhythms across languages.' In Y. Tohkura, E. Vatikiotis-Bateson, and Y. Sagisaka (eds.), pp. 457–63.

—— and EDWARDS, Jan (1990). 'Lengthenings and shortenings and the nature of prosodic constituency.' In J. Kingston and M. E. Beckman (eds.), pp. 152–78.

—— and PIERREHUMBERT, Janet B. (1986). 'Intonational structure in Japanese and English.' *Phonology Yearbook* 3: 255–310.

BELL, Alexander Melville (1867). *Visible Speech: the Science of Universal Alphabetics.* London: Simpkin Marshall.

—— (1886). *Essays and Postscripts on Elocution.* New York.

BENDER, Ernest and HARRIS, Zellig S. (1946). 'The phonemes of North Carolina Cherokee.' *International Journal of American Linguistics* 12: 14–21.

BENEDIKTSSON, Hreinn (1963). 'The non-uniqueness of phonemic solutions: quantity and stress in Icelandic.' *Phonetica* 10: 133–53.

BERGSVEINSSON, S. (1941). *Grundfragen der isländischen Satzphonetik.* Berlin: Metten.

BERMAN, A. and SZAMOSI, M. (1972). 'Observations on sentential stress.' *Language* 48: 304–28.

BICKMORE, Lee S. (1995a). 'Tone and stress in Lamba.' *Phonology* 12: 307–41.

—— (1995b). 'Accounting for compensatory lengthening in the CV and moraic frameworks.' In J. Durand and F. Katamba (eds.), pp. 119–48.

BIERWISCH, Manfred (1966). 'Regeln für die Intonation deutscher Sätze.' *Studia Grammatica* 7: 99–178.

BJÖRKHAGEN, Im (1944). *Modern Swedish Grammar.* Stockholm: Svenska Bokförlaget.

BLAKE, Norman (ed.) (1992). *The Cambridge History of the English Language, II, 1066–1476.* Cambridge: Cambridge University Press.

BLANCQUAERT, Edgaed and PÉE, Willem (eds.) (1939). *Proceedings of the Third International Congress of Phonetic Sciences.* Ghent: University of Ghent.

BLEVINS, Juliette (1995). 'The syllable in phonological theory.' In J. A. Goldsmith (ed.), pp. 206–44.

BLOCH, Bernard (1946). 'Studies in colloquial Japanese II: syntax.' *Language* 22: 200–48.

—— (1950). 'Studies in Colloquial Japanese IV: phonemics.' *Language* 26: 86–125. Also in M. Joos (ed.), pp. 329–48.

—— and TRAGER, George L. (1942). *Outline of Linguistic Analysis.* Baltimore: Linguistic Society of America.

BLOOMFIELD, Leonard (1935). *Language.* London: George Allen and Unwin.

BOGERS, Koen, HULST, Harry van der, and MOUS, Maarten (eds.) (1986). *The Phonological Representation of Suprasegmentals.* Dordrecht: Foris.

BOLINGER, Dwight L. (1948). 'The intonation of accosting questions.' *English Studies* 29: 109–14.

—— (1951). 'Intonation: levels versus configurations.' *Word* 7: 199–210.

—— (1955). 'Intersections of stress and intonation.' *Word* 11: 195–203.

—— (1957). 'On certain functions of Accents A and B.' *Litera* 4: 80–9.

—— (1958a). 'A theory of pitch accent in English.' *Word* 14: 109–49.

—— (1958b). 'Stress and information.' *American Speech* 33: 5–20.

—— (1958c). 'On intensity as a qualitative improvement of pitch accent.' *Lingua* 7: 175–82.

—— (1961). *Generality, Gradience, and the All-or-None.* The Hague: Mouton.

—— (1962). '"Secondary stress" in Spanish.' *Romance Philology* 15: 273–9.

—— (1964). 'Intonation as a universal.' In H. Lunt (ed.), pp. 833–44.

—— (1965). 'Pitch accent and sentence rhythm.' In *Forms of English: Accent, Morpheme, Order.* Cambridge, MA: Harvard University Press.

—— (1972). 'Accent is predictable (if you're a mind reader).' *Language* 48: 633–44.

—— (1978). 'Intonation across languages.' In J. H. Greenberg (ed.), pp. 471–524.

—— (1981). *Two Kinds of Vowels, Two Kinds of Rhythm.* Bloomington: Indiana University Linguistics Club.

—— (ed.) (1972). *Intonation.* Harmondsworth: Penguin.

BORGSTRØM, Carl Hj. (1962). 'Tonemes and phrase intonation in Southeastern Standard Norwegian.' *Studia Linguistica* 16: 34–7.

BRADSHAW, Joel (1979). 'Obstruent harmony and tonogenesis in Jabêm.' *Lingua* 49: 189–205.

BRAME Michael K. (1973). 'On stress assignment in two Arabic dialects.' In S. R. Anderson and P. Kiparsky (eds.), pp. 14–25.

—— (1974). 'The cycle in phonology: stress in Palestinian, Maltese, and Spanish.' *Linguistic Inquiry* 5: 39–60.

—— (ed.) (1972). *Contributions to Generative Phonology.* Austin: University of Texas Press.

BRAZIL, David (1975). *Discourse Intonation.* Birmingham: Birmingham University.

—— (1997). *The Communicative Value of Intonation in English.* Cambridge: Cambridge University Press.

—— COULTHARD, Malcolm, and JOHNS, Catherine (1980). *Discourse Intonation and Language Teaching.* London: Longman.

BREND, Ruth M. (ed.) (1974). *Advances in Tagmemics.* Amsterdam: North Holland.

—— and PIKE, Kenneth L. (eds.) (1976). *Tagmemics, Vol. 1, Aspects of the Field.* The Hague: Mouton.

BRENTARI, Diane and BOSCH, Anna (1990). 'The mora: Autosegment or syllable constituent.' In M. Ziolkowski, M. Noske, and K. Deaton (eds.) *Chicago Linguistic Society Papers 26: Parasession on the Syllable in Phonetics and Phonology.* Chicago: Chicago Linguistic Society, pp. 1–16.

BRESNAN, Joan (1971). 'Sentence stress and syntactic transformations.' *Language* 47: 257–81.

—— (1972). 'Stress and syntax: a reply.' *Language* 48: 326–42.

BROWN, Gillian, CURRIE, Karen, and KENWORTHY, Joanne (1980). *Questions of Intonation.* London: Croom Helm.

BROWN, J. Marvin (1965). *From Ancient Thai to Modern Dialects.* Bangkok: Social Science Association.

BROWNE, E. W. and McCAWLEY, James D. (1965). 'Srpskohrvatski akcenat.' *Zbornik za Filologiju Lingvistiku* 8: 147–51. English translation: 'Serbo-Croatian accent.' In E. Fudge (ed.) (1973), pp. 330–5.

BRUCE, Gösta (1977). 'Swedish word-accents in sentence perspective.' *Working Papers* 12. Lund: Dept. of Linguistics, Lund University, pp. 61–70.

—— and GÅRDING, Eva (1978). 'A prosodic typology for Swedish dialects.' In E. Gårding, G. Bruce, and R. Bannert (eds.), pp. 219–28.

BRUCK, Anthony, FOX, Robert A., and LA GALY, Michael W. (eds.) (1974). *Papers from the Parasession on Natural Phonology.* Chicago: Chicago Linguistic Society.

BRÜCKE, Ernst W. von (1856). *Grundzüge der Physiologie und Systematik der Sprachlaute für Linguisten und Taubstummenlehrer.* Vienna: Gors.

BRUGMANN, Karl (1886–90), *Grundriss der vergleichenden Grammatik der indogermanischen Sprachen.* Strassburg: Teubner.

BUTTERWORTH, B. Brian (ed.) (1980). *Language Production, Vol. I, Speech and Talk.* New York: Academic Press.

BUXTON, Hilary (1983). 'Temporal predictability in the perception of English speech.' In A. Cutler and D. R. Ladd (eds.), pp. 111–21.

BYARUSHENGO, Ernest Rugwa, HYMAN, Larry M., and TENENBAUM, Sarah (1976). 'Tone, accent and assertion in Haya.' In L. M. Hyman (ed.) (1976), pp. 185–205.

CARNOCHAN, Jack (1951). 'A study of quantity in Hausa.' *Bulletin of the School of Oriental and African Studies* 13: 1032–44. Also in F. R. Palmer (ed.), pp. 91–103.

—— (1957). 'Gemination in Hausa.' In: *Studies in Linguistic Analysis,* London: Philological Society, pp. 149–81.

CARRELL, Patricia (1966). *A Transformational Grammar of Igbo.* Cambridge: Cambridge University Press.

CATFORD, J. C. (1966). 'English phonology and the teaching of pronunciation.' *College English* 27: 605–13.

—— (1977). *Fundamental Problems in Phonetics.* Edinburgh: Edinburgh University Press.

CHAMBERLAIN, James R. (1979). 'Tone in Thai: a new perspective.' In T. W. Gething and Ng. D. Liem (eds.) *Tai Studies in Honor of William J. Gedney* (Papers in S. E. Asian Linguistics 6). Australian National University, Canberra, pp. 119–23.

CHANG, Kun (1973). 'The reconstruction of proto–Miao–Yao tones.' *Bulletin of the Institute of History and Philology, Academica Sinica* 44: 541–628.

CHAO, Yuan-Ren (1924). 'Singing in Chinese.' *Le maître phonétique* 39: 9–10.

—— (1930). 'A system of tone-letters.' *Le maître phonétique* 45: 24–7.

—— (1956). 'Tone, intonation, singsong, chanting, recitative, tonal composition, and atonal composition in Chinese.' In M. Halle *et al.* (eds.), pp. 52–9.

—— (1968). *A Grammar of Spoken Chinese.* Berkeley: University of California Press.

CHAPLIN, Hamako Ito and MARTIN, Samuel E. (1967). *A Manual of Japanese Writing.* New Haven: Yale University Press.

CHAPMAN, Carol (1993). 'Überlänge in North Saxon Low German: evidence for the metrical foot.' *Zeitschrift für Dialektologie und Linguistik* 60: 129–57.

CHEN, Matthew Y. (1996). 'Tonal geometry—A Chinese perspective.' In C.-T. J. Huang and Y.-H. A. Li (eds.), pp. 21–48.

CHENG, Chin-Chuan (1973). *A synchronic phonology of Mandarin Chinese.* The Hague: Mouton.

CHIBA, Tsutomu (1935). *A Study of Accent. Research into its nature and scope in the light of experimental phonetics.* Tokyo: Fuzanbo.

CHIU, Bien-Ming (1930). 'Chinese (Amoy dialect).' *Le maître phonétique* 45: 38–40.

CHOMSKY, Noam (1957). *Syntactic Structures.* The Hague: Mouton.

—— (1964). *Current issues in Linguistic Theory.* The Hague: Mouton.

—— (1965). *Aspects of the Theory of Syntax.* Cambridge, MA: MIT Press.

—— (1981). *Lectures on Government and Binding.* Dordrecht: Foris.

—— and HALLE, Morris (1968). *The Sound Pattern of English.* New York: Harper and Row.

—— —— and LUKOFF, Fred (1956). 'On accent and juncture in English.' In M. Halle *et al.* (eds.), pp. 65–80.

CHRISTALLER, J. G. (1875). *A Grammar of the Asante and Fante Languages called Tshi (Chwee, Twi)*. Basel.

CLARK, Mary (1988). 'An accentual analysis of the Zulu noun.' In H. van der Hulst and N. Smith (eds.) (1988a), pp. 51–79.

CLEMENTS, George N. (1983). 'The hierarchical representation of tone features.' In I. R. Dihoff (ed.), pp. 145–76.

—— (1985). 'The geometry of phonological features.' *Phonology Yearbook* 2: 225–52.

—— (1986). 'Compensatory lengthening and consonant gemination in Luganda.' In L. Wetzels and E. Sezer (eds.), pp. 37–77.

—— (1990). 'The status of register in intonation theory: comments on the papers by Ladd and by Inkelas and Leben.' In J. Kingston and M. E. Beckman (eds.), pp. 58–71.

—— (ed.) (1977). *Harvard Studies in Phonology I*. Cambridge, MA, Harvard University Press.

—— and FORD, Kevin C. (1977). 'On the phonological status of downstep in Kikuyu.' In G. N. Clements (ed.), pp. 187–272.

—— —— (1979). 'Kikuyu tone shift and its synchronic consequences.' *Linguistic Inquiry* 10: 179–210.

—— and GOLDSMITH, John A. (1984). 'Autosegmental Studies in Bantu Tone: Introduction.' In G. N. Clements and J. A. Goldsmith (eds.), pp. 1–17.

—— —— (eds.) (1984). *Autosegmental Studies in Bantu Tone*. Dordrecht: Foris.

—— and KEYSER, Samuel Jay (1983). *CV Phonology. A Generative Theory of the Syllable*. Cambridge, MA: MIT Press.

COHEN, Antonie and 't HART, Johan (1967). 'On the anatomy of intonation.' *Lingua* 19: 177–92.

—— COLLIER, René, and 't HART, Johan (1982). 'Declination: construct or intrinsic feature of speech pitch?' *Phonetica* 39: 254–73.

COLE, Jennifer and KISSEBERTH, Charles (eds.) (1994). *Perspectives in Phonology*. Stanford, CA: Centre for the Study of Language and Information.

COLEMAN, H. O. (1914). 'Intonation and emphasis.' *Miscellanea Phonetica I*, International Phonetics Association, 6–26.

—— (1924). 'Chinese singing.' *Le maître phonétique* 39: 10–11.

COMRIE, Bernard (1981). *The Languages of the Soviet Union*. Cambridge: Cambridge University Press.

—— (ed.) (1990). *The Major Languages of Eastern Europe*. London: Routledge.

CONNELL, Bruce and ARVANITI, Amalia (eds.) (1995). *Phonology and Phonetic Evidence. Papers in Laboratory Phonology IV*. Cambridge: Cambridge University Press.

COOPER, W. E. and EADY, S. J. (1986). 'Metrical phonology in speech production.' *Journal of Memory and Language* 25: 369–84.

COPE, Anthony T. (1970). 'Zulu tonal morphology.' *Journal of African Languages* 9.3: 111–52.

CORBETT, Greville (1990). 'Serbo–Croat.' In B. Comrie (ed.), pp. 125–43.

COUPER-KUHLEN, Elizabeth (1986). *An Introduction to English Prosody*. Tübingen/London: Niemeyer/Edward Arnold.

COUSTENOBLE, Hélène N. and ARMSTRONG, Lilias E. (1934). *Studies in French Intonation.* Cambridge: Heffer.

CRUTTENDEN, Alan (1981). 'Falls and rises: meaning and universals.' *Journal of Linguistics* 17: 77–91.

—— (1997). *Intonation.* 2nd edn. Cambridge: Cambridge University Press.

CRYSTAL, David (1969). *Prosodic Systems and Intonation in English.* Cambridge: Cambridge University Press.

—— (1997). *A Dictionary of Linguistics and Phonetics.* 4th edn. Oxford: Blackwell.

—— (ed.) (1982). *Linguistic Controversies.* London: Edward Arnold.

—— and QUIRK, Randolph (1964). *Systems of Prosodic and Paralinguistic Features in English.* The Hague: Mouton.

CUTLER, Anne (1980). 'Syllable omission errors and isochrony.' In H. W. Dechert and M. Raupach (eds.), pp. 183–90.

—— (1984). 'Stress and accent in language production and understanding.' In D. Gibbon and H. Richter (eds.), pp. 77–90.

—— (1990). 'From performance to phonology. Comments on Beckman and Edwards' paper.' In J. Kingston and M. E. Beckman (eds.), pp. 208–14.

—— and ISARD, Stephen D. (1980). 'The production of prosody.' In B. Butterworth (ed.), pp. 245–69.

—— and LADD, D. Robert (1983). 'Comparative notes on terms and topics in the contributions.' In A. Cutler and D. R. Ladd (eds.), pp. 141–6.

—— —— (eds.) (1983). *Prosody: Models and Measurements.* Berlin: Springer.

DASHER, Richard and BOLINGER, Dwight L. (1982). 'On preaccentual lengthening.' *Journal of the International Phonetic Association* 12: 58–71.

DAUER, R. M. (1983). 'Stress-timing and syllable-timing reanalysed.' *Journal of Phonetics* 11: 51–62.

De ANGULO, Jaime (1926). 'Tone patterns and verb forms in a dialect of Zapoteco.' *Language* 2: 238–50.

—— (1937). 'Cantonese dialect of Chinese.' *Le maître phonétique* 52: 69–70.

De CHENE, Brent Eugene and ANDERSON, Stephen R. (1979). 'Compensatory lengthening.' *Language* 55: 505–35.

DECHERT, H. W. and RAUPACH, M. (eds.) (1980). *Temporal Variables in Speech. Studies in Honour of Frieda Goldman-Eisler.* The Hague: Mouton.

DELATTRE, Pierre (1965). *Comparing the Phonetic Features of English, French, German and Spanish: an Interim Report.* Heidelberg: Julius Gross.

—— POENACK, E., and OLSEN, C. (1965). 'Some characteristics of German intonation for the expression of continuation and finality.' *Phonetica* 13: 134–61.

DENES, Peter E. and PINSON, Elliot N. (1993). *The Speech Chain. The Physics and Biology of Spoken Language.* 2nd edn. New York: Freeman.

DIHOFF, Ivan R. (ed.) (1983). *Current Approaches to African Linguistics (vol. 1).* Dordrecht: Foris.

DIMMENDAAL, Gerrit J. and BREEDVELD, Anneke (1986). 'Tonal influence on vocalic quality.' In K. Bogers et al. (eds.), pp. 1–33.

DOBSON E. J. (1962). 'Middle English lengthening in open syllables.' *Transactions of the Philological Society,* 124–48.

DOKE, Clement M. (1923). 'A dissertation on the phonetics of the Zulu language.' *Bulletin of the School of Oriental Studies* 2: 685–729.

—— (1926). *The Phonetics of the Zulu Language.* Special Number of *Bantu Studies*, Johannesburg: University of Witwatersrand.

—— (1931). *A Comparative Study in Shona Phonetics.* Johannesburg: University of Witwatersrand.

DOOREN, K. van and EYNDE, K. van den (1982). 'A structure for the intonation of Dutch.' *Linguistics* 20: 203–35.

DOWNING, Bruce T. (1970). *Syntactic Structure and Phonological Phrasing in English.* PhD., University of Texas.

DRESSLER, W. U. et al. (eds.), *Phonologica 1984.* Cambridge: Cambridge University Press.

DUANMU, San (1990). *A Formal Study of Syllable, Tone, Stress, and Domain in Chinese Languages.* Doctoral Dissertation, MIT.

DUNSTAN, Elizabeth (ed.) (1969). *Twelve Nigerian Languages. A Handbook on their Sound Systems for Teachers of English.* London: Longman.

DURAND, Jacques (1990). *Generative and Non-linear Phonology.* London: Longman.

—— and KATAMBA, Francis (eds.) (1995). *Frontiers of Phonology: Atoms, Structures, Derivations.* London: Longman.

DURAND, Marguerite (1939). 'Durée phonétique et durée phonologique.' In E. Blancquaert and W. Pée (eds.), pp. 261–5.

—— (1946). *Voyelles longues et voyelles brèves. Essai sur la nature de la quantité vocalique.* Paris: Klincksieck.

EGEROD, Søren (1971). 'Phonation types in Chinese and South East Asian languages.' *Acta Linguistica Hafniensis* 13.2: 159–71.

ELERT, Claes-Christian, JOHANSSON, Iréne, and STRANGERT, Eva (eds.) (1984). *Nordic Prosody III. Papers from a Symposium.* Stockholm: Almqvist and Wiksell International.

ELIMELECH, Baruch (1974). 'On the reality of underlying contour tones.' In I. Maddieson (ed.), pp. 74–83.

ELLIS, Alexander J. (1848). *The Essentials of Phonetics.* London.

EMENANJO, E. Nolue (1987). *Elements of Modern Igbo Grammar.* Ibadan: University Press.

ESSEN, Otto von (1962). 'Trubetzkoys "fester" und "loser Anschluß" in experimentalphonetischer Sicht.' *Proceedings of the 4th International Congress of Phonetic Sciences*, The Hague: Mouton, pp. 590–7.

FAIRBANKS, Grant and PRONOVOST, W. (1939). 'An experimental study of the pitch characteristics of the voice during the expression of emotion.' *Speech Monographs* 6: 87–104.

FÉRY, Caroline (1993). *German Intonational Patterns.* Tübingen: Niemeyer.

FIRTH, John Rupert (1948). 'Sounds and prosodies.' *Transactions of the Philological Society,* 127–52.

FISCHER-JØRGENSEN, Eli (1940–1), 'Neuere Beiträge zum Quantitätsproblem.' *Acta Linguistica II*: 175–81.

FONAGY, Ivan (1958). 'Elektrophysiologische Beiträge zur Akzentfrage.' *Phonetica* 2: 12.

—— and MAGDICS, Klara (1963). 'Emotional patterns in intonation and music.' *Zeitschrift für Phonetik* 16: 293–326.

FORCHHAMMER, Jørgen (1939). 'Länge und Kürze.' *Archiv für vergleichende Phonetik* III: 19–27.

FOWLER, Carol A. (1990). 'Lengthening and the nature of prosodic constituency: comments on Beckman and Edwards's paper.' In J. Kingston and M. E. Beckman (eds.), pp. 201–7.

FOX, Anthony (1973). 'Tone sequences in English.' *Archivum Linguisticum* 4 (new series): 17–26.

—— (1978). *A Comparative Study of English and German Intonation*. PhD, University of Edinburgh.

—— (1981). 'Falling–rising intonations in English and German.' In C. V. J. Russ (ed.), pp. 55–72.

—— (1982). 'Remarks on intonation and "Ausrahmung" in German.' *Journal of Linguistics* 18: 89–106.

—— (1984a). *German Intonation: an Outline*. Oxford: Clarendon Press.

—— (1984b). 'Subordinating and co-ordinating intonation structures in the articulation of discourse.' In D. Gibbon and H. Richter (eds.), pp. 120–33.

—— (1985). 'Aspects of prosodic typology', *Working Papers in Linguistics and Phonetics* (University of Leeds) 3: 60–119.

—— (1990). *The Structure of German*. Oxford: Oxford University Press.

—— (1995). 'Principles of intonational typology.' In J. W. Lewis (ed.), pp. 187–10.

FRAISSE, P. (1956). *Les structures rhythmiques*. Louvain: Publications Universitaires de Louvain.

—— (1963). *The Psychology of Time*. New York: Harper and Row.

FROMKIN, Victoria A. (1974). 'On the phonological representation of tone.' In I. Maddieson (ed.), pp. 1–17.

—— (ed.) (1978). *Tone: a Linguistic Survey*. New York, Academic Press.

FRY, Dennis B. (1955). 'Duration and intensity as physical correlates of linguistic stress.' *Journal of the Acoustical Society of America* 27: 765–9.

—— (1958). 'Experiments in the perception of stress.' *Language and Speech* 1: 126–52.

—— (1964). 'The functions of the syllable.' *Zeitschrift für Phonetik, Sprachwissenschaft und Kommunikationsforschung* 17: 215–37.

—— (1968). 'Prosodic phenomena.' In B. Malmberg (ed.), pp. 364–410.

FUDGE, Erik C. (1969). 'Syllables.' *Journal of Linguistics* 5: 253–86.

—— (1984). *English Word-Stress*. London: George Allen and Unwin.

—— (ed.) (1973). *Phonology*. Harmondsworth: Penguin.

FUJISAKI, Hiroya and NAGASHIMA, S. (1969). 'A model for the synthesis of pitch contours of connected speech.' *Annual Report of the Engineering Research Institute*. Tokyo: Faculty of Engineering, University of Tokyo.

—— and SUDO, Hiroshi (1971). 'A generative model for the prosody of connected speech in Japanese.' *Annual Report of the Engineering Research Institute*. Tokyo: Faculty of Engineering, University of Tokyo, 30: 75–80.

—— HIROSE, Keikichi, and OHTA, Kazuhiko (1979). 'Acoustic features of the fundamental frequency contours of declarative sentences in Japanese.' *Annual Bulletin of the Research Institute of Logopaedics and Phoniatrics*, University of Tokyo: 13: 163–73.

GANDOUR, Jackson T. (1974a). 'The features of the larynx: N-ary or binary?' In I. Maddieson (ed.), pp. 147–59.

—— (1974b). 'Consonant types and tone in Siamese.' In I. Maddieson (ed.). pp. 92–117.

—— (1974c). 'On the representation of tone in Siamese.' In I. Maddieson (ed.), pp. 118–46.

—— (1974d). 'The glottal stop in Siamese: predictability in phonological description.' In I. Maddieson (ed.), pp. 84–91.

—— (1977). 'On the interaction between tone and vowel length: evidence from Thai dialects.' *Phonetica* 34: 54–65.

GARDE, Paul (1965). 'Accentuation et morphologie.' *Linguistique* 1: 25–39.

—— (1967). 'Principes de description synchronique des faits d'accent.' In J. Hamm (ed.), pp. 32–43.

—— (1968). *L'Accent*. Paris: Presses Universitaires de France.

GÅRDING, Eva (1977). *The Scandinavian Word Accents*. Lund: CWK Gleerup.

—— (1981). 'Contrastive prosody. A model and its application.' *Studia Linguistica* 35: 146–65.

—— (1983). 'A generative model of intonation.' In A. Cutler and D. R. Ladd (eds.), pp. 11–25.

—— (1984). 'Chinese and Swedish in a generative model of intonation.' In C. C. Elert *et al.* (eds.), pp. 79–91.

—— BRUCE, Gösta, and BANNERT, R. (eds.) (1978). *Nordic Prosody*. Gleerup.

GARNES, S. (1973). 'Phonetic evidence supporting a phonological analysis.' *Journal of Phonetics* 1: 273–83.

GARVIN, Paul L. (ed.) (1970). *Method and Theory in Linguistics*. The Hague: Mouton.

GEORGE, Isaac (1970). 'Nupe tonology.' *Studies in African Linguistics* 1: 100–21.

GIBBON, Dafydd (1976). *Perspectives of Intonation Analysis*. Berne.

—— and RICHTER, Helmut (eds.) (1994). *Intonation, Accent and Rhythm. Studies in Discourse Phonology*. Berlin: de Gruyter.

GIEGERICH, Heinz J. (1980). 'On stress-timing in English phonology.' *Lingua* 51: 187–221.

—— (1983). 'On English sentence-stress and the nature of metrical structure.' *Journal of Linguistics* 19: 1–28.

—— (1984). *Relating to Metrical Structure*. Bloomington: Indiana University Linguistics Club.

—— (1985). *Metrical Phonology and Phonological Structure: German and English*. Cambridge: Cambridge University Press.

GILDERSLEVE, B. L. and LODGE, Gonzalez (1895). *Latin Grammar*. 3rd edn. London: Macmillan.

GIMSON, A. C. (1945–9). 'Implications of the phonemic/chronemic grouping of English vowels.' *Acta Linguistica* V.

—— (1956). 'The linguistic relevance of stress in English.' *Zeitschrift für Phonetik* 9.2: 113–49.

—— (1980). *An Introduction to the Pronunciation of English*. 3rd edn. London: Edward Arnold.

GLEASON, H. A., Jr. (1961). *An Introduction to Descriptive Linguistics*. 2nd edn. New York: Holt, Rinehart, & Winston.

GOLDSMITH, John A. (1976). *Autosegmental Phonology*. Doctoral Dissertation, MIT. Distributed by Indiana University Linguistics Club, Bloomington.

—— (1978). 'English as a tone language.' *Communication and Cognition* 11, 3/4: 453–76.

GOLDSMITH, John A. (cont.) (1981). 'English as a tone language.' In D. L. Goyvaerts (ed.) (1981), pp. 287–308.

—— (1982). 'Accent systems.' In H. van der Hulst and N. Smith (eds.) (1982), pp. 47–63.

—— (1983). 'Accent in Tonga: an autosegmental approach.' In I. R. Dihoff (ed.), pp. 227–34.

—— (1984a). 'Tone and accent in Tonga.' In G. N. Clements and J. A. Goldsmith (eds.), pp. 19–51.

—— (1984b). 'Meussen's rule.' In M. Aronoff and R. Oehrle (eds.), pp. 245–59.

—— (1987a). 'The rise of rhythmic structure in Bantu.' In *Phonologica 1984*. Cambridge: Cambridge University Press.

—— (1987b). 'Tone and accent and getting the two together.' *Berkeley Linguistic Society: Proceedings* 13: 88–104.

—— (1990). *Autosegmental and Metrical Phonology*. Oxford: Blackwell.

—— (1994). 'A dynamic computational theory of accent systems.' In J. Cole and C. Kisseberth (eds.), pp. 1–28.

—— (ed.) (1995). *The Handbook of Phonological Theory*. Oxford: Blackwell.

GOYVAERTS, Didier L. (ed.) (1981). *Phonology in the 1980s*. Ghent: Storia-Scientia.

—— (ed.) (1985). *African Linguistics. Essays in Memory of M. W. K. Semikenke*. Amsterdam: John Benjamins.

—— and PULLUM, Geoffrey K. (eds.) (1975). *Essays on the Sound Pattern of English*. Ghent: Storia-Scientia.

GREENBERG, Joseph H. (1941). 'Some problems in Hausa phonology.' *Language* 17: 316–23.

—— (ed.) (1978). *Universals of Language, Vol. 2*. Palo Alto: Stanford University Press.

GRIMM, Jakob (1822). *Deutsche Grammatik*. 2nd edn. Repr. 1870–98. Göttingen: Dietrich.

GRØNNUM, Nina (see also THORSEN, Nina) (1991). 'Prosodic parameters in a variety of regional Danish standard languages, with a view towards Swedish and German.' *Phonetica* 47: 188–214.

GRUBER, Jeffrey (1964). 'The distinctive features of tone.' Unpublished MS. Cited in Anderson, 1978.

GRUNDT, Alice W. (1976). *Compensation in Phonology: Open Syllable Lengthening*. Bloomington, Indiana: Indiana University Linguistics Club.

GRÜTZMACHER, M. (1939). 'Ein neuer Tonhöhenschreiber, seine Anwendung auf mathematische, phonetische und musikalische Probleme, nach gemeinsamen Versuchen mit W. Lottermoser.' In E. Blancquaert and W. Pée (eds.), p. 105.

GUERSSEL, Mohammed (1977). 'Constraints on phonological rules.' *Language* 53: 267–305.

GUSSENHOVEN, Carlos (1983). 'Stress shift and the nucleus.' *Linguistics* : 303–39. Also in *On the Grammar and Semantics of Sentence Accents*. Dordrecht: Foris, pp. 291–332.

—— and JACOBS, Haike (1998). *Understanding Phonology*. London: Arnold.

HADDING-KOCH, Kerstin (1962). 'Notes on the Swedish word-tones.' In *Proceedings of the Fourth International Congress of Phonetic Sciences*. The Hague: Mouton, pp. 630–8.

HAÏK, Isabelle and TULLER, Laurice (eds.) (1989). *Current Approaches to African Linguistics, Vol. 6*. Dordrecht: Foris.

HALLE, Morris (1973). 'Stress rules in English: a new version.' *Linguistic Inquiry* 4: 451–64.

—— (1977). 'Tenseness, vowel shift, and the phonology of the back vowels in Modern English.' *Linguistic Inquiry* 8: 611–25.

—— *et al.* (eds.) (1956). *For Roman Jakobson.* The Hague: Mouton.

—— and KEYSER, Samuel Jay (1971). *English Stress, its Form, its Growth, and its Role in Verse.* New York: Harper and Row.

—— and MOHANAN, Karuvannur P. (1985). 'Segmental phonology of modern English.' *Linguistic Inquiry* 16: 57–116.

—— and STEVENS, Kenneth (1969). 'On the Feature "Advanced Tongue Root".' *Quarterly Progress Report* 94: 209–15.

—— —— (1971). 'A note on laryngeal features.' *Quarterly Progress Report* 101: 198–213. Research Laboratory of Electronics, MIT.

—— and VERGNAUD, Jean-Roger (1982). 'On the framework of autosegmental phonology.' In H. van der Hulst and N. Smith (eds.), pp. 65–82.

—— —— (1987a). *An Essay on Stress.* Cambridge, MA: MIT Press.

—— —— (1987b). 'Stress and the cycle.' *Linguistic Inquiry* 18: 45–84.

HALLIDAY, Michael A. K. (1961). 'Categories of the theory of grammar.' *Word* 17: 241–92.

—— (1963a). 'The tones of English.' *Archivum Linguisticum* 15: 1–28.

—— (1963b). 'Intonation in English grammar.' *Transactions of the Philological Society,* 143–69.

—— (1966). 'The concept of rank: a reply.' *Journal of Linguistics* 2: 110–18.

—— (1967). *Intonation and Grammar in British English.* The Hague: Mouton.

—— (1970). *A Course in Spoken English: Intonation.* London: Oxford University Press.

—— (1985). *An Introduction to Functional Grammar.* London: Edward Arnold.

—— MCINTOSH, Angus, and STREVENS, Peter (1964). *The Linguistic Sciences and Language Teaching.* London: Longman.

HAMM, Josef (ed.) (1967). *Phonologie der Gegenwart. Vorträge und Diskussionen anläßlich der Internationalen Phonologie-Tagung in Wien.* Graz: Bohlau.

HAMMERICH, L. L. *et al.* (eds.) (1971). *Form and Substance: Phonetic and Linguistic Papers presented to Eli Fischer-Jørgensen.* Odense: Akademisk Forlag.

HAMMOND, Michael (1997). 'Optimality Theory and prosody.' In D. Archangeli and D. T. Langendoen (eds.), pp. 33–58.

HARAGUCHI, Shosuke (1977). *The Tone Pattern of Japanese: an Autosegmental Theory of Tonology.* Tokyo: Kaitakusha.

HARMS, Robert T. (1962). *Estonian Grammar.* Bloomington: Indiana University Publications, Uralic and Altaic Series 12.

—— (1968). *Introduction to Phonological Theory.* Englewood Cliffs, NJ: Prentice-Hall.

HARRIS, James W. (1969). *Spanish Phonology.* Cambridge, MA: MIT Press.

—— (1983). *Syllable Structure and Stress in Spanish: a Nonlinear Analysis.* Cambridge, MA: MIT Press.

HARRIS, Jimmy G. and NOSS, Richard B. (eds.) (1972). *Tai Phonetics and Phonology.* Bangkok: Central Institute of English Language.

HARRIS, Zellig S. (1944). 'Simultaneous components in phonology.' *Language* 20: 181–205.

HART, John (1569). *An orthographie, conteyning the due order and reason, how to write or point thimage of mannes voice, most like to the life of nature.* London: Serres.

't HART, Johan and COHEN, Antonie (1973). 'Intonation by rule: a perceptual quest.' *Journal of Phonetics* 1: 309–27.

—— and COLLIER, René (1975). 'Integrating different levels of intonation analysis.' *Journal of Phonetics* 3: 235–55.

't HART, Johan, COLLIER, René, and COHEN, Antonie (1990). *A Perceptual Study of Intonation. An experimental-phonetic approach to speech melody.* Cambridge: Cambridge University Press.

HATTORI, Shiro (1967). 'Descriptive linguistics in Japan.' In *Current Trends in Linguistics II.* The Hague: Mouton, pp. 530–84.

HAUDRICOURT, André G. (1954). 'De l'origine des tons en viêtnamien.' *Journal Asiatique* 242: 69–82.

—— (1961). 'Bipartition et tripartition des systèmes de tons dans quelques langues de l'extréme-orient.' *Bulletin de la société linguistique de Paris* 56: 163–80. English translation: 'Two-way and three-way splitting of tonal systems in some far-Eastern languages.' In J. G. Harris and R. B. Noss (eds.) (1972), pp. 58–86.

HAUGEN, Einar (1949). 'Phoneme or prosodeme?' *Language* 25: 278–82.

—— (1958). 'The phonemics of Modern Icelandic.' *Language* 34: 55–88.

—— (1963). 'Pitch accent and tonemic juncture in Scandinavian.' *Monatshefte für den Deutschunterricht* 55: 157–61.

—— (1967). 'On the rules of Norwegian tonality.' *Language* 43: 185–202.

—— and JOOS, Martin (1952). 'Tone and intonation in East Norwegian.' *Acta Philologica Scandinavica* 22: 51–64.

HAYES, Bruce (1981). *A Metrical Theory of Stress Rules.* Doctoral dissertation, MIT. Distributed by Indiana University Linguistics Club, Bloomington.

—— (1984). 'The phonology of rhythm in English.' *Linguistic Inquiry* 15: 33–74.

—— (1989). 'Compensatory lengthening in moraic phonology.' *Linguistic Inquiry* 20: 253–306.

—— (1995). *Metrical Stress Theory.* Chicago: University of Chicago Press.

HEGEDÜS, L. (1959). 'Beitrag zur Frage der Geminaten.' *Zeitschrift für Phonetik* 12: 68–106.

HENDERSON, Eugénie J. A. (1949). 'Prosodies in Siamese.' *Asia Minor* (New Series) 1: 189–215.

—— (1952). 'The main features of Cambodian pronunciation.' *Bulletin of the School of Oriental and African Studies* 14: 149–74.

—— (1979). 'Bwe Karen as a two-tone language? An enquiry into the interrelationships of pitch, tone and initial consonant.' *S. E. Asian Linguistic Studies (Pacific Linguistics,* C45) 3: 301–26.

HERZOG, George (1934). 'Drum signalling in a West African tribe.' *Word* 1: 217–38.

HEWSON, John (1980). 'Stress in English: four levels or three?' *Canadian Journal of Linguistics* 25.2: 197–203.

HILL, Archibald A. (1961). 'Suprasegmentals, prosodies, prosodemes. Comparison and discussion.' *Language* 37: 457–68.

HILL, L. A. (1960). 'Stress, pitch, and prominence.' *Le maître phonétique* 114: 22–4.

HIRANBURANA, Samang (1972). 'Changes in the pitch contours of unaccented syllables in Spoken Thai.' In J. G. Harris and R. B. Noss (eds.), pp. 23–7.

HIRAYAMA, Teruo (1961). 'A study of Japanese accent.' *Study of Sounds* 9: 141–53.

HIRST, Daniel J. (1976). 'A distinctive feature analysis of English intonation.' *Linguistica* 168: 27–42.

—— (1983). 'Structures and categories in prosodic representations.' In A. Cutler and D. R. Ladd (eds.), pp. 93–109.

—— (1988). 'Tonal Units as constituents of prosodic structure: the evidence from English and French intonation.' In H. van der Hulst and N. Smith (eds.) (1988a), pp. 151–65.

HJELMSLEV, Louis (1937). 'Accent, intonation, quantité.' *Studi Baltici* 6: 1–58. Also in *Essais linguistiques* II, = *Travaux du cercle linguistique de Copenhague XIV*, 1973: 181–222.

HOARD, James E. (1971). 'The new phonological paradigm.' *Glossa* 5: 222–68.

HOCK, Hans-Henrich (1986). 'Compensatory lengthening: in defense of the concept "mora".' *Folia Linguistica* 20: 431–60.

HOCKETT, Charles F. (1947). 'Peiping phonology.' *Journal of the American Oriental Society* 67: 253–67.

—— (1955). *A Manual of Phonology*. Baltimore: Waverly Press.

HODGE, Carelton Taylor (1958). 'Serbo–Croatian stress and pitch.' *General Linguistics* 3: 43–54.

—— and HAUSE, H. E. (1944). 'Hausa tone.' *Journal of the American Oriental Society* 64: 51–2.

HOEQUIST C., Jr. (1983). 'Durational correlates of linguistic rhythm categories.' *Phonetica* 40: 19–31.

HOGG, Richard M. (1992). *A Grammar of Old English*. Oxford: Blackwell.

—— and McCULLY, Christopher B. (1987). *Metrical Phonology: a Coursebook*. Cambridge: Cambridge University Press.

HOIJER, Harry (1938). *Chiracahua and Mescalero Texts*. Chicago: University of Chicago Press.

—— (1943). 'Pitch accent in the Apachean languages.' *Language* 19: 38–41.

—— (1945). *Navaho Phonology*. Albuquerque: University of New Mexico Press.

HOMBERT, Jean-Marie (1974). 'Universals of downdrift: their phonetic basis and significance for a theory of tone.' *Studies in African Linguistics*, Suppl. 5: 69–83.

—— (1977). 'Consonant types, vowel height, and tone in Yoruba.' *Studies in African Linguistics* 8: 173–90.

—— (1978). 'Consonant types, vowel quality, and tone.' In V. A. Fromkin (ed.), pp. 77–111.

—— O'HALA, John J., and EWAN, William G. (1979). 'Phonetic explanations for the development of tones.' *Language* 55: 37–58.

HOOGSHAGEN, Searle (1959). 'Three contrastive vowel lengths in Mixe.' *Zeitschrift für Phonetik* 12: 111–15.

HUANG, C.-T. James (1985). 'The autosegmental and metrical nature of tone terracing.' In D. L. Goyvaerts (ed.), Amsterdam: Benjamins, pp. 209–38.

—— and LI, Y.-H. Audrey (eds.) (1996). *New Horizons in Chinese Linguistics*. Dordrecht, Kluwer.

HUDDLESTON, Rodney D. (1965). 'Rank and depth.' *Language* 41: 574–86.

HULST, Harry van der and SMITH, Norval (1982). 'An overview of autosegmental and metrical phonology.' In H. van der Hulst and N. Smith (eds.), pp. 1–45.

—— —— (eds.) (1982). *The Structure of Phonological Representations Pt I*. Dordrecht: Foris.

—— —— (eds.) (1988a). *Autosegmental Studies on Pitch Accent*. Dordrecht: Foris.

—— —— (eds.) (1988b). *Features, Segmental Structure and Harmony Processes, Part I*. Dordrecht: Foris.

HULST, Harry van der and SMITH, Norval (cont.) (1988c). 'The variety of Pitch Accent systems: Introduction.' In H. van der Hulst and N. Smith (eds.) (1988a), pp. ix–xxiv.

—— and SNIDER, Keith (eds.) (1992). *The Phonology of Tone. The Representation of Tonal Register.* Berlin: Mouton de Gruyter.

HYMAN, Larry M. (1973). 'The role of consonant types in natural tonal assimilations.' In L. M. Hyman (ed.), pp. 151–79.

—— (1977). 'On the nature of linguistic stress.' In L. M. Hyman (ed.), pp. 37–82.

—— (1978). 'Tone and/or accent', In D. J. Napoli (ed.), pp. 1–20.

—— (1981). 'Tonal accent in Somali.' *Studies in African Linguistics* 12: 169–203.

—— (1982). 'Globality and the accentual analysis of Luganda tone.' *Journal of Linguistic Research* 2.3: 1–40.

—— (1985). *A Theory of Phonological Weight.* Dordrecht: Foris.

—— (1986). 'The representation of multiple tone heights.' In K. Bogers *et al.* (eds.), pp. 109–52.

—— (1992). 'Register tones and tonal geometry.' In H. van der Hulst and K. Snider (eds.), pp. 75–108.

—— (ed.) (1973). *Consonant Types and Tone.* Los Angeles: University of Southern California.

—— (ed.) (1976). *Studies in Bantu Tonology* (Southern California Occasional Papers in Linguistics 3). Los Angeles: Department of Linguistics: University of Southern California.

—— (ed.) (1977). *Studies in Stress and Accent.* Los Angeles: Department of Linguistics, University of Southern California.

—— and BYARUSHENGO, Ernest Rugwa (1984). 'A model of Haya tonology.' In G. N. Clements and J. A. Goldsmith (ed.), pp. 53–103.

—— and KATAMBA, Francis X. (1993). 'A new approach to tone in Luganda.' *Language* 69.1: 34–67.

—— and LI, Charles N. (eds.) (1988). *Language, Speech and Mind: Studies in Honour of Victoria A. Fromkin.* London: Routledge.

—— and PULLEYBLANK, Douglas (1988). 'On feature copying: parameters of tone rules.' In L. M. Hyman and C. N. Li (eds.), pp. 30–48.

—— and SCHUH, Russell G. (1972). 'Universals of tone rules.' *Working Papers in Language Universals* 10: 1–50.

—— —— (1974). 'Universals of tone rules: evidence from West Africa.' *Linguistic Inquiry* 5: 81–115.

—— and TADADJEU, Maurice (1976). 'Floating tones in Mbam-Nkam.' In L. M. Hyman (ed.), pp. 57–111.

INGRIA, R. (1980). 'Compensatory lengthening as a metrical phenomenon.' *Linguistic Inquiry* 11: 465–95.

INKELAS, Sharon (1987). 'Tone feature geometry.' In *Proceedings of North-Eastern Linguistics Society* 18: 223–37.

—— (1989). 'Register tone and the phonological representation of downstep.' In I. Haïk and L. Tuller (eds.), pp. 65–82.

—— and LEBEN, William R. (1990). 'Where phonology and phonetics intersect: the case of Hausa intonation.' In J. Kingston and M. E. Beckman (eds.), pp. 17–34.

—— and ZEC, Draga (1990). 'Introduction.' In S. Inkelas and D. Zec (eds.), pp. xiii–xv.

—— —— (eds.) (1990). *The Phonology–Syntax Connection*. Chicago: University of Chicago Press.

ISACENKO, Alexander V. and SCHÄDICH, Hans-Joachim (1966). 'Untersuchungen über die deutsche Satzintonation.' In *Untersuchungen über Akzent und Intonation im Deutschen, Studia Grammatica* 7: 7–67.

ÎTO, Junko (1986). *Syllable Theory in Prosodic Phonology*. Doctoral Dissertation, University of Massachusetts, Amherst. Published New York: Garland.

JACKENDOFF, Ray (1977). *X′ Syntax: a Study of Phrase Structure*. Cambridge, MA: MIT Press.

JACOBS, Roderick A. and ROSENBAUM, Peter S. (eds.) (1970). *Readings in Transformational Grammar*. Waltham, MA: Ginn.

JAKOBSON, Roman (1931). 'Über die Betonung und ihre Rolle in der Wort und Syntagmaphonologie.' *Traveaux du Cercle Linguistique de Prague IV*. Also in R. Jakobson *Selected Writings I*, The Hague: Mouton, pp. 117–36.

—— (1937). 'Über die Geschaffenheit der prosodischen Gegensätze.' In *Mélanges de linguistique et de philologie offerts à J. van Ginneken*, Paris. 25–33. Also in R. Jakobson *Selected Writings I*, The Hague: Mouton, pp. 254–61.

—— FANT, C. Gunnar, and HALLE, Morris (1952). *Preliminaries to Speech Analysis. The distinctive features and their correlates*. Cambridge, MA: MIT Press.

—— and HALLE, Morris (1956). *Fundamentals of Language*. The Hague: Mouton.

—— —— (1964). 'Tenseness and laxness.' In D. Abercrombie *et al.* (eds.), pp. 96–101.

—— and KAWAMOTI, Shigeo (eds.) (1970). *Studies in General and Oriental Linguistics Presented to Shirô Hattori*. Tokyo: TEC Co.

JASANOFF, Jay H. (1966). 'Remarks on the Scandinavian word tones.' *Lingua* 16: 71–81.

JASSEM, Wiktor (1952). *The Intonation of Conversational English*. Warsaw: La Société des Sciences et des Lettres.

—— (1959). 'The phonology of Polish stress.' *Word* 15: 252–69.

—— and GIBBON, Dafydd (1980). 'Re-defining English accent and stress.' *Journal of the International Phonetic Association* 10: 2–16.

—— HILL, D. R., and WITTEN, I. H. (1984). 'Isochrony in English speech: its statistical validity and linguistic relevance.' In D. Gibbon and H. Richter (eds.), pp. 203–25.

JENSEN, Martin Kloster (1958). 'Recognition of word-tones in whispered speech.' *Word* 14: 187–96.

—— (1961). *Tonemicity. A Technique for Determining the Phonemic Status of Suprasegmental Patterns in Pairs of Lexical Units, Applied to a Group of West Norwegian Dialects, and to Faroese*. Bergen: Norwegian Universities Press.

JESPERSEN, Otto (1912). *Elementarbuch der Phonetik*. Leipzig: Teubner.

—— (1913). *Lehrbuch der Phonetik*. 2nd edn. Leipzig: Teubner.

JIMBO, K. (1925). 'The word-tone of the Standard Japanese Language.' *Bulletin of the School of Oriental and African Studies* 3: 660–7.

JOHNSON, Lawrence (1976). 'Devoicing, tone and stress in Runyankore.' In L. M. Hyman (ed.), pp. 207–16.

JONES, Charles (1989). *A History of English Phonology*. London: Longman.

JONES, Daniel (1909). *Intonation Curves*. Leipzig: Teubner.

—— (1913). 'Chinese tones.' *Le maître phonétique* 28: 95–6.

JONES, Daniel (cont.) (1944). 'Chronemes and tonemes.' *Acta Linguistica* 4: 1–10. Also in W. E. Jones and J. Laver (eds.), pp. 159–67.

—— (1956). *An Outline of English Phonetics.* 8th edn. Cambridge: Heffer.

—— (1967). *The Phoneme. Its nature and use.* 3rd edn. Cambridge: Heffer.

—— and PLAATJE, S. (1916). *A Sechuana Reader.* London: University of London Press.

—— and WOO, Kwing-Tong (1912). *A Cantonese Phonetic Reader.* London: University of London Press.

JONES, Stephen (1932). 'The accent in French—what is accent?' *Le maître phonétique* 40: 74–5.

JONES, William E. and LAVER, John (eds.) (1973). *Phonetics in Linguistics: a Book of Readings.* London: Longman.

JOOS, Martin (ed.) (1957). *Readings in Linguistics I.* Chicago: Chicago University Press.

JORDEN, Eleanor Harz (1955). *The Syntax of Modern Colloquial Japanese.* Language Dissertation No. 52. Supplement to *Language* 31.

—— and CHAPLIN, Hamako Ito (1963). *Beginning Japanese.* New Haven: Yale University Press.

KAGER, René (1995). 'The metrical theory of word stress.' In J. A. Goldsmith (ed.), pp. 367–402.

KAHN, Daniel (1976). *Syllable-based Generalizations in English Phonology.* PhD Dissertation, MIT.

KARCEVSKIJ, Serge (1931). 'Sur la phonologie de la phrase.' *Traveaux du Cercle Linguistique de Prague* 4: 188–228.

KARLGREN, Bernard (1926). *Études sur la phonologie chinoise.* Uppsala: Appelberg.

KAWAKAMI, Shin (1961). 'On the relation between word-tone and phrase tone in Japanese language.' *Study of Sounds* 9: 169–77.

KAYE, Jonathan, KOOPMAN, Hilda, SPORTICHE, Dominique, and DUGAS, André (eds.) (1983). *Current Approaches to African Linguistics (vol. 2).* Dordrecht: Foris.

KELLER, Rudolf E. (1961). *German Dialects: Phonology and morphology.* Manchester: Manchester University Press.

KELLY, M. H. and BOCK, J. K. (1988). 'Stress in time.' *Journal of Experimental Psychology, Human Perception and Performance* 14: 389–403.

KENSTOWICZ, Michael (1970). 'On the notation of vowel length in Lithuanian.' *Papers in Linguistics* 3: 73–113.

—— (1994). *Phonology in Generative Grammar.* Oxford: Blackwell.

—— and KISSEBERTH, Charles (1979). *Generative Phonology.* Orlando, FL: Academic Press.

—— —— (eds.) (1973). *Issues in Phonological Theory.* The Hague: Mouton.

—— and PYLE, Charles (1973). 'On the phonological integrity of geminates.' In M. Kenstowicz and C. Kisseberth (eds.), pp. 27–43.

KINGDON, Roger (1939). 'Tonetic stress marks for English.' *Le maître phonétique* 68: 60–4.

—— (1958a). *The Groundwork of English Stress.* London: Longman.

—— (1958b). *The Groundwork of English Intonation.* London: Longman.

KINGSTON, John and BECKMAN, Mary E. (eds.) (1990). *Papers in Laboratory Phonology I. Between the grammar and physics of speech.* Cambridge: Cambridge University Press.

KIPARSKY, Paul (1979). 'Metrical structure assignment is cyclical.' *Linguistic Inquiry* 10: 421–41.

—— (1982). 'From cyclic phonology to Lexical Phonology.' In H. van der Hulst and N. Smith (eds.), pp. 131–75.

KISSEBERTH, Charles W. (1970). 'On the functional unity of phonological rules.' *Linguistic Inquiry* 1: 291–306.

—— and ABASHEIKH, M. I. (1974). 'Vowel length in Chi Mwi:ni—a case study of the rôle of grammar in phonology.' In A. Bruck *et al.* (eds.), pp. 193–209.

KLATT, D. (1975). 'Vowel lengthening is syntactically determined in a connected discourse.' *Journal of Phonetics* 3: 129–40.

—— (1976). 'Linguistic uses of segmental duration in English: acoustic and perceptual evidence.' *Journal of the Acoustical Society of America* 59: 1208–21.

KLINGHARDT, Hermann (1927). *Übungen im deutschen Tonfall. Für Lehrer und Studierende, auch für Ausländer.* Leipzig: Quelle und Meyer.

—— and FOURMESTRAUX, M. de (1911). *Französische Intonationsübungen.* Leipzig: Cöthen.

—— and KLEMM, G. (1920). *Übungen im englischen Tonfall.* Leipzig, Cöthen.

KOELLE, Sigismund W. (1854). *Africa Polyglotta; or, A comparative vocabulary of nearly three hundred words and phrases in more than one hundred distinct African languages.* London: Church Missionary House.

KUBOZONO, Haruo (1989). 'The mora and syllable structure in Japanese: evidence from speech errors.' *Language and Speech* 32: 249–78.

—— (1995). 'Perceptual evidence for the mora in Japanese.' In B. Connell and A. Arvaniti (eds.), pp. 141–56.

KURYŁOWICZ, Jerzy (1948). 'Contribution à la théorie de la syllabe.' *Biuletyn polskiego towarzystwa jezykoznawczego* 8: 80–114. Also in *Esquisses linguistiques.* Warsaw, 1960, pp. 193–220.

—— (1966). 'Accent and quantity as elements of rhythm.' In Roman Jakobson *et al.* (eds.) *Poetics II.* Warsaw: Polish Scientific Publishers, pp. 163ff.

LADD, D. Robert (1978). 'Stylized intonation.' *Language* 54: 517–39.

—— (1981). 'On intonational universals.' In T. Myers *et al.* (eds.), pp. 389–97.

—— (1983). 'Peak features and overall slope.' In A. Cutler and D. R. Ladd (eds.), pp. 39–52.

—— (1984). 'Declination: a review and some hypotheses.' *Phonology Yearbook* 1: 53–74.

—— (1990). 'Metrical representation of pitch register.' In J. Kingston and M. E. Beckman (eds.), pp. 35–57.

—— (1996). *Intonational Phonology.* Cambridge: Cambridge University Press.

LADEFOGED, Peter (1964). *A Phonetic Study of West African Languages. An auditory-instrumental survey.* Cambridge: Cambridge University Press.

—— (1967). 'Stress and respiratory activity.' In *Three areas of experimental phonetics.* London: Oxford University Press, pp. 1–49.

—— (1971). *Preliminaries to Linguistic Phonetics.* Chicago: Chicago University Press.

—— (1973). 'The features of the larynx.' *Journal of Phonetics* 1: 73–83.

—— (1975). *A Course in Phonetics.* New York: Harcourt, Brace, Jovanovich.

—— DRAPER, M. H., and WHITTERIDGE, D. (1958). 'Syllables and stress.' International Phonetic Association *Miscellanea Phonetica* 3: 1–14.

LADEFOGED, Peter and MADDIESON, Ian (1996). *The Sounds of the World's Languages.* Oxford: Blackwell.

LAKOFF, George (1972). 'The global nature of the nuclear stress rule.' *Language* 48: 285–303.

LARSON, Jerry (1971). 'Downstep, downdrift, and diacritics.' *Studies in African Linguistics*, Supplement 2: 171–81.

LASS, Roger (1984). *Phonology: an Introduction to Basic Concepts.* Cambridge: Cambridge University Press.

—— (1992). 'Phonology and morphology.' In N. Blake (ed.), pp. 23–155.

—— (1994). *Old English: a Historical Linguistic Companion.* Cambridge: Cambridge University Press.

—— and ANDERSON, John M. (1975). *Old English Phonology.* Cambridge: Cambridge University Press.

LAUGHREN, Mary (1984). 'Tone in Zulu nouns.' In G. N. Clements and J. A. Goldsmith (ed.), pp. 183–234.

LAVER, John (1994). *Principles of Phonetics.* Cambridge: Cambridge University Press.

—— and HUTCHESON, Sandy (1972). 'Introduction.' In J. Laver and S. Hutcheson (eds.), pp. 11–15.

—— —— (eds.) (1972). *Communication in Face to Face Interaction.* Harmondsworth: Penguin.

LAZICZIUS, Gyula (1939). 'Zur Lautquantität.' *Archiv für Vergleichende Phonetik* 3: 245–9. Also in Sebeok (ed.) (1966) *Selected Writings of Gyula Laziczius.* The Hague: Mouton, pp. 71–6.

LEA, Wayne (1973). 'Segmental and suprasegmental influences on fundamental frequency contours.' In L. M. Hyman (ed.), pp. 15–70.

LEBEN, William R. (1971). 'Suprasegmental and segmental representation of tone.' *Studies in African Linguistics*, Suppl. 2: 183–200.

—— (1973a). *Suprasegmental Phonology.* Bloomington: Indiana University Linguistics Club.

—— (1973b). 'The role of tone in segmental phonology.' In L. M. Hyman (ed.), pp. 115–49.

—— (1976). 'The tones of English intonation.' *Linguistic Analysis* 2: 69–107.

—— (1977). 'Length and syllable structure in Hausa.' *Studies in African Linguistics*, Suppl. 7: 137–43.

—— (1978). 'The representation of tone.' In V. A. Fromkin (ed.), pp. 177–219.

—— (1980). 'A metrical analysis of length.' *Linguistic Inquiry* 11: 497–509.

—— (1996). 'Tonal feet and the adaptation of English borrowings into Hausa.' *Studies in African Linguistics* 25: 139–54.

LEHISTE, Ilse (1960). 'Segmental and syllabic quantity in Estonian.' *American Studies in Uralic Linguistics.* Bloomington: Indiana University Press, pp. 21–82.

—— (1965). 'The function of quantity in Finnish and Estonian.' *Language* 41: 447–56.

—— (1966). *Consonant Quantity and Phonological Units in Estonian.* Bloomington: Indiana University Press.

—— (1970). *Suprasegmentals.* Cambridge, MA: MIT Press.

—— (1971). 'Temporal organization of spoken language.' In L. L. Hammerich *et al.* (eds.), pp. 159–69.

—— (1977). 'Isochrony reconsidered.' *Journal of Phonetics* 5: 253–63.

—— (1982). 'Some phonetic characteristics of discourse.' *Studia Linguistica* 36(2): 117–30.

—— and IVIĆ, Pavle (1978). 'Interrelationship between word tone and sentence intonation in Serbocroatian.' In D. J. Napoli (ed.), pp. 100–28.

—— OLIVE, J. P. and STREETER, L. A. (1976). 'The role of duration in disambiguating syntactically ambiguous sentences.' *Journal of the Acoustical Society of America* 60: 1199–1202.

—— and PETERSON, Gordon E. (1961). 'Some basic considerations in the analysis of intonation.' *Journal of the Acoustical Society of America* 33: 419–25.

LEHMANN, Winfred P. (1955). *Proto-Indo-European Phonology*. Austin: University of Texas Press.

—— (1993). *Theoretical Bases of Indo-European Linguistics*. London: Routledge.

—— (ed.) (1967). *A Reader in Nineteenth Century Historical Indo-European Linguistics*. Bloomington: Indiana University Press.

LEPSCHY, Giulio (ed.) (1994). *History of Linguistics, vol. I. The eastern traditions of linguistics*. London: Longman.

LERDAHL, Fred and JACKENDOFF, Ray (1983). *A Generative Theory of Tonal Music*. Cambridge, MA: MIT Press.

LEVELT, Willem J. M. (1989). *Speaking. From intention to articulation*. Cambridge, MA: MIT Press.

LEVIN, Juliette (1985). *A Metrical Theory of Syllabicity*. PhD, MIT.

LEWIS, Jack Windsor (ed.) (1995). *Studies in General and English Phonetics. Essays in honour of Professor J. D. O'Connor*. London: Routledge.

LI, Fang-Kuei (1948). 'The distribution of initials and tones in the Sui language.' *Language* 24.2: 160–7.

LIBERMAN, Mark (1975). *The Intonational System of English*. Dissertation, MIT. Distributed by Indiana University Linguistics Club, Bloomington, 1978.

—— and PRINCE, Alan S. (1977). 'On stress and linguistic rhythm.' *Linguistic Inquiry* 8: 249–336.

—— and SAG, Ivan (1974). 'Prosodic form and discourse function.' *Chicago Linguistic Society Papers* 10: 416–27.

LIEBERMAN, Philip (1960). 'Some acoustic correlates of word stress in American English.' *Journal of the Acoustical Society of America* 35: 344–53.

—— (1965). 'On the acoustic basis of the perception of intonation by linguists.' *Word* 21: 40–54.

—— (1967). *Intonation, Perception, and Language*. Cambridge, MA, MIT Press.

—— and BLUMSTEIN, Sheila E. (1988). *Speech Physiology, Speech Perception, and Acoustic Phonetics*. Cambridge: Cambridge University Press.

LIIV, Georg (1962). 'On the quantity and quality of Estonian vowels of three phonological degrees of length.' *Proceedings of the 4th International Congress of Phonetic Sciences*. The Hague: Mouton, pp. 682–7.

LINKE, G. (1939). 'Problemgeschichtlicher Überblick über Quantitäts- und Lautdauermessungen.' *Archiv für vergleichende Phonetik* III: 108–16.

LIST, George (1961). 'Speech melody and song melody in Central Thailand.' *Ethnomusicology* 5.1: 16–32.

LLOYD, James A. (1925). 'The tones of Yoruba.' *Bulletin of the School of Oriental Studies* 3: 119–28.

LONGACRE, Robert E. (1952). 'Five phonemic pitch levels in Trique.' *Acta Linguistica* 7: 62–82.

—— (1970). 'Hierarchy in language.' In P. L. Garvin (ed.).

LORENTZ, Owe (1984). 'Stress and tone in an accent language.' In C. C. Elert *et al.* (eds.), pp. 165–78.

LOWENSTAMM, Jean and KAYE, Jonathan (1986). 'Compensatory lengthening in Tiberian Hebrew.' In L. Wetzels and E. Sezer (eds.), pp. 97–132.

LUNT, Horace (ed.) (1964). *Proceedings of the 9th International Congress of Linguists*. The Hague: Mouton.

McCARTHY, John J. (1979). *Formal Properties of Semitic Phonology and Morphology*. PhD dissertation, MIT. Distributed by Indiana University Linguistics Club.

—— (1986). 'OCP effects: gemination and antigemination.' *Linguistic Inquiry* 17: 207–63.

—— and PRINCE, Alan S. (1986). *Prosodic Morphology*. MS. Amherst, MA: University of Massachusetts.

—— —— (1993). *Prosodic Morphology 1: Constraint Interaction and Satisfaction*. MS. Amherst, MA: University of Massachusetts and New Brunswick, NJ: Rutgers University.

—— —— (1995). *Prosodic Morphology*. In J. A. Goldsmith (ed.), pp. 318–66.

MacCARTHY, Peter (1975). *The Pronunciation of German*. London: Oxford University Press.

McCAWLEY, James D. (1964). 'What is a tone language?.' Unpublished paper, Linguistic Society of America.

—— (1968). *The Phonological Component of a Grammar of Japanese*. The Hague: Mouton.

—— (1970). 'Some tonal systems that come close to being pitch-accent systems but don't quite make it.' In *Papers from the 6th regional meeting, Chicago Linguistic Society*, pp. 526–32.

—— (1973). 'Some Tonga tone rules.' In S. R. Anderson and P. Kiparsky (eds.), pp. 140–52.

—— (1977). 'Accent in Japanese.' In L. M. Hyman (ed.) pp. 261–302.

—— (1978). 'What is a tone language?' In V. A. Fromkin (ed.), pp. 113–31.

MacPHERSON, Ian R. (1975). *Spanish Phonology, Descriptive and Historical*. Manchester: Manchester University Press.

MADDIESON, Ian (1972). 'Tone system typology and distinctive features.' In *Proceedings of the Seventh International Congress of Phonetic Sciences*. The Hague: Mouton, pp. 957–61.

—— (1974). 'A note on tone and consonants.' In I. Maddieson (ed.), pp. 18–27.

—— (1978). 'Universals of tone.' In J. H. Greenberg (ed.), pp. 335–66.

—— (ed.) (1974). *The Tone Tome. Studies on tone from the UCLA Tone Project* (Working Papers in Phonetics 27). Los Angeles: University of California.

MALMBERG, Bertil (ed.) (1968). *Manual of Phonetics*. Amsterdam: North Holland.

MALMQVIST, Göran (1994). 'Chinese Linguistics.' In G. Lepschy (ed.), pp. 1–24.

MALONE, Kemp (1953). 'Long and short in Icelandic phonemics.' *Language* 29: 61–2.

MARAN, La Raw (1973). 'On becoming a tone language: a Tibeto-Burman model of tonogenesis.' In L. M. Hyman (ed.), pp. 97–114.

MARTIN, Samuel E. (1952). *Morphophonemics of Standard Colloquial Japanese*. Baltimore: Waverly Press.
—— (1967). 'On the accent of Japanese adjectives.' *Language* 43: 246–77.
—— (1970). 'Junctural cues to ellipsis in Japanese.' In R. Jakobson and S. Kawamoti (eds.), pp. 429–46.
MARTINET, André (1949). *Phonology as Functional Phonetics*. Oxford: Blackwell.
—— (1954). 'Accents et tons.' *Miscellanea Phonetica* II: 13–24.
—— (1964). *Elements of General Linguistics*. London: Faber. (Translation of *Éléments de linguistique générale*. Paris: Armand Collin, 1960.)
—— (1968). 'Accents et tons.' In A. Martinet (ed.), pp. 141–61.
—— (ed.) (1968). *La Linguistique synchronique, études et recherches*. Paris: Presses Universitaires de France.
MATEŠIĆ, Josip (1970). *Der Wortakzent in der Serbokroatischen Schriftsprache*. Heidelberg: Winter.
MATISOFF, James A. (1970). 'Glottal dissimilation and the Lahu high-rising tone: a tonogenetic study.' *Journal of the American Oriental Society* 90.1: 13–44.
—— (1973). 'Tonogenesis in Southeast Asia.' In L. M. Hyman (ed.), pp. 71–95.
MATTHEWS, Peter H. (1966). 'The concept of rank in "Neo-Firthian" grammar.' *Journal of Linguistics* 2: 101–10.
MEINHOF, Carl (1915). *An Introduction to the Study of African Languages*. London: Dent.
MEUSSEN, A. E. (1963). 'Morphotonology of the Tonga verb.' *Journal of African Languages* 2: 72–92.
—— (1970). 'Tone typologies for West African Languages.' *African Language Studies* 11: 266–71.
MEYER, Ernst A. (1903). *Englische Lautdauer, eine Experimentalphonetische Untersuchung*. Uppsala: Akademiska Bokhandeln (= Skrifter utgifna af K. Humanistiska Vetenskaps-Samsfundet i Uppsala, VIII, 3).
MEYER-EPPLER, W. (1948). 'Tonhöhenschreiber.' *Zeitschrift für Phonetik* 2: 16–38.
MILLER, Roy A. (ed.) (1970). *Bernard Bloch on Japanese*. New Haven: Yale University Press.
MINKOVA, Donka (1982). 'The environment for open syllable lengthening in Middle English.' *Folia Linguistica Historica* 3: 29–58.
MITCHELL, Terrence F. (1957). 'Long consonants in phonology and phonetics.' In *Studies in Linguistic Analysis*, pp. 182–205. London: Philological Society.
MIYATA, K. (1927). 'New view on the Japanese accent and its notation.' *Study of Sounds* 1: 18–22.
MOHANAN, Karuvannur P. (1982). *Lexical Phonology*. Bloomington: Indiana University Linguistics Club.
—— (1986). *The Theory of Lexical Phonology*. Dordrecht: Reidel.
MOL, H. and UHLENBECK, E. M. (1956). 'The linguistic relevance of intensity in stress.' *Lingua* 5: 205–13.
MORTON, John and JASSEM, Wiktor (1965). 'Acoustic correlates of stress.' *Language and Speech* 8: 159–87.
—— MARCUS, S. M., and FRANKISH, C. (1976). 'Perceptual Centres (P-centres).' *Psychological Review* 83: 405–8.

MOULTON, William G. (1962). *The Sounds of English and German.* Chicago: Chicago University Press.

MUST, H. (1959). 'Duration of speech sounds in Estonian.' *Orbis* 8: 213–23.

MUYSKENS, John H. (1931). 'An analysis of accent in English from kymograph records.' *Vox* 17.2: 55–65.

MYERS, Terry, LAVER, John, and ANDERSON, John (eds.) (1981). *The Cognitive Representation of Speech.* Amsterdam: North Holland.

NAERT, P. (1943). 'Sur la nature phonologique de la quantité.' *Cahiers Ferdinand de Saussure* 3: 15–25.

NAKATANI, Lloyd H., O'CONNOR, Kathleen D., and ASTON, Carletta H. (1981). 'Prosodic aspects of American English speech rhythm.' *Phonetica* 38: 84–106.

NAPOLI, Donna J. (ed.) (1978). *Elements of Tone, Stress, and Intonation.* Washington DC: Georgetown University Press.

NAVARRO TOMÁS, Tomás (1936). *Manual de pronunciación española.* Consejo Superior de Investigaciones Científicas, Madrid.

NESPOR, Marina and VOGEL, Irene (1979). 'Clash avoidance in Italian.' *Linguistic Inquiry* 10.1: 467–82.

—— —— (1982). 'Prosodic domains of external sandhi rules.' In H. van der Hulst and N. Smith (eds.), pp. 225–55.

—— —— (1983). 'Prosodic structure above the word.' In A. Cutler and D. R. Ladd (eds.), pp. 123–40.

—— —— (1986). *Prosodic Phonology.* Dordrecht: Foris.

NEWMAN, Paul (1973). 'Syllable weight as a phonological variable. The nature and function of the contrast between "heavy" and "light" syllables.' *Studies in African Linguistics* 3: 301–23.

—— (1975). 'The non-correlation of tone and vowel height in Hausa.' *Studies in African Linguistics* 6: 207–13.

—— (1986a). 'Contour tones as phonemic primes in Grebo.' In K. Bogers *et al.* (eds.), pp. 175–93.

—— (1986b). 'Tone and affixation in Hausa.' *Studies in African Linguistics* 17: 249–67.

—— (1995). 'Hausa Tonology: Complexities in an "Easy" Tone Language.' In J. A. Goldsmith (ed.), pp. 762–81.

NEWMAN, Stanley S. (1946). 'On the stress system of English.' *Word* 2: 171–87.

NISHINUMA, Yukihiro (1979). *Un modèle d'analyse automatique de la prosodie. Accent et intonation en japonais.* Paris: Éditions du Centre National de la Recherche Scientifique.

NORMAN, Jerry (1988). *Chinese.* Cambridge: Cambridge University Press.

O'CONNOR, J. D. and ARNOLD, G. F. (1961). *Intonation of Colloquial English.* London: Longman.

ODDEN, David (1982). 'Tonal phenomena in KiShambaa.' *Studies in African Linguistics* 13: 177–208.

—— (1985). 'An accentual approach to tone in Kimatuumbi.' In D. L. Goyvaerts (ed.), pp. 345–419.

—— (1986). 'On the role of the obligatory contour principle in phonological theory.' *Language* 62: 353–83.

—— (1988). 'Predictable tone systems in Bantu.' In H. van der Hulst and N. Smith (eds.) (1988a), pp. 225–51.

—— (1995). 'Tone: African languages.' In J. A. Goldsmith (ed.), pp. 444–75.

OHALA, John J. (1973). 'The physiology of tone.' In L. M. Hyman (ed.) (1973), pp. 1–14.

—— (1977). 'The Physiology of Stress.' In L. M. Hyman (ed.) (1977), pp. 145–68.

—— (1978). 'Production of tone.' In V. A. Fromkin (ed.), pp. 5–39.

—— (1983). 'Cross-language use of pitch—an ethological view.' *Phonetica* 40: 1–18.

PALMER, Frank R. (1957). 'Gemination in Tigrinya.' In *Studies in Linguistic Analysis.* London: Philological Society, pp. 139–48.

—— (1970). 'Introduction.' In F. R. Palmer (ed.), pp. ix–xvi.

—— (ed.) (1970). *Prosodic Analysis.* London: Oxford University Press.

PALMER, Harold E. (1922). *English Intonation with Systematic Exercises.* Cambridge: Heffer.

—— (1924). *A Grammar of Spoken English.* Cambridge: Heffer.

—— (1933). *A New Classification of English Tones.* Tokyo: Kaitakusha.

PANCONCELLI-CALZIA, G. (1917). 'Über das Verhalten von Dauer und Höhe im Akzent.' *Vox* 27: 127 ff.

PANKRATZ, Leo and PIKE, Eunice V. (1967). 'Phonology and morphotonemics of Ayutla Mixtec.' *International Journal of American Linguistics* 33: 287–99.

PARMENTER, C. E. and BLANC, A. V. (1933). 'An experimental study of accent in French and English.' *Publications of the Modern Language Association of America* 48: 598–607.

PETERS, Ann M. (1973). 'A new formalization of downdrift.' *Studies in African Linguistics* 4: 139–53.

PIERREHUMBERT, Janet B. (1980). *The Phonology and Phonetics of English Intonation.* PhD, MIT.

—— and BECKMAN, Mary E. (1988). *Japanese Tone Structure.* Cambridge, MA: MIT Press.

PIJPER, Jan Roelof de (1983). *Modelling British English Intonation.* Dordrecht: Foris.

PIKE, Eunice V. (1974). 'A multiple stress system versus a tone system.' *International Journal of American Linguistics* 40: 169–75.

—— (1976). 'Phonology.' In R. M. Brend and K. L. Pike (eds.).

—— and ORAM, Joy (1976). 'Stress and tone in the phonology of Diuxi Mixtec.' *Phonetica* 33: 321–33.

—— and SMALL, Priscilla (1974). 'Downstepping terrace tone in Coatzospan Mixtec.' In R. M. Brend (ed.), pp. 105–34.

—— and WISTRAND, Kent (1974). 'Step-up terrace tone in Acatlán Mixtec (Mexico).' In R. M. Brend (ed.), pp. 81–104, .

PIKE, Kenneth L. (1943). *Phonetics. A critical analysis of phonetic theory and a technic for the practical description of sounds.* Ann Arbor: University of Michigan Press.

—— (1945). *The Intonation of American English.* Ann Arbor: University of Michigan Press.

—— (1947). *Phonemics. A technique for reducing languages to writing.* Ann Arbor: University of Michigan Press.

—— (1948). *Tone Languages. A technique for determining the number and type of pitch contrasts in a language, with studies in tonemic substitution and fusion.* Ann Arbor: University of Michigan Press.

PIKE, Kenneth L. (cont.) (1967). *Language in Relation to a Unified Theory of the Structure of Human Behaviour*. The Hague: Mouton.

—— (1970). *Tagmemic and Matrix Linguistics Applied to Selected African Languages*. Norman, OK: Summer Institute of Linguistics.

—— and PIKE, Eunice V. (1947). 'Immediate constituents of Mazateco syllables.' *International Journal of American Linguistics* 13: 78–91.

PILSZCZIKOWA-CHODAK, N. (1972). 'Tone-vowel height correlation and tone assignment in the patterns of verb and noun plurals in Hausa.' *Studies in African Linguistics* 3: 399–421.

PITRELLI, John F., BECKMAN, Mary E., and HIRSCHBERG, Julia (1994). 'Evaluation of prosodic transcription labelling reliability in the ToBI framework.' In *Proceedings of the 1994 International Conference on Spoken Language Processing*, 1. Yokohama, pp. 123–6.

POINTON, Graham E. (1980). 'Is Spanish really syllable timed?' *Journal of Phonetics* 8: 293–304.

POLLAK, H. W. (1911). 'Zur Schlußkadenz im deutschen Aussagesatz.' *Phonetische Untersuchungen I*, Vienna.

POPPERWELL, R. G. (1963). *The Pronunciation of Norwegian*. Cambridge: Cambridge University Press.

POSER, William J. (1984). *The Phonetics and Phonology of Tone and Intonation in Japanese*. Dissertation, MIT.

—— (1990). 'Evidence for foot structure in Japanese.' *Language* 66: 78–105.

POSTI, Lauri (1950). 'On quantity in Estonian.' *Journal de la société Finno-Ougrienne* 54: 1–14.

PRINCE, Alan S. (1980). 'A metrical theory for Estonian quantity.' *Linguistic Inquiry* 11: 511–62.

—— (1983). 'Relating to the grid.' *Linguistic Inquiry* 14: 19–100.

—— and SMOLENSKY, Paul (1993). *Optimality Theory: Constraint Interaction in Generative Grammar*. Piscataway, NJ: Rutgers University Centre for Cognitive Science.

PULLEYBLANK, Douglas (1983). 'Accent in Kimatuumbi.' In J. Kaye *et al.* (eds.), pp. 195–215.

—— (1986). *Tone in Lexical Phonology*. Dordrecht: Reidel.

PYLE, C. (1970). 'West Greenlandic Eskimo and the representation of vowel length.' *Papers in Linguistics* 3: 115–46.

RAVEN, David S. (1962). *Greek Metre*. London: Faber and Faber.

RAVILA, Paavo (1962). 'Quantity and phonemic analysis.' In *Proceedings of the 4th International Congress of Phonetic Sciences*. The Hague: Mouton, pp. 490–3.

REES, Martin (1975). 'The domain of isochrony.' *Work in Progress* 8: 14–28. Edinburgh: Edinburgh University Linguistics Department.

RICHTER, Elise (1938). 'Länge und Kürze.' *Archiv für Vergleichende Phonetik* 2.

RIGAULT, A. (1962). 'Rôle de la fréquence, de l'intensité et de la durée vocaliques dans la perception de l'accent en français.' In *Proceedings of the 4th International Congress of Phonetic Sciences*. The Hague: Mouton, pp. 735–48.

RISCHEL, Jørgen (1960). 'Über die phonematische und morphophonematische Funktion der sogenannten Worttöne im Norwegischen.' *Zeitschrift für Phonetik* 13: 177–85.

—— (1963). 'Morphemic tone and word tone in Eastern Norwegian.' *Phonetica* 10: 154–64.

—— (1964). 'Stress, juncture and syllabification in phonemic description.' In H. Lunt (ed.), pp. 85–93.

ROACH, Peter J. (1982). 'On the distinction between stress-timed and syllable-timed languages.' In D. Crystal (ed.), pp. 73–9.

—— (1994). 'Conversion between prosodic transcription systems: Standard British and ToBI.' *Speech and Communication* 15: 91–9.

ROBINS, R. H. (1957). 'Aspects of prosodic analysis.' *Proceedings of the University of Durham Philosophical Society I*, Series B (Arts), 1: 1–12.

—— (1997). *A Short History of Linguistics.* 4th edn. London: Longman.

ROCA, Iggy (1986). 'Secondary stress and metrical rhythm.' *Phonology Yearbook* 3: 341–70.

—— (1994). *Generative Phonology.* London: Routledge.

ROSS, John Robert (1970). 'On declarative sentences.' In R. A. Jacobs and P. S. Rosenbaum (eds.), pp. 222–72.

—— (1972). 'A reanalysis of English word stress (Part I).' In M. K. Brame (ed.), pp. 229–323.

RUSS, Charles V. J. (ed.) (1981). *Contrastive Aspects of English and German.* Heidelberg: Julius Gross.

SAGEY, Elizabeth (1986). *The Representation of Features and Relations in Non-linear Phonology.* PhD Dissertation, MIT.

SAMPSON, Geoffrey (1969). 'A note on Wang's "Phonological features of tone".' *International Journal of American Linguistics* 35: 62–6.

—— (1973). 'Duration in Hebrew consonants.' *Linguistic Inquiry* 4: 101–4.

SAPIR, Edward (1931). 'Notes on the Gweabo language of Liberia.' *Language* 7: 30–41.

SARAN, Franz (1907). *Deutsche Verslehre.* München: Beck.

SAUSSURE, Ferdinand de (1967 [1916]). *Cours de linguistique générale.* Paris: Payot.

SCHACHTER, Paul (1961). 'Phonetic similarity in tonemic analysis, with notes on the tone system of Akwapim Twi.' *Language* 37: 231–8.

—— and FROMKIN, Victoria A. (1968). *A Phonology of Akan.* Los Angeles: UCLA Working Papers in Phonetics 9.

SCHADENBERG, Thilo C. (1973). 'Kinga: a restricted tone system.' *Studies in African Linguistics* 4: 23–47.

SCHANE, Sanford A. (1973). *Generative Phonology.* Englewood Cliffs: Prentice Hall.

—— (1975). 'Non-cyclic English word stress.' In D. L. Goyvaerts and G. K. Pullum (eds.), p. 249.

—— (1979a). 'The rhythmic nature of English word accentuation.' *Language* 55.3: 559–602.

—— (1979b). 'Rhythm, accent and stress in English words.' *Linguistic Inquiry* 10: 483–502.

SCHEIN, Barry and STERIADE, Donca (1986). 'On geminates.' *Linguistic Inquiry* 17: 691.

SCHMITT, Alfred (1924). *Untersuchungen zur allgemeinen Akzentlehre, mit einer Anwendung auf den Akzent des Griechischen und Lateinischen.* Heidelberg: Winter.

SCHRAMM, W. L. (1937). 'The acoustical nature of accent in American speech.' *American Speech* 12: 49–56.

SCHUBIGER, Maria (1935). *The Role of Intonation in Spoken English.* Cambridge: Heffer.

—— (1958). *English Intonation, its form and function.* Tübingen: Niemeyer.

SCHUH, Russell G. (1978). 'Tone rules.' In V. A. Fromkin (ed.), pp. 221–56.

392 Prosodic Features and Prosodic Structure

SCOTT, Donia R., ISARD, Stephen D., and BOYSSON-BARDIES, Bénédicte de (1985). 'Perceptual isochrony in English and French.' *Journal of Phonetics* 13: 155–62.

SCOTT, Norman C. (1938). 'Stress as a distinctive feature.' *Le maître phonétique* 63: 42–3.

—— (1939). 'An experiment on stress perception.' *Le maître phonétique* 67: 44–5.

—— (1940). 'Distinctive rhythm.' *Le maître phonétique*: 6.

SELKIRK, Elisabeth O. (1978). 'On prosodic structure and its relation to syntactic structure.' Bloomington: Indiana University Linguistics Club.

—— (1980). 'The role of prosodic categories in English word-stress.' *Linguistic Inquiry* 11: 563–605.

—— (1984). *Phonology and Syntax. The relation between sound and structure.* Cambridge, MA: MIT Press.

SHEN, Xiao-Nan Susan (1989). *The Prosody of Mandarin Chinese.* Berkeley/Los Angeles: University of California Press.

SHEN, Y. and PETERSON, G. C. (1962). 'Isochronism in English.' *University of Buffalo Studies in Linguistics*, Occasional Papers 9: 1–36.

SHIBATANI, Masayoshi (1972). 'The non-cyclic nature of Japanese accentuation.' *Language* 48: 584–95.

—— (1973). 'The role of surface phonetic constraints in generative phonology.' *Language* 49: 87–106.

—— (1990). *The Languages of Japan.* Cambridge: Cambridge University Press.

SIERTSEMA, Berta (1959a). 'Problems of phonemic analysis II. Long vowels in a tone language.' *Lingua* 8: 42–64.

—— (1959b). 'Stress and tone in Yoruba word composition.' *Lingua* 8: 385–402.

SIEVERS, Eduard (1901). *Grundzüge der Phonetik.* 3rd edn. Leipzig: Breitkopf and Härtel.

SILVERMAN, Kim E. A. and PIERREHUMBERT, Janet B. (1990). 'The timing of prenuclear high accents in English.' In J. Kingston and M. E. Beckman (eds.), pp. 72–106.

—— BECKMAN, Mary E., PITRELLI, John (1992). 'ToBI: a standard for labeling English prosody.' In *Proceedings of the Second International Conference on Spoken Language Processing*, 2. Banff, Canada, pp. 867–70.

SINCLAIR, Donald E. and PIKE, Kenneth L. (1948). 'The tonemes of Mesquital Otomi.' *International Journal of American Linguistics* 14: 91–8.

SLEDD, James (1962). 'Notes on English stress.' In *First Texas Conference on problems of Linguistic Analysis in English.* Austin: University of Texas, pp. 33–44.

SLOAT, Clarence (1974). 'Stress in English.' *Glossa* 8.1: 121–38.

SMITH, Nielsen V. (1967). 'The phonology of Nupe.' *Journal of African Languages* 6: 153–69.

SNIDER, Keith (1988). 'Towards the representation of tone: a three-dimensional approach.' In H. van der Hulst and N. Smith (eds.) (1988b), pp. 237–67.

—— (1990). 'Tonal upstep in Krachi: evidence for a register tier.' *Language* 66: 453–74.

—— and HULST, Harry van der (1992). 'Introduction.' In H. van der Hulst and K. Snider (eds.), pp. 1–27.

SOMMERFELT, Alf (1951). 'The development of quantity as evidence of Western European linguistic interdependence.' *English Studies Today.* Also in A. Sommerfelt (ed.) (1962), *Diachronic and Synchronic Aspects of Language.* The Hague: Mouton, pp. 81–6.

SPAANDONCK, Marcel van (1971). 'On the so-called reversing tonal system of Ciluba: a case for restructuring.' *Studies in African Linguistics* 2: 131–44.

SPEARS, R. A. (1967). 'Tone in Mende.' *Journal of African Languages* 6: 231–44.

SPENCE N. C. W. (1965). 'Quantity and quality in the vowel system of Vulgar Latin.' *Word* 21: 1–18.

SPENCER, Andrew (1996). *Phonology.* Oxford: Blackwell.

SPIERS, L., HALLOWELL, A. Irving, and NEWMAN, Stanley S. (eds.) (1941). *Language, Culture and Personality.* Menasha, WI: Sapir Memorial Publication Fund.

SPRIGG, R. K. (1955). 'The tonal system of Tibetan (Lhasa dialect) and the nominal phrase.' *Bulletin of the School of Oriental and African Studies* 17: 134–53.

—— (1968). 'Junction in spoken Burmese.' In *Studies in Linguistic Analysis.* Oxford: Blackwell, pp. 104–38.

STAHLKE, H. (1977). 'Some problems with binary features for tone.' *International Journal of American Linguistics* 43: 1–10.

STEELE, Joshua (1775), *An Essay towards establishing the melody and measure of speech, to be expressed and perpetuated by peculiar symbols.* London: Boyer and Nichols. (2nd edn. *Prosodia Rationalis*, 1779, London: Nichols).

STERIADE, Donca (1982). *Greek prosodies and the nature of syllabification.* PhD Dissertation. Cambridge, MA: MIT Press.

STETSON, R. H. (1928). 'Motor Phonetics.' The Hague (= *Archives néerlandaise de phonétique expérimentale* 3).

STEVICK, Earl W. (1965). 'Pitch and duration in two Yoruba dialects.' *Journal of African Languages* 4: 85–101.

—— (1969a). 'Tone in Bantu.' *International Journal of American Linguistics* 35: 330–41.

—— (1969b). 'Pitch and duration in Ganda.' *Journal of African Languages* 8: 1–28.

STEWART, John M. (1966). 'The typology of the Twi tone system.' Preprint from *Bulletin of the Institute of African Studies* 1. Cited by Voorhoeve, 1968.

—— (1992). 'Dschang and Ebrie as Akan-type total downstep languages.' In H. van der Hulst and K. Snider (eds.), pp. 185–244.

STOCKWELL, Robert P. (1960). 'The role of intonation in a generative grammar of English.' *Language* 36: 360–7.

—— (1972). 'The role of intonation: reconsiderations and other considerations.' In D. Bolinger (ed.) *Intonation.* Harmondsworth: Penguin, pp. 87–109.

—— BOWEN, J. Donald, and SILVA-FUENZALIDA, I. (1956). 'Spanish juncture and intonation.' *Language* 32: 641–5.

SUÁREZ, Jorge A. (1983). *The Mesoamerican Indian languages.* Cambridge: Cambridge University Press.

SWADESH, Morris (1937). 'The phonemic interpretation of long consonants.' *Language* 13: 1–10.

SWEET, Henry (1877). *A Handbook of Phonetics.* Repr. (1970) by McGrath Publishing Co., College Park, Maryland, pp. 59–60.

—— (1889). 'On English stress.' *Le maître phonétique* 4: 18.

—— (1906). *A Primer of Phonetics.* 3rd edn. Oxford: Clarendon Press.

TADADJEU, Maurice (1974). 'Floating tones, shifting rules, and downstep in Dschang-Bamileke.' *Studies in African Linguistics*, Supplement 5: 283–90.

TAULI, Valter (1966). 'On quantity and stress in Estonian.' *Acta Linguistica Hafniensia* 9: 145–62.

TAYLOR, L. F. (1920). 'On the tones of certain languages of Burma.' *Bulletin of the School of Oriental Studies* 1.4: 91–106.

TENCH, Paul (1976). 'Double ranks in a phonological hierarchy.' *Journal of Linguistics* 12: 1–20.

THORSEN, Nina (1983). 'Two issues in the prosody of Standard Danish.' In A. Cutler and D. R. Ladd (eds.), pp. 27–38.

THRÁINSSON, Hoskuldur (1978). 'On the phonology of Icelandic pre-aspiration.' *Nordic Journal of Linguistics* 1: 3–54.

TOGEBY, Knut (1965). *Structure immanente de la langue française*. Paris: Larousse.

TOHKURA, Y., VATIKIOTIS-BATESON, E., and SAGISAKA, Y. (eds.) (1992). *Speech Perception, Production, and Linguistic Structure*. Tokyo: Ohmsha.

TRAGER, George L. (1939). 'The phonemes of Castilian Spanish.' *Traveaux du Cercle Linguistique de Prague* 8.

—— (1940). 'Serbo–Croatian accents and quantities.' *Language* 16: 29–32.

—— (1941). 'The theory of accentual systems.' In L. Spiers, A. I. Hallowell, And S. S. Newman (eds.), pp. 131–45.

—— and BLOCH, Bernard (1941). 'The syllabic phonemes of English.' *Language* 17: 223–46.

—— and SMITH, Henry Lee, Jr. (1951). *An Outline of English Structure*. Washington, DC: American Council of Learned Societies.

TRANEL, Bernard (1991). 'CVC light syllables, geminates, and Moraic Theory.' *Phonology* 8.2: 291–302.

TRASK, R. Larry (1996). *A Dictionary of Phonetics and Phonology*. London: Routledge.

TRIM, John L. M. (1959). 'Major and minor tone-groups in English.' *Le maître phonétique* 112: 26–9.

—— (1964). 'Tonetic stress marks for German.' In D. Abercrombie *et al.* (eds.), pp. 374–83.

—— (1969). 'Some continuously variable features in British English intonation.' *Actes de 10e. Congrès International des Linguistes*. The Hague: Mouton, pp. 267–72.

TRUBETZKOY, Nikolai S. (1935). *Anleitung zu phonologischen Beschreibungen*. Repr. (1958) Göttingen: Vandenhoek and Ruprecht.

—— (1936). 'Die phonologischen Grundlagen der sogenannten Quantität in den verschiedenen Sprachen.' *Scritti in onore di A. Trombetti*. Milan, 155 ff.

—— (1938). 'Die Quantität als phonologisches Problem.' *Actes du 4e. Congrès International des Linguistes*, pp. 117–22. Copenhagen.

—— (1939). *Grundzüge der Phonologie*. = *Traveaux du Cercle Linguistique de Prague* 7. Repr. (1968) Göttingen: Vandenhoek and Ruprecht.

TSUJIMURA, Natsuko (1996). *An Introduction to Japanese Linguistics*. Oxford: Blackwell.

TUCKER, Archibald N. (1929). *The Comparative Phonetics of the Suto-Chuana Group of Bantu Languages*. London: Longman.

—— (1935). 'Survey of the language groups in the Southern Sudan.' *Bulletin of the School of Oriental Studies* 7: 861–96.

—— (1940). *The Eastern Sudanic Languages*. London: Oxford University Press.

ULDALL, Elizabeth T. (1971). 'Isochronous stresses in R.P.' In L.L. Hammerich *et al.* (eds.), pp. 205–10.

UPSON, Jessamine (1968). 'Chatino length and tone.' *Anthropological Linguistics* 10.2: 1–7.

VACHEK, Josef (1959). 'Notes on the quantitative correlation of vowels in the phonematic development of English.' *Mélanges de linguistique et de philologie*. Paris: Didier, pp. 444–56.

VAGO, Robert M. (1985). 'The treatment of long vowels in word-games.' *Phonology* 2: 329–42.

—— (1987). 'On the representation of length.' In W. U. Dressler *et al.* (eds.): *Phonologica 1984*. Cambridge: Cambridge University Press.

VALDMAN, Albert (ed.) (1970). *Studies in Linguistics and Phonetics in Memory of Pierre Delattre*. The Hague: Mouton.

VANCE, Timothy J. (1987). *An Introduction to Japanese Phonology*. Albany, NY: State University of New York.

VANDERSLICE, Ralph and LADEFOGED, Peter (1972). 'Binary suprasegmental features and transformational word-accentuation rules.' *Language* 48: 819–38.

VANVIK, Arne J. (1955a). 'Stress and gestures.' *Le maître phonétique* 103: 8.

—— (1955b). *On Stress in Present-Day English (R.P.)*. Bergen/Oslo: Norwegian Universities' Press.

—— (1961). 'Three tonemes in Norwegian?' *Studia Linguistics* 15: 22–8.

—— (1963). 'Some problems in Scandinavian tonemics.' *Phonetica* 10: 165–73.

VERNER, Karl (1875). 'Eine Ausnahme der ersten Lautverschiebung.' *Zeitschrift für vergleichende Sprachforschung* 23: 97–130.

VIËTOR, Wilhelm (1894). *Elemente der Phonetik des Deutschen, Englischen und Französischen*. 3rd edn. Leipzig: Reisland.

VOGEL, Irene and SCALISE, S. (1982). 'Secondary stress in Italian.' *Lingua* 58: 213–42.

VOORHOEVE, Jan (1968). 'Towards a typology of tone systems.' *Linguistics* 46: 99–114.

—— (1973). 'Safwa as a restricted tone system.' *Studies in African Linguistics* 4: 1–22.

WALKER, J. (1787), *The Melody of Speaking Delineated*. London: Published for the author.

WANG, William S.-Y. (1967). 'Phonological features of tone.' *International Journal of American Linguistics* 33: 93–105.

—— (1970). 'The many uses of Fo.' In A. Valdman (ed.), pp. 487–504.

—— and LI, K. P. (1967). 'Tone 3 in Pekinese.' *Journal of Speech and Hearing Research* 10.3: 629–36.

WÄNGLER, Hans-Heinrich (1963). *Zur Tonologie des Hausa*. Berlin: Akademie.

WARD, Ida C. (1933). *The Phonetic and Tonal Structure of Efik*. Cambridge: Heffer.

—— (1936). *An Introduction to the Ibo Language*. Cambridge: Heffer.

—— (1939). *The Phonetics of English*. 3rd edn. Cambridge: Heffer.

—— (1952). *An Introduction to the Yoruba Language*. Cambridge: Heffer.

WEIDERT, Alfons (1987). *Tibeto-Burman Tonology*. Amsterdam: Benjamins.

WEINRICH, H. (1958). *Phonologische Studien zur Romanischen Sprachgeschichte*. Münster: Aschendorf.

WELLS, Rulon S. (1945). 'The pitch phonemes of English.' *Language* 21: 27–39.

—— (1947). 'Immediate constituents.' *Language* 23: 81–117. Also in M. Joos (ed.), 1957: pp. 186–207.

WELMERS, William E. (1959). 'Tonemics, morphotonemics, and tonal morphemes.' *General Linguistics* 4: 1–9.

—— (1973). *African Language Structures.* Berkeley: University of California Press.

WENK, B. J. and WIOLAND, F. (1982). 'Is French really syllable-timed?' *Journal of Phonetics* 10: 193–216.

WESTERMANN, Diedrich and WARD, Ida C. (1933). *Practical Phonetics for Students of African Languages.* London: Oxford University Press.

WETZELS, Leo (1986). 'Phonological timing in ancient Greek.' In L. Wetzels and E. Sezer (eds.), pp. 297–344.

—— and SEZER, E. (eds.) (1986). *Studies in Compensatory Lengthening.* Dordrecht: Foris.

WIJK, Nikolaas van (1940). 'Quantiteit en intonatie.' *Mededeelingen van der Koninklijke Akademie van Wetenschappen,* III.1.

WILLIAMS, Edwin (1976). 'Underlying tone in Margi and Ibgo.' *Linguistic Inquiry* 7: 463–84.

WILSON, W. A. A. (1968). 'An interpretation of the Temne tone system.' *Journal of West African Languages* 5.1: 5–12.

WINSTON, Denis (1960). 'The "mid tone" in Efik.' *African Language Studies* 1: 185–92.

WITHGOTT, Meg and HALVORSEN, Per-Kristian (1988). 'Phonetic and phonological considerations bearing on representation of East Norwegian Accent.' In H. van der Hulst and N. Smith (eds.) (1988a), pp. 279–94.

WOO, Nancy (1969). *Prosody and Phonology.* Bloomington: Indiana University Linguistics Club.

YIP, Moira (1980). *The Tonal Phonology of Chinese.* Bloomington: Indiana University Linguistics Club.

—— (1989). 'Contour tones.' *Phonology* 6: 149–74.

—— (1992). 'Tonal register in East Asian languages.' In H. van der Hulst and K. Snider (eds.), pp. 245–68.

—— (1995). 'Tone in East Asian Languages.' In J. A. Goldsmith (ed.), pp. 477–94.

YORIO, Carlos Alfredo (1973). 'The generative process of intonation.' *Linguistics* 97: 111–25.

YOSHIBA, Hiroshi (1981). 'The mora constraint in Japanese phonology.' *Linguistic Analysis* 7: 241–62.

YOSHIDA, Shohei (1990). 'A government-based analysis of the "mora" in Japanese.' *Phonology* 7.2: 331–51.

YULE, George (1980). 'The functions of phonological prominence.' *Archivum Linguisticum* 11: 31–46.

ZEE, E. and MADDIESON, Ian (1980). 'Tones and tone sandhi in Shanghai: phonetic evidence and phonological analysis.' *Glossa* 14: 45–88.

ZIMMERMAN, S. A. and SAPON, S. M. (1958). 'Note on vowel duration seen cross-linguistically.' *Journal of the Acoustical Society of America* 30: 152–3.

ZWIRNER, Eberhard (1932). 'Quantität, Lautdauerschätzung und Lautkurvenmessung.' *Proceedings of the International Congress of Phonetic Sciences,* 145–55. Amsterdam.

—— (1939). 'Phonologische und phonometrische Probleme der Quantität.' In E. Blancquaert and W. Pée (eds.), pp. 57–66.

General Index

accent 86, 111–12, 114–78, 359–60
  level 1 vs. level 2 145–50, 167–8, 177–8,
    359–60
  tonal 21, 215, 246–53
  and tone 243–67
advanced tongue root (ATR) 30–1
ambisyllabic 52, 65

bottom-up approach 362–4
bracketing, minimal vs. maximal 352–3
British School of intonation 277–80

category, prosodic 156
chroneme 77–8
classical tradition 15, 46, 115–16
clitic-group 358
compression, of intonation patterns 322–3
configuration, in intonation 298–301
constituents, immediate vs. ranked 352–3
contact 25–7, 29
cyclical rules 171–5

declination 189, 297, 307–10
  see also downdrift
domain, prosodic 333–5
downdrift 189–90, 212–13, 230–1, 297
downstep 190–2, 198–200, 212–13, 218–19, 221,
    230, 294, 307–10
duration 22
Dutch School of intonation 285–7

extendibility 24–7, 29

features:
  diacritic 13
  distinctive 7, 28–31, 151–2, 194–5, 200–15,
    314–15
  envelope 324–6
  intersyllabic vs. intrasyllabic 7
  laryngeal 213–15
  modality 324, 327–8
  paralinguistic 10, 270–1
  prosodic 1–11
  prominence 324, 326–7
foot 87–94, 104–7, 109–11, 145, 156, 167–8,
  253–4, 337, 355–7
frequency, fundamental 182–3

geminate 35, 38–40, 41–2, 63

gesture, vocal 271
glide 36–8
gradation 44–6
Greeks 1, 15, 46, 115–16
grid, metrical 155, 158–61, 163–7

head, of intonation pattern 295, 302–4
hierarchy:
  accentual 149–50, 178
  paired 350–1
  primary vs. secondary 344–7
  prosodic 335–40
hypercharacterization 53, 56

iamb(ic) 88 n., 113, 162–3
Iambic-Trochaic Law 163
intensity 25
intonation 132–4, 146–9, 179, 269–329, 361
  and accentuation 290–1
intonation-unit 288–90, 337, 355
IPO, *see* Dutch School of intonation
isochron(icit)y 87–94, 145

juncture 171–2, 200

key 316–17

language:
  contour tone vs. register tone 192–3
  monotonic vs. polytonic 111
  mora(-counting) 24, 47, 55–6, 111–12, 356
  syllable(-counting) 24, 111–12, 356
  terraced-level 191
  tone-harmony 263–4
larynx 3–4
left-to-right approach 363–4
length 12–113, 360–1
  analytic 24, 34–6
  of consonants 41–2, 57–8, 63, 65–7
  intrinsic vs. extrinsic 12–13
  of syllable 15–16, 21–2, 85–6, 92–4, 96–7
lengthening:
  compensatory 71–6, 100–4
  open syllable 67–71
level, in intonation 298–301
Lund School 283–5

markedness 24, 204, 249
mora 6, 24, 46–50, 79–85, 97–9, 240–1, 355–6

Index of Languages

.

Lightning Source UK Ltd.
Milton Keynes UK
19 May 2010

9 780199 253968